AF183816

Patient Safety Coaching

Susanne Knowles

Patient Safety Coaching

Transforming Healthcare Culture

Springer

Susanne Knowles
Independent Researcher
Brisbane, QLD, Australia

ISBN 978-3-031-68721-1 ISBN 978-3-031-68722-8 (eBook)
https://doi.org/10.1007/978-3-031-68722-8

© The Editor(s) (if applicable) and The Author(s), under exclusive license to Springer Nature Switzerland AG 2024
This work is subject to copyright. All rights are solely and exclusively licensed by the Publisher, whether the whole or part of the material is concerned, specifically the rights of translation, reprinting, reuse of illustrations, recitation, broadcasting, reproduction on microfilms or in any other physical way, and transmission or information storage and retrieval, electronic adaptation, computer software, or by similar or dissimilar methodology now known or hereafter developed.
The use of general descriptive names, registered names, trademarks, service marks, etc. in this publication does not imply, even in the absence of a specific statement, that such names are exempt from the relevant protective laws and regulations and therefore free for general use.
The publisher, the authors and the editors are safe to assume that the advice and information in this book are believed to be true and accurate at the date of publication. Neither the publisher nor the authors or the editors give a warranty, expressed or implied, with respect to the material contained herein or for any errors or omissions that may have been made. The publisher remains neutral with regard to jurisdictional claims in published maps and institutional affiliations.

This Springer imprint is published by the registered company Springer Nature Switzerland AG
The registered company address is: Gewerbestrasse 11, 6330 Cham, Switzerland

If disposing of this product, please recycle the paper.

Acknowledgment

I wish to acknowledge the valued contribution to this work of my Subject Matter Expert, Sara Thorn. Sara originally trained as a doctor and specialized in health service management. Her roles in public health services were predominantly in the areas of clinical governance. Her interest in patient safety stems from her long-standing commitment to continuous improvement and patient-centered care. She holds a Bachelor of Medical Science (Sydney University), MBBS (Sydney University), and Master of Health Management (UNSW) and is a retired prize-winning fellow of the Royal Australasian College of Medical Administrators (RACMA). Sara has also been a faculty member for the Clinical Skills Development Service, Queensland Health, delivering their Improvement Science Courses over a number of years.

In recent years, Sara completed a Diploma in Leadership Coaching with the *Australian Institute of Professional Coaches* (AIPC). Now, as an Education Manager and Head of Operations with the AIPC, Sara combines her wealth of knowledge and experience in healthcare with her commitment to personal and professional growth, and applies this enthusiasm to her position as well as to her work with clients in her own private coaching practice.

About the Book

This book offers invaluable insights for clinical leaders in healthcare organizations, empowering them to cultivate a patient safety culture based on evidence-based research. Prioritizing patient safety at every stage of healthcare is fundamental, from prevention to rehabilitation.

By adopting a coaching approach and fostering a psychologically safe work environment where near-misses are openly discussed, leaders can enhance team performance and mitigate risks effectively. The strategies outlined in the book emphasize the importance of stakeholder collaboration and interdisciplinary teamwork to achieve patient-centric goals.

Furthermore, the book delves into strategies for promoting staff well-being, emphasizing the role of leaders in supporting their teams through stress reduction, mindfulness practice, and resilience building. This coaching approach not only fosters trust and compassion but also enhances patient care by understanding and addressing staff challenges effectively.

Patient safety stands as the bedrock of quality healthcare, and this book equips executives and clinical leaders with governance insights and best practices to enhance patient safety as a quality improvement strategy. It prompts leaders to reflect on organizational factors and decisions impacting patient safety culture, emphasizing the critical role of governance in staffing and resourcing decisions.

Contents

List of Figures

List of Tables

About the Author

Susanne Knowles was awarded a PhD in Management from the University of Queensland, Australia, in 2020, specializing in how organizations embed a coaching culture into their everyday operations to achieve transformational cultural change. She also holds three master's degrees in Education, Psychology, and Business Administration. Based on her PhD research, Susanne authored two previous books, which have been published by Springer: *Positive Psychology Coaching* (2021) and *Coaching Culture* (2022). Her research interest now lies in how clinical and governance leaders can improve the patient safety culture within healthcare organizations through coaching.Susanne has held teaching positions at the University of Queensland, Queensland University of Technology and Griffith University, as well as senior executive positions in government and private sector organizations. She has served as a Board member on several government, not-for-profit, and professional service firms. Her experience as an Executive Coach was gained from 20 years as a consultant to national and international organizations. In 2012, as a former practicing educational, organizational and counselling psychologist, Susanne founded the *Australian Institute of Professional Coaches* to support individuals achieve their personal and professional goals, and organizations to increase employee engagement, retain talent, and improve profitability. She now leads a quiet life as an independent researcher and keen observer of nature and the human condition.

Chapter 1
Introduction

This chapter introduces the background and context for patient safety coaching within healthcare organizations. As a global imperative of the World Health Organization (WHO), patient safety is *the* number one priority of every healthcare organization worldwide. Traditionally, when an adverse event occurred, it was investigated and blame apportioned—an employee was fired, and the organization fined. However, these practices of investigation and reprisal have done little to stop incidents from occurring—some with fatal consequences. A paradigm shift is necessary to rethink healthcare organizations' approaches to patient safety. This shift is toward a Safety-11 [1] perspective that goes beyond compliance and provides the mechanisms by which organizations and staff learn from mistakes. A particularly helpful developmental approach to support this cultural change in healthcare organizations is *coaching*. Patient safety coaching increases leadership capability so leaders can better support staff well-being and develop a patient safety culture within their team. Executives with a governance responsibility learn how coaching practices enhance clinical practice and promote the creation of a patient safety culture across the entire organization.

1.1 Patient Safety

The WHO has defined patient safety as "the absence of preventable harm to a patient and reduction of risk of unnecessary harm associated with health care to an acceptable minimum" [2]. Within the broader healthcare context, patient safety has been defined as "a framework of organized activities that creates cultures, processes, procedures, behaviors, technologies and environments in healthcare that consistently and sustainably lower risks, reduce the occurrence of avoidable harm, make error less likely, and reduce its impact when it does occur" [3]. With approximately 42.1 million admissions to hospitals worldwide each year, causing harm to

© The Author(s), under exclusive license to Springer Nature Switzerland AG 2024

S. Knowles, *Patient Safety Coaching*,
https://doi.org/10.1007/978-3-031-68722-8_1

approximately 10% of patients [4], patient safety is a major global concern. The incidence levels remain relatively stable in the published literature, with a median rate of fatal events of 7.3% [5]. While some success has been noted in the reduction of hospital-acquired infection and medication safety, the frequency of preventable harm remains too high [6]. Not only do adverse events lead to care complications for patients, but they also increase the costs of healthcare provision system-wide.

1.2 Adverse Events

Definitions of adverse events vary by jurisdiction; however, there is agreement on the following elements in most definitions. Adverse events:

- Cause harm to the patient (which can take the form of complications, prolonged stay, injury, death, and disability—permanent or temporary)
- Are unintended in nature

Terms such as "sentinel events" [7] describe adverse events of the highest severity—those events that result in death or permanent disability or that should never occur (e.g., wrong-side operations, sponges retained after surgery).

There are multiple causes of adverse events in healthcare which can be attributed to human error, systems failure, cultural issues, or a combination of these factors. Specifically, cultural issues relating to communication failures are a leading cause and contributing factor to the occurrence of adverse events since miscommunication or communication breakdown can result in deteriorating relationships, lack of role clarity, task overlap, and workplace conflict [8–10]. Effective communication is critical to safe patient care to prevent adverse events from occurring and to effectively discover, manage, and learn from the adverse events that occur. At best, the outcome of an adverse event for a patient may be the need for prolonged or extended care or, at worst, disablement or death.

In an attempt to classify the adverse events that continue to occur in healthcare organizations and learn from them, the WHO published draft *Guidelines for Adverse Event Reporting and Learning Systems: From information to action* (2005) [11]. In 2009, the *International Classification for Patient Safety* was developed which consists of ten high-level classes based on the conceptual framework for the classification [12]. The framework provided a comprehensive overview of the key domains related to patient safety. It represented a continuous learning and improvement cycle emphasizing the identification of risk; the prevention, detection, and reduction of risk; and aspects regarding incident recovery and system resilience—all of which occur throughout and at any point within the conceptual framework. In 2020, the classification system was simplified to distinguish between three different levels of patient harm:

1. Near-miss: an incident that did not reach the patient (e.g., a unit of blood being connected to the wrong patient's intravenous line but the error was detected before the transfusion started).
2. No harm incident: one in which an event reached a patient but no discernible harm resulted (e.g., if the unit of blood was transfused but was not incompatible).
3. Harmful incident: an incident that results in harm to a patient (e.g., the wrong unit of blood was transfused and the patient died from a hemolytic reaction).

1.2.1 The Statistics

Healthcare is a complex, adaptive system with many interactions and patients, each with different physiological, cultural, emotional, and social needs and circumstances. Every step in the healthcare process has the potential for practices to result in unintended harm by virtue of this complexity. According to the WHO, the risk of patient death occurring due to a preventable medical accident while receiving healthcare is estimated to be 1 in 300; this is unacceptable compared with an estimated risk of 1 in 3,000,000 from dying in a plane crash. When patient harm originates in ambulatory care as well, the figure increases to 4 out of 10 patients experiencing a safety issue in their interactions in these settings [13].

Research has also highlighted the enormous consequences of errors. For example, in the United States (USA), at least 210,000 deaths per annum associated with medical errors were reported in hospitals [14]. In Australia, 18,000 preventable deaths are attributable to medical errors every year, and at least 50,000 patients are disabled [15]. In Germany, the number of deaths resulting from 100,000 medical errors per year was reported to be 25,000 [16]. In addition to the tremendous harm caused to patients and their families by these adverse events, from a systems perspective, perceptions of quality of care are negatively affected, and reputational damage occurs, not to mention the resulting increase in the cost of medical care provision that affects all patients [17].

The risk to life and limbs is particularly acute in emergency departments as these are generally pressurized, overcrowded places of work that may lack sufficient staff or equipment. Patients can present with life-threatening illnesses which increases the likelihood of medical errors [18]. Studies have shown that medical errors occur in 46.8% of nurse interactions in emergency departments [19]. In the USA, nearly 3% of all hospital accidents are related to the emergency department [20]. In less developed countries such as Iran, the rate of medical errors in emergency departments is alarming [21].

Global statistics reveal a tale of even larger proportions:

- In OECD countries, 15% of the total hospital activity and expenditures are a direct result of adverse events [22].

- As many as 4 in 10 patients are harmed in primary hospitals and outpatient facilities, with the most detrimental errors related to diagnosis, prescription, and the use of medicines [23].
- The occurrence of adverse events due to unsafe care is one of the leading causes of death and disability worldwide [24]:
  - In high-income countries, it is estimated that 1 in every 10 patients is harmed while receiving hospital care, caused by a range of adverse events, with nearly 50% of them being preventable [22, 25, 26].
  - In low- and middle-income countries, it is estimated that 134 million adverse events occur in hospitals each year, with approximately two-thirds due to unsafe care, resulting in 2.6 million deaths and years lost to disability [27, 28].

Care for patients who have experienced complications as a result of errors usually requires more therapy and a longer hospital stay, resulting in lost opportunities for new patients to occupy beds and receive the treatment they need. Research into the financial benefits of reducing patient harm indicates that investing more in patient safety not only results in better patient outcomes, but can also lead to significant financial savings for organizations and their shareholders [22]. One example of prevention (more engagement with patients in their own healthcare) has shown that this strategy alone can reduce the burden of harm by up to 15% [23].

Medical errors are costly. For example, preventable adverse events in Canadian acute care systems result in $397 million in extra healthcare costs annually [29]. In Australia, the costs of hospital-acquired complications were estimated in 2021 to be $4.1 million [30]; when this figure was added to estimates of direct costs due to safety lapses in primary and ambulatory care—additional tests, treatments and healthcare—this number represented approximately 2.5% of the total expenditure on healthcare. In OECD countries, it is estimated that safety lapses resulting in hospitalizations each year may account for 6% of all hospital bed days and more than seven million admissions [13]. In addition, the cost of harm associated with the loss of life or permanent disability, which results in lost capacity and productivity of the affected patients and families, amounts to trillions of US dollars every year. Furthermore, the psychological cost to the patient and their family associated with the loss or disabling of a loved one is significant, although more difficult to measure.

1.3 That Pivotal Report

> *...the biggest challenge to moving toward a safer health system is changing the culture from one of blaming individuals for errors to one in which errors are treated not as personal failures, but as opportunities to improve the system and prevent harm.* (Kohn et al., *To Err is Human*, 2000)

The whole patient safety landscape changed for first-world countries with the release of the Institute of Medicine's (IOM) seminal paper, *To Err Is Human: Building a Safer Health System* [15]. The release of the IOM paper exposed the impact of the harm caused by adverse events. It started the conversation about how to keep patients safe in healthcare organizations and created the impetus for change to a patient safety agenda. Ways of categorizing adverse events, investigating them, and governing them were the result.

The original intent of the report was to address not the entire quality of care agenda but rather an important element of it, namely, patient safety. For the first time, the spotlight was on systemic factors that contributed to errors rather than on investigating the "frailty" of human beings—their competence, intentions, or hard work. The report recommendations were intended to be applied within multiple jurisdictions such as hospitals, primary care clinics, nursing homes, retail pharmacies, and in-home care.

The overarching message of the IOM report was that preventing death and injury from medical errors requires extensive, system-wide changes in strategy to first recognize and then mitigate harm from error. This message was based on the premise that early intervention provides the greatest potential for curbing patient harm. Moreover, the report proposed that new tools and patient care systems should be developed to make it easier for staff to do things *right* and reduce the incidence of things going *wrong*.

Subsequently, from an extensive literature review and based on the collective background and experience of WHO Committee members, principles of care were developed for the provision of quality healthcare to prevent patient harm [31]. These included simplification of processes; standardization of equipment; making procedures visible so that steps can be checked and back-tracked if necessary; attending to work factors that contribute to fatigue and distraction such as workloads, staffing ratios, and shift changes; and avoiding long shifts and rotating staff. Furthermore, it recommended the following: establishing interdisciplinary team training so that staff can learn how to work well together; placing patients' history, medications, charts, etc. at their bedside to assist immediate decision-making; and involving patients in their care. It recommended that critical functions be duplicated in case of initial failure and that procedures be designed to expect unexpected changes, especially at times of restructuring and other organization-wide changes.

Furthermore, the Committee recommended a four-part plan that would apply to all frontline workers, clinical administrators and boards of directors, regulators, accrediting agencies, licensing groups, and government agencies. The plan included: establishing a National Center for Patient Safety; instigating mandatory and voluntary reporting systems; recognizing the role of consumers, professionals, and accreditation groups in patient safety; and building a *culture* of patient safety. Although significant progress has been made in the first three areas over the past two decades, establishing a culture of patient safety in healthcare organizations remains elusive.

The Committee suggested that the implementation of their recommendations would necessitate the development of "a new field of health care research, a new taxonomy of error, and new tools for addressing problems" [31]. Moreover, they noted that the responsibility for implementation needed to be borne not by single individuals but by multiple parties involved in patient care—healthcare organizations, government agencies, education and training providers, and patients and their families. Currently, two decades after the release of *To Err is Human*, the key message remains the same:

> *The greatest challenge we all face is to learn, use, and share better information about how to prevent harm to patients.* [31]

1.4 Universal Health Coverage

The WHO believes that the provision of patient safety and quality health services is a prerequisite for strengthening healthcare systems globally and making progress toward effective universal health coverage (UHC). Under their *Sustainable Development Goal 3*: *To ensure healthy lives and promote health and well-being for all at all ages*, UHC includes "financial risk protection, access to quality essential healthcare services, and access to safe, effective, quality and affordable essential medicines and vaccines for all" [32]. For the WHO, working toward UHC is the most effective approach for achieving better health globally and ensuring that quality services are delivered to patients safely [33]. The provision of safe services will not only keep patients from harm but also reduce costs related to patient care and improve overall efficiency in healthcare systems. In addition, safe health systems restore community confidence and trust in the system [34].

Over the past two decades, in response to the growing demand for increased patient safety from professionals, consumer groups, and healthcare organizations, the WHO has established a series of discussion forums and policy think-tanks to address the issue of patient safety, including the following:

1. In 2004, the WHO recognized the importance of patient safety with the launch of the *World Alliance for Patient Safety*. Since then, they have facilitated improvements in the safety of healthcare within member states through the establishment of global patient safety challenges, e.g.:

    - *Clean Care is Safer Care* (2005)—with the goal of reducing healthcare-associated infection by focusing on improved hand hygiene.
    - *Safe Surgery Saves Lives* (2008)—dedicated to reducing risks associated with surgery.
    - *Medication without Harm* (2017)—with the aim of reducing the level of severe, avoidable harm related to medications globally by 50% over 5 years.

2. In 2019, the WHO's *72nd World Health Assembly* recognized patient safety as a global health priority by adopting resolution WHA72.6 on *Global Action on Patient Safety*, which endorsed the establishment of the *World Patient Safety Day* to be observed every year on September 17. Its purpose is to promote patient safety by increasing public awareness and engagement, enhancing global understanding, and working toward global solidarity and action.

3. The resolution also requested that the WHO's Director General "formulate a global patient safety action plan in consultation with Member States, regional economic integration organizations and all relevant stakeholders including in the private sector" [32]. This plan was to be based on the guiding principles of equity, sustainability, and accountability.
4. In February 2020, in response to the unprecedented global patient safety movement, the need for urgent and concerted action in this area, and to align with the *Sustainable Developmental Goals*, the WHO launched its flagship initiative: *A Decade of Patient Safety 2020–2030*.
5. Since 2011, the WHO has been pivotal in the production of technical guidance and resources such as the *Multi-Professional Patient Safety Curriculum Guide* [35], *Safe Childbirth Checklist*, *Surgical Safety Checklist*, *Patient Safety Solutions*, and *5 Moments for Medication Safety*. Interprofessional collaboration and teamwork among all health professional groups are important so that these frameworks can be implemented as planned [36].
6. To prompt global action, the WHO has created networking and collaborative initiatives such as the *Global Patient Safety Network* and the *Global Patient Safety Collaborative*. Recognizing the importance of patients' active involvement in healthcare governance, health policy and system improvement, and their own care, the WHO also established the *Patients for Patient Safety* program to foster the engagement of patients and families.
7. The WHO continues to provide strategic guidance and leadership to countries through the annual *Global Ministerial Summit on Patient Safety*, which seeks to advance the patient safety agenda at the political leadership level with the support of health ministers, high-level delegates, experts, and representatives from international organizations. The *Patient Safety and Risk Management* Unit at the WHO has been instrumental in advancing and shaping the patient safety agenda globally by a number of means, including conducting research in areas of strategic importance and driving improvements in these areas, setting global priorities and providing global leadership for action, fostering collaboration between member states and relevant stakeholders to build member state capacity, and providing guidelines and technical expertise to develop tools that support and monitor improvements in patient safety.

By focusing on these key areas to facilitate sustainable improvements in patient safety, the WHO aims to enhance the patient experience worldwide, reduce risk and harm, achieve better health outcomes, and lower costs.

1.5 Healthcare System Attempts to Reduce Errors

Within developed nations, governments have mandated that health authorities implement quality measures in accordance with the WHO's guidelines for patient safety, customized to meet the consumer needs and interests of their constituents.

In the USA, the Joint Commission (TJC) is the authority that sets quality health standards, accredits health organizations and monitors their performance, and provides resources and tools to ensure that quality and safe care is delivered to patients to support continuous improvement. It is an independent, not-for-profit organization created in 1951 that accredits more than 20,000 US healthcare programs and organizations [37]. Its mission is to "continuously improve health care for the public, in collaboration with other stakeholders, by evaluating health care organizations and inspiring them to excel in providing safe and effective care of the highest quality and value."[1] Its vision is that "all people always experience the safest, highest quality, best-value health care across all settings."[2] The TJC aims to assist all healthcare organizations in achieving zero harm by utilizing contemporary knowledge, resources, and practices delivered to the highest standards of patient care across the continuum of care. It interfaces with the federal government and other stakeholders on key legislative, regulatory, and public policy issues to promote safe and high-quality healthcare.

In the United Kingdom (UK), the National Health Service (NHS) is the authority responsible for the delivery of comprehensive, universal, and free health services across England, Scotland, Wales, and Northern Ireland. Established in 1948 as part of the social reform agenda after the war, the NHS's role is to ensure that healthcare organizations receiving public funds improve the health and well-being of patients in their care. Their role in preventing poor health and promoting healthy living is essential for reducing health inequalities and sustaining quality healthcare for future generations. In their report from the NHS Future Forum, Soni and Bailey (2023) [38] recorded several recommendations, including the following:

1. Every healthcare professional should use every contact with an individual to maintain or improve their mental and physical health and well-being where possible.
2. In partnership with their staff, NHS organizations and their delivery partners should design and implement a strategy for improving staff mental and physical health and well-being.
3. All providers of NHS-funded care should prevent poor health and promote healthy living in their day-to-day business and be recognized for achieving excellence.
4. NHS commissioners and providers of NHS-funded care should use partnerships with other local services to improve the health and well-being of communities that the local NHS finds difficult to reach, providing training where appropriate.
5. Healthcare professionals, NHS commissioners, and providers of NHS-funded care should share learning about improving the public's health and well-being and reducing health inequalities, and seek to learn from others.

[1] https://www.jointcommission.org/who-we-are/#a8d46e698e644267bc9193ef844bfa07

[2] https://www.jointcommission.org/who-we-are/#a8d46e698e644267bc9193ef844bfa07

In June of that same year, the NHS *Long-term Workforce Plan* was announced. It aims to train more doctors and nurses and add new roles to their health services [39]. Leaders who can deliver patient safety coaching[3] may be well regarded in the future vision of the NHS.

In Australia, the Australian Commission on Safety and Quality in Health (ACSQH) is the relevant healthcare authority. In 2005, it produced a *National Patient Safety Education Framework* followed by a detailed *Australian Patient Safety Education Framework* [40]. The framework provides a simple, flexible and accessible approach that identifies the knowledge, skills, behaviors, attitudes, and performance required by all healthcare workers in relation to patient safety in Australia. In addition, in 2009, the ACSQH developed a *Patient Safety Curriculum Guide* based on the WHO document of the same name, which was designed to be used by all health professions in Australia not just doctors. Following the Australian lead, the WHO's later document, the *Patient Safety Curriculum Guide*: *Multi-Professional Edition* (2011), included guidelines for training in patient safety in other disciplines such as dentistry, midwifery, nursing, and pharmacy [35]. Each of these professional associations endorsed the principles of patient safety contained in the *Guide* and supported the importance of multidisciplinary education and multi-disciplinary care teams.

Furthermore, in November 2017, the National Safety and Quality Health Service (NSQHS), in collaboration with the Australian government, states and territories, private sector providers, clinical experts, patients, and carers, developed a series of eight *Standards.*[4] The primary aim of the *Standards* is to protect the public from harm and improve the quality of health service provision. Each of the *Standards* provides a nationally consistent statement of the level of care patients can expect from healthcare providers. They were updated in May 2021 (second edition) [33] and provide guidance to clinical staff in a number of areas that can significantly affect patient care:

- Medication safety
- Communicating for safety
- Preventing and controlling infection
- Blood management
- Comprehensive care
- Clinical governance
- Partnering with consumers
- Recognizing and responding to acute deterioration

[3] Healthcare workers can be trained to deliver patient safety coaching by the Australian Institute of Professional Coaches. www.professionalcoachtraining.com.au

[4] https://www.safetyandquality.gov.au/standards/nsqhs-standards

The *Safety and Quality Advice Centre* of the NSQHS provides support for healthcare organizations, assessors, and accrediting agencies in relation to the following initiatives[5]:

- NSQHS Standards
- National Safety and Quality Primary and Community Healthcare Standards
- Australian Health Service Safety and Quality Accreditation Scheme
- National General Practice Accreditation Scheme
- National Pathology Accreditation Scheme
- National Diagnostic Imaging Accreditation Scheme

The State of Patient Safety and Quality in Australian Hospitals, a 2019 NSQHS report, provides comprehensive information on the performance of the Australian healthcare system at that time and the state of Australian leadership in relation to patient safety and quality of care.

1.6 Contemporary Approaches to Reduce Patient Harm

Standard procedures to keep patents safe (e.g., risk management strategies, investigations of adverse events, root cause analysis) rely on a backward examination of incidents and adverse events once patients have been harmed. They identify the source of the harm and determine who is to blame. The solution is to "fix" the situation or person so that a similar event does not occur in the future. However, patients keep dying! Therefore, these procedures, while constructive in their findings post-event, are insufficient to prevent incidents from occurring in the future. Something different has to be done!

Cultural change was recommended by the WHO Committee as the ultimate solution to keep patients safe [31]. However, before cultural change can occur, people often need to change their mindset, which requires a paradigm shift. Rather than focusing time, effort, and finances on finding retrospective solutions to what went *wrong*, contemporary proponents of change propose an emphasis on looking forward to ways that are already working and can easily be replicated—to what's going *right*. Looking forward can preempt the occurrence of adverse events and incidents because systems can be adjusted as circumstances arise, and people can be trained in preventative measures.

[5] https://www.safetyandquality.gov.au/standards/nsqhs-standards/safety-and-quality-advice-centre

1.6.1 Paradigm Shift: From Safety-1 to Safety-11

When an adverse event occurs, much of the investigation data arise from retrospective reviews of medical charts and indirect or lagging indicators such as readmission rates. These techniques are focused on improving isolated processes within a complex, adaptive system. They were introduced into high-risk industries following the Chernobyl disaster in 1986 and represent what Hollnagel et al. [1] call a Safety-1 approach to keeping people safe. Subsequent to this event and that of similar others, contemporary research in healthcare has demonstrated the causal relationship between poor safety and quality culture and the occurrence of adverse patient events [36]. Hence, it is time to focus on changing the culture of healthcare organizations by utilizing the power of the greatest resource within these systems—the staff themselves—to transform the environment in which healthcare is provided into a Safety-11 approach to patient care [1].

In 2015, Hollnagel et al. [1] proposed a Safety-11 approach to addressing incidents and adverse events. Instead of finding what went *wrong* and someone to blame, they espoused identifying all the things going *right* in a workplace and replicating them. They encouraged concentrating on identifying systemic issues rather than apportioning individual blame. The Safety-11 approach does not negate the need for compliance with legislation and protocols; rather, it focuses on how situations and individuals can be systemically set up for success each and every time compliance protocols are in place. Therefore, in terms of patient safety, this means identifying how patients can receive the very best of care without harm befalling them by staff who are not stressed because they have everything they need to do their job well.

In a Safety-11 environment, staff feel confident that they are providing the best possible care to patients when:

1. They work in a psychologically safe workplace in which they feel able to report near misses without fear of being blamed and losing their job.
2. They have leaders focused on excellence who adopt and can demonstrate contemporary clinical practices from which they learn.
3. They are supported emotionally when trauma strikes, so they are able to overcome adversity more quickly and become more resilient.

This book addresses how staff can do their job *well* when these three conditions prevail. It also addresses how clinical leaders and organizational executives can exercise good clinical governance in relation to both staff and patients in their care. Specifically, it discusses how executives can:

- Change the culture of their organization to develop a patient safety culture in which near misses are reported without fear or blame, recrimination, or reprisal.
- Learn from excellence by identifying and utilizing contemporary clinical practices to save lives.

- Utilize coaching as a developmental approach to increase leader capability, support staff well-being, and create psychological safety within teams to bring about cultural change.

1.6.2 Cultural Change

Getting all healthcare organization executives on the same page, ready to implement initiatives to achieve a patient safety culture, requires the dedication and commitment of a chief executive officer who can work well with their team. Understanding the dimensions of the task before them starts with a reality check of the facts and possible consequences resulting from patient harm. Next, executives must be willing to establish a shared vision and goals in relation to patient safety. They need to be prepared to extend standard procedures to embrace new processes and technologies and acquire the nontechnical, coaching skills that are vital to the creation of a person-centered cultural approach to patient safety in healthcare settings.

1.6.3 Coaching for Patient Safety

A key component of the Safety-11 solution for better patient care is effective leadership, which supports individuals and teams as they strive to manage workplace dilemmas and prevent adverse events. Well-functioning staff can focus meaningfully and purposefully on the job at hand, be mindful of doing their job well, and relate and communicate effectively with colleagues. Remaining centered and emotionally regulated in an often-changing work environment is of utmost importance for delivering exceptional patient care, especially in situations in which split-second decisions are needed.

Coaching is a developmental process in which leaders engage in reflection to discover greater self-awareness of how they lead, how they support team members in their daily clinical practice, and how they create the environment and conditions in which a patient safety culture can flourish (Fig. 1.1). Patient safety coaching is a Safety-11 process that supports leaders, team members, and interdisciplinary teams to ensure the presence of the necessary preconditions for a positive patient safety culture to thrive and flourish.

Clinicians add nontechnical, coaching skills to their repertoire when they become educated and trained in patient safety coaching.[6] This nontechnical skillset—patient safety coaching—works in concert with their primary functional expertise to support the development of a patient safety culture within their team. As the team

[6] A course to train clinical leaders and team members in patient safety coaching is delivered by the Australian Institute of Professional Coaches. https://professionalcoachtraining.com.au/

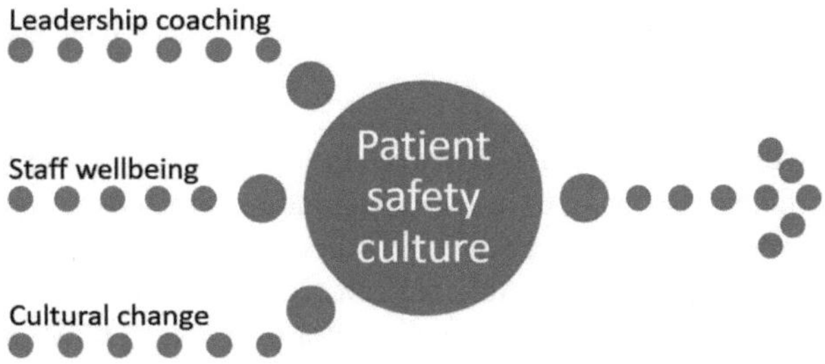

Fig. 1.1 How coaching supports the development of a patient safety culture

culture changes from the ground up, the culture of the organization as a whole transforms as well, into a patient safety culture.

1.7 Chapter Overviews

Chapter 1: Introduction This chapter introduces the background and context for patient safety coaching within healthcare organizations. As a global imperative of the WHO, patient safety is *the* number one priority of every healthcare organization. In the past, when adverse events occurred, they were investigated and blame apportioned. Usually, an employee was fired, and the organization fined. However, these practices of investigation and reprisal have done little to stop incidents from occurring—some with fatal consequences. A paradigm shift is necessary to rethink healthcare organizations' approaches to patient safety. Enter Safety-11 [1]—a philosophical, cultural mindset change that underpins contemporary mechanisms by which organizations and staff can prevent adverse events from occurring in the first place by learning from mistakes as they arise.

Chapter 2: The Future of Healthcare Healthcare systems worldwide operate in increasingly complex environments: people are living longer, often with multiple presentations; hospital workforces are shrinking; advanced technology is impacting multiple treatment areas; budgets cannot keep pace with demand; and patient expectations are changing with increased access to medical information on the Internet. These factors will shift future healthcare agendas from the provision of the full range of services for everyone within fixed facilities to the delivery of care in community settings where less intensive treatments are available for common illnesses, with the support of general practitioners, pharmacists, and allied health professionals and in-home care services. Healthcare services will increasingly be delivered in clinics at the local level or at home using personalized treatment plans and options supported by internal monitoring equipment and external wearable technology. Within fixed facilities, the shift will be toward active patient partnerships and proactive patient care, assisted by advanced technologies such as robotics and customized medical treatment regimens.

Chapter 3: Adverse Events in Healthcare Finding ways to avoid adverse events presents a significant challenge to healthcare organizations and a compelling rationale for the deployment of extensive, resource-intensive initiatives to improve patient safety. Adverse events in healthcare can occur due to a number of causes that may relate to clinical factors, human factors, or systemic/cultural factors. Traditionally, adverse events have been addressed using a Safety-1 [1] investigative approach to discover what happened and who was to blame. More recently, a shift in thinking has caused clinical leaders, healthcare administrators, and executives to operationalize their efforts and direct their budgets to prevent adverse events from occurring in the first place, i.e., toward a Safety-11 approach to patient care [1]. Safety-11 clinical practices focus on doing more of what is going *right* to identify excellence rather than looking backward at what could have or should have been done to prevent the incident from occurring. Of course, investigations into major incidents must still occur, but could these adverse events have been prevented by learning from contemporary procedures that showcase the very latest and best in clinical practice and healthcare technology?

Chapter 4: Patient Safety Coaching in Healthcare Coaching is a developmental, relational, and social process that motivates and supports coachees to solve their own problems and achieve their goals [41]. The coaching process helps individuals and teams gain greater self-awareness and insight into their current situation and guides them toward behavioral change, which leads to better outcomes. In a healthcare setting, coaching supports the utilization of strengths and learning from excellence, develops staff capability in nontechnical interpersonal skills, reduces stress, and promotes resilience and well-being. When adopted by all leaders and teams as a better way of behaving, communicating with, and relating to others, coaching leads to transformational cultural change [42]. Coaching of teams post-incident results in improved clinical practices that are utilized in the future. Coaching preemptively highlights learning from observations and feedback as a result of exceptional clinical practice.

Chapter 5: Coaching to Increase Leader Capability This chapter explores the first purpose of coaching in a healthcare setting—to increase leadership capability so leaders can prevent the occurrence of adverse events and keep patients safe from harm. Staff in healthcare organizations are critically aware of the importance of keeping patients safe. They have the clinical (technical) skills to do so but not always the personal (nontechnical) skills to render compassionate, person-centered care, especially in difficult situations or when working in interdisciplinary teams. Coaching can increase leaders' nontechnical capability to communicate and relate better with patients and other staff members. Leaders who are emotionally intelligent and adopt a coaching leadership style [42–44] are better able to motivate and inspire staff to emulate excellent clinical practice and learn from adverse events.

Communication is enhanced when leaders actively engage in dialog with staff and patients and encourage others to do the same. Leaders who adopt a coaching leadership style listen to what staff members are saying and utilize the strengths of interdisciplinary teams. They encourage staff to analyze situations, think critically about possible outcomes, and take preventative action in relation to potentially adverse outcomes that may cause patients harm.

Chapter 6: Coaching for Staff Well-Being This chapter explores the second purpose of patient safety coaching in a healthcare setting—to improve staff well-being and job satisfaction so that staff are fully "present" with patients and alert to their care needs. Keeping patients safe from harm relies on clinical staff being focused and on-purpose every minute of their shift. A concentration failure could result in dire consequences. Leaders have an obligation to ensure that all staff are fully present as they work, mindful of patient needs and concerns, and aware of any organizational barriers or constraints that may impede progress or cause patients harm. Staff who present to shift alert, self-aware, and confident in their ability to perform well are able to navigate through the trauma that may result following an adverse event. Coaching is a developmental process that helps staff overcome this trauma. It nurtures physical, mental, and emotional well-being so that staff can provide excellent patient care. Staff well-being is the sum of their resourcefulness, resilience, and emotional commitment to compassionate care. Staff who are motivated, enthusiastic, and empowered demonstrate the emotional strength that inspires confidence in all around them. Patients benefit when staff operate "in the flow" on a daily basis, supported by leaders who coach them when necessary to help them learn, grow, and develop to become excellent clinical practitioners.

Chapter 7: Coaching to Develop a Patient Safety Culture This chapter explores the third purpose of patient safety coaching in a healthcare setting—to develop a patient safety culture within frontline teams and across the entire healthcare organization. In a psychologically safe workplace in which there is no blame or recrimination, near misses are reported, and staff learn from their mistakes. Routinely, they pay attention to, and observe and learn from, excellent clinical practices to prevent the occurrence of adverse events. A patient safety culture is formed when all staff members share the values of patient safety, understand and share the meaning behind the words, are focused on a common purpose, and behave in ways that demonstrate commitment to patient safety. As a subculture of organizational culture, a patient safety culture is developed when healthcare leaders display patient safety behaviors in every situation, utilize a coaching leadership style, and support a bottom-up approach to cultural change within their team.

Chapter 8: Measuring Patient Safety Culture Assessing the patient safety culture of a healthcare organization at the beginning of a cultural change program is essential to its success. Baseline data can be collected using several validated instruments, principally the *Hospital Survey of Patient Safety Culture* (HSOPSC) which gathers staff perceptions of a patient safety culture in eight areas, including how staff communicate with and relate to each other and how *well* teams work together. Gaps in survey results become the focus of targeted interventions to improve patient safety culture. Medical and nonmedical staff may be selected to complete the survey. The results may be analyzed by ward or staff unit, occupation or position within the organization, and/or seniority within the ward or hospital. Other assessment instruments are available that measure staff attitudes toward patient safety, job satisfaction, and staff assessment of working conditions. Strategies to develop a patient safety culture based on a Safety-11 approach [1] include *coaching* to develop leadership capability, support staff well-being, and create a psychologically safe working environment. When the organization is ready for cultural change, measurements can be taken and strategies implemented, as part of a quality management strategy to improve its patient safety record.

Chapter 9: Governance in Healthcare Executives in healthcare organizations are responsible for the effective and efficient operation of their facility. They must ensure compliance with all government legislation and associated regulations. They have a fiduciary duty of care as well as a moral obligation to manage the best possible healthcare system for their patients. Society expects that patients can turn to healthcare staff to look after them in their hours of need. However, managerial and clinical staff perceptions of patient safety may vary significantly in terms of prioritizing interventions that can improve patient care and safety, as well as in relation to their perceived roles in establishing and maintaining a patient safety culture [45, 46]. Research has shown that hospital executives and managers, by failing to recognize their role in supporting patient safety, may actually hinder error reporting and learning from excellence, particularly at critical times such as patient handovers [47, 48].

Key Takeaways

- Patients continue to be harmed in healthcare facilities and during transit on a daily basis despite advances and changes at an unacceptable rate.
- Finding blame as an approach to addressing adverse events when they occur unfortunately still exists. This is a Safety-1 approach to patient safety.
- A Safety-11 [1] approach examines the systemic factors which led to the adverse event occurring in the first place. This strategy pre-emptively manages risk by focusing on what the organization is doing *well* and how it reinforces *excellent* clinical practices.
- Coaching is a nontechnical skill that leaders can learn to use to support staff well-being and create a patient safety culture within their team.

1.8 Case Study 1: Anatomy of an Adverse Event

A typical day in the general medical unit of a major metropolitan teaching hospital begins with the nursing shift handover. The night shift team briefs the incoming day shift on patient statuses, new admissions, and significant overnight events. This ensures continuity of care and prepares the team for the day ahead.

The bulk of the day's activity starts with multidisciplinary team rounds, including doctors, nurses, and allied health professionals. Together, they review patient progress, update treatment plans, and address any concerns from patients or their families.

Morning activities involve administering medications, performing routine assessments, and conducting diagnostic tests. Patients receive care from physiotherapists, occupational therapists, and other specialists. The unit buzzes with activity as staff attend to the diverse needs of their patients and coordinate care. Families might visit, and patients might leave the ward for assessments and diagnostic tests. Junior medical staff work busily to ensure that everything discussed on the ward round is documented and actioned.

In the afternoon, the focus shifts to patient admissions and discharges. New patients arriving from inter-hospital transfers or the emergency department are assessed, oriented to the ward, and care commenced. Simultaneously, junior medical staff work to prepare discharge summaries and medication scripts and coordinate with community services to ensure continuity of care for departing patients. This becomes increasingly important as the ward fills up and pressure mounts to discharge patients.

Late in the afternoon, due to pressure from a busy emergency department, the ward accepts four patients at once, which is outside the planned admission policy. These patients are placed in a four-bed bay at the end of the corridor that was closed earlier in the day due to low nursing staff availability.

One of the new patients in the four-bed bay, unsteady on their feet, attempts to go to the bathroom. Unable to call for help and with the bed rail up, they climb over the rail and fall, sustaining a hip injury, head injury, and multiple skin tears. The other patients, either delirious or behind drawn curtains, are unaware of the fall, leading to a prolonged delay before the patient is found injured and confused on the floor.

The nurse in charge of the new four-bed bay had just started his shift; he was taking a handover and assisting colleagues when the event occurred. When it is discovered by chance by a nurse seeking an infusion pump, immediate measures are taken to stabilize the patient, who is placed in a warm blanket and carefully assisted back to bed. The evening registrar is called, examines the patient, and refers them for an X-ray of the hip and a CT brain scan. Senior medical staff on call are alerted, and the family is notified of the fall and the management plan. Detailed documentation of the event, including the time, nature, immediate actions, and patient's response, is recorded in the patient chart.

Later that evening, it is clear that the patient sustained a neck of femur fracture and a moderate head injury. They will need to undergo unplanned surgery to fix the neck of femur fracture. Transparent communication with the patient's family is essential; an update is made by the evening medical registrar. The next day, a senior medical staff member meets with the family to explain what happened, the steps taken to address the issue, and the current status of the patient. This conversation is conducted with compassion and honesty, acknowledging the distress the event may have caused.

After care is started, the nursing staff document the event in the hospital's incident reporting system. Eventually an investigation is conducted to identify underlying causes, using analysis tools such as a root cause analysis. Based on the findings, recommendations are developed to prevent recurrence. At the organizational level, policies and protocols may be updated to address identified weaknesses. New training programs may be implemented to ensure staff are fully equipped to prevent similar events in the future.

Communication with the family continues, offering regular updates on the patient's condition, the steps being taken to address the situation, and any deficits that come to light from the investigation. The hospital offers apologies and takes responsibility where appropriate, emphasizing their commitment to rectifying the issue and preventing future occurrences.

For Discussion

1. Why is patient safety important?
   - What happened in this case study, and what could have been done differently?
2. What has been the traditional way to address adverse events?
   - What happened in this case study, and what could have been done differently?
3. What cultural or systemic factors may be at play in this case study?
   - What could have been done differently?
4. In what ways do you think that coaching can be part of a cultural change process?

References

1. Hollnagel, E., Wears, R., & Braithwaite, J. (2015). *From safety-I to safety-II: A white paper*. University of Southern Denmark, University of Florida, USA, and Macquarie University.
2. WHO. (2019). *Medication safety in high-risk situations; Technical report*. World Health Organization.
3. WHO. (2021). *Global Patient Safety Action Plan 2021–2030: Towards eliminating avoidable harm in health care*. World Health Organization, Licence: CC BY-NC-SA 3.0 IGO.
4. WHO. (2020). *Patient Safety Assessment Manual, Third Edition*. World Health Organization. Regional Office for the Eastern Mediterranean. License: CC BY-NC-SA 3.0 IGO.

5. Schwendimann, R., et al. (2018). The occurrence, types, consequences and preventability of in-hospital adverse events—A scoping review. *BMC Health Services Research, 18*, 521.
6. Bates, D. W., & Singh, H. (2018). Two decades since 'To err is human': An assessment of progress and emerging priorities in patient safety. *Health Affairs (Millwood), 37*(11).
7. TJC. (2021). Sentinel event alert 63: Optimizing smart infusion pump safety with DERS. *The Joint Commission Journal on Quality and Patient Safety, 47*, 394–397.
8. Verhaegh, K. J., et al. (2017). An exploratory study of healthcare professionals' perceptions of interprofessional communication and collaboration. *Journal of Interprofessional Care, 31*(3), 397–400.
9. Latvis, L., Fick, J., & Dishman, L. (2021). What senior healthcare leadership competencies matter most to affect positive patient experiences in United States inpatient acute care hospitals? *Michigan Academician, 48*(1), 51–52.
10. Collins, D., et al. (2018). Integration of health coaching concepts and skills into clinical practice among VHA providers: A qualitative study. *Global Advances in Health and Medicine, 7*, 2164957X18757463.
11. WHO. (2005). *Draft guidelines for adverse event reporting and learning systems: From information to action, in World Alliance for Patient Safety*. World Health Organization.
12. WHO. (2009). *Conceptual framework for the International Classification for Patient Safety, Version 1.1: Final technical report*. World Health Organization.
13. Auraaen, A., Slawomirski, L., & Klazinga, N. (2018). *The economics of patient safety in primary and ambulatory care- Flying blind*. OECD Health Working Papers (No. 106).
14. James, J. T. (2013). A new, evidence-based estimate of patient harms associated with hospital care. *Journal of Patient Safety, 9*(3), 122–128.
15. Kohn, L. T., Corrigan, J. M., & Donaldson, M. S. (2000). Errors in health care: A leading cause of death and injury. In *To err is human: Building a safer health system*. National Academies Press.
16. Durmus, S. Ç., et al. (2013). Medical errors: An important indicator of quality of care and patient safety. *Holistic Nursing Practice, 27*(4), 225–232.
17. Chen, L.-C., et al. (2018). A study on the reporting intention of medical incidents: A nursing perspective. *Clinical Nursing Research, 27*(5), 560–578.
18. Asadi, E. M., & Dadashpour, N. (2018). Medical errors in emergency department; A letter to editor. *Emergency, 6*(1), e33.
19. Ehsani, S. R., et al. (2013). Medication errors of nurses in the emergency department. *Journal of Medical Ethics, 6*(11).
20. Pham, J. C., et al. (2011). National study on the frequency, types, causes, and consequences of voluntarily reported emergency department medication errors. *Journal of Emergency Medicine, 40*(5), 485–492.
21. Vazin, A., Zamani, Z., & Hatam, N. (2014). Frequency of medication errors in an emergency department of a large teaching hospital in southern Iran. *Drug Health Patient Safety, 6*, 179–184.
22. Slawomirski, L., A. Auraaen, and N. Klazinga, The economics of patient safety: Strengthening a value-based approach to reducing patient harm at national level. 2017.
23. Slawomirski, L., Auraaen, A., & Klazinga, N. (2018). *The economics of patient safety in primary and ambulatory care: Flying blind*. Organisation for Economic Co-operation and Development.
24. Jha, A. K. (2018). Presentation at the "patient safety—A grand challenge for healthcare professionals and policymakers alike": A roundtable at the grand challenges meeting of the Bill & Melinda Gates Foundation.
25. Thomas, E. J., et al. (2000). Incidence and types of adverse events and negligent care in Utah and Colorado. *Medical Care, 38*(3), 261–271.
26. de Vries, E. N., et al. (2008). The incidence and nature of in-hospital adverse events: A systematic review. *Quality & Safety in Health Care, 17*, 216–223.

27. National Academies of Sciences, Engineering, and Medicine, *Crossing the global quality chasm: Improving health care worldwide*. 2018: .
28. Jha, A. K., et al. (2013). *The global burden of unsafe medical care: Analytic modelling of observational studies*. BMJ Qual Saf Published Online First.
29. Etchells, E., et al. (2012). *The economics of patient safety in acute care: Technical report*. Patient Safety Institute.
30. Thompson, L., et al. (2021). Clinical coaches and patient safety—Just in time: A descriptive exploratory study. *Nurse Education in Practice, 54*, 103134.
31. WHO. (2010). *Learning from error: Patient safety workshop*. World Health Organization.
32. WHO. (2019). *Global action on patient safety. Report by the Director-General*. World Health Organization.
33. NSQHS. (2021). National safety and quality health service standards. *Second edition*. In *Australian Commission on Safety and Quality in Health Care*.
34. Leape, L. (1997). Testimony before the President's advisory commission on consumer production and quality in the health care industry.
35. WHO. (2011). *Patient safety curriculum guide—Multi-professional Edition*. World Helath Organization.
36. Davis, E., & Beale, N. (2015). It's time: The poor culture regarding safety and quality in Australian hospitals must be addressed! *Asia Pacific Journal of Health Management, 10*(3), GS36–GS41.
37. Patterson, C. H. (1995). Joint commission on accreditation of healthcare organizations. *Infection Control and Hospital Epidemiology, 16*(1), 36–42.
38. Soni, A., & Bailey, V. (2023). *The NHS's role in the public's health: A report from the NHS Future Forum*. National Health Service.
39. BBC. (2023, June 30). *Plan to train and retain more NHS doctors and nurses*.
40. Walton, M. (2006). Developing a national patient safety education framework for Australia. *Quality Safety Healthcare, 15*, 437–442.
41. Knowles, S. (2021). *Positive psychology coaching*. Springer Nature.
42. Knowles, S. (2022). *Coaching culture*. Springer Nature.
43. Karlsen, J. T., & Berg, M. E. (2020). Coaching leadership style: A learning process. *International Journal of Knowledge and Learning, 13*(4), 356–368.
44. Goleman, D. (2000). Leadership that gets results. *Harvard Business Review, 78*(2), 78–90.
45. Parand, A., et al. (2014). The role of hospital managers in quality and patient safety: A systematic review. *BMJ Open, 4*(9), e005055.
46. Quenon, J.-L., et al. (2020). Exploring the role of managers in the development of a safety culture in seven French healthcare facilities: A qualitative study. *BMC Health Services Research, 20*(1), 517.
47. Richter, J. P., McAlearney, A. S., & Pennell, M. L. (2016). The influence of organizational factors on patient safety: Examining successful handoffs in health care. *Health Care Management Review, 41*(1), 32.
48. Richter, J. P., McAlearney, A. S., & Pennell, M. L. (2015). Evaluating the effect of safety culture on error reporting: A comparison of managerial and staff perspectives. *American Journal of Medical Quality, 30*(6), 550–558.

Chapter 2
The Future of Healthcare

Healthcare systems worldwide operate in increasingly complex environments: people are living longer, often with multiple presentations; hospital workforces are shrinking; advanced technology is impacting multiple treatment areas; budgets cannot keep pace with demand; and patient expectations are changing with increased access to medical information on the Internet. These factors will shift future healthcare agendas from the provision of the full range of services for everyone within fixed facilities to the delivery of care in community settings where less intensive treatments are available for common illnesses, with the support of general practitioners, pharmacists, and allied health professionals and in-home care services. Healthcare services will increasingly be delivered in clinics at the local level or at home using personalized treatment plans and options supported by internal monitoring equipment and external wearable technology. Within fixed facilities, the shift will be toward active patient partnerships and proactive patient care, assisted by advanced technologies such as robotics and customized medical treatment regimens.

2.1 The Global Landscape

The global landscape of the healthcare industry has changed in the last two decades as risks to patients have increased in a more complex, global environment. Since 2005, patient safety has been recognized by the World Health Organization (WHO) as a large and growing global public health challenge and a fundamental principle of healthcare [1]. Studies have reported adverse events resulting from 4 to 17% of hospital admissions, with 5–21% of these adverse events resulting in death—half of which could have been prevented [2]. Despite global efforts, the incidence of adverse events has not decreased substantially over the past two decades. However, the focus on patient safety has intensified as a result of increasing reports of patient harm not only while in hospitals but also while on waiting lists or being transported

© The Author(s), under exclusive license to Springer Nature Switzerland AG 2024

S. Knowles, *Patient Safety Coaching*,
https://doi.org/10.1007/978-3-031-68722-8_2

to and from hospitals. Moreover, the need for hospital care has increased over the past 5 years as the pressures of pandemics and natural disasters have impacted service delivery not only in hospitals but also in other healthcare organizations, such as aged care facilities and community healthcare settings. Developed nations agree that quality healthcare services should be effective, safe, people-centered, timely, equitable, integrated, and efficient [3].

In response to this increasing concern over the number of adverse events in healthcare, governments, governance organizations, medical authorities, and professionals have sought to significantly reduce this occurrence. The historical approach to managing risk investigated adverse events after they had occurred, using root cause analysis to identify what went *wrong*. Although this approach continues to be an expectation of governments and legislators and an important part of healthcare compliance systems, it can, when solely relied upon or performed in environments with poor cultures, produce negative results such as a blame focus, avoidance behaviors, defensiveness, and fear, as the WHO noted in its 2014 report:

> *Patient safety is challenged by not only the complexity of health care processes but also the culture of denial and blame, the two characteristics that have dominated the environment of problem solving and learning that the health care service is. In addition, inconsistencies in the reporting and learning systems prevent collection and dissemination of information in a meaningful way.* [4]

Hence, in recent years, there have been increasing calls for a more proactive approach to managing risks in healthcare and improving patient outcomes. These calls have been for the development of a positive patient safety culture in all healthcare organizations.

2.1.1 The Context for Future Healthcare

There is no doubt that healthcare systems worldwide operate in increasingly complex environments:

- *People are living longer.* The need to provide care for an aging population is an additional burden on an already strained health system. Moreover, as people age, their care needs increase and become more complicated, often requiring specialized diagnosis and treatment. Comorbidities and polypharmacy are increasing.
- *Aging workforce.* The average age of nurses is declining. The workforce increasingly consists of older workers. Many new graduates do not remain in nursing as a lifetime career because of remuneration, the cost of living expenses, and housing issues. Finding accommodation close to work is an increasingly difficult task for shift workers. Working beyond traditional scope (i.e., more use of nurse practitioners) and the introduction of electronic medical records (EMRs) are common concerns of nurses.
- *Hospital workforces are shrinking.* Clinical staff are trying to provide the same level of service with fewer staff and, at times, inadequate resources and equip-

ment. This is occurring both on an absolute and relative level to the population. The recent strain of the pandemic on the healthcare workforce has led many people to leave their profession.
- *Advanced technologies*. New treatments and technologies can offer better outcomes but may have unintended consequences or interact with the current system in ways that can lead to patient harm. Issues relate to how technological advances can seamlessly integrate with existing systems and concerns regarding methods of delivering care (such as telehealth, personalized genomic therapeutics, and wearable technology for diagnostics).
- *Budgets for healthcare are static*. Having to do more with less is a common experience of staff in both developed and developing nations. The provision of care beyond fixed facilities and funding for community partnerships are now common agenda items in many healthcare organizations.
- *Internet access*. The ready availability of health information on the Internet has given rise to increased patient expectations about their care. Patients now expect to be better involved in decision-making about treatment options and planning their short- and long-term health outcomes.

The COVID-19 pandemic focused worldwide attention on the need for a universal approach to healthcare. It imposed an additional burden on already stretched hospital systems. Staff were asked to give more, resulting in fatigue and stress from working long hours. Exhaustion and burnout caused many staff to leave the profession, which imposed an even greater burden on those remaining. Since the release of damning statistics such as the following, healthcare organizations have been forced to rethink their workforce and clinical practice models [5]:

- Between February 2020 and February 2021, the healthcare workforce declined 3.5%, from 16.49 million to 15.92 million (American Hospital Association's *2022 Health Care Talent Scan*).
- Thirty-two percent of registered nurses indicated that they may leave their current position within the next year, citing insufficient staffing levels as the top factor influencing their decision to leave (2021 McKinsey survey of frontline staff).
- Demand for healthcare talent is predicted to grow to 30% higher than current levels in the next decade (Shubham Singhal, senior partner at McKinsey, Detroit).

2.1.2 The Operational Environment for Future Healthcare

Contemplating the complexity of the operating environment for healthcare and the ever-increasing threat of climate-related impacts, coupled with the effects of overpopulation, urbanization, and globalization, raises the following question: What is the future for the provision of healthcare services in developed countries? Radick [5] posits three predictions that may significantly influence the way care is delivered in the future and the impact on healthcare:

1. The delivery of healthcare will transition from fixed facility treatment to community-based and home care, supported by healthcare professionals such as pharmacists, general practitioners, and other allied health professionals. This change was accelerated by the pandemic and is likely to continue because of the positive responses of the community to localized healthcare access. This prediction suggests that acute care facilities such as hospitals, while still needed for those requiring surgery and high-end care, will constitute a smaller proportion of the overall delivery of patient care in the future.
2. Governments will increasingly be called upon to allocate additional funding for the provision of healthcare services such as Medicare-funded prescriptions and services. However, since governments tend not to increase the size of the funding budget for healthcare, what is likely to occur into the future is merely a redistribution of existing expenditures.
3. There will be a shift from providing healthcare services for everyone for everything in healthcare organizations and community settings to providing value for the delivery of services that will maximize the dollars spent from the public purse. The focus will increasingly be on funding outcomes instead of on the number of procedures performed or services provided.

If these three predictions are realized, healthcare services will increasingly be delivered at the local level, resulting in a need for more staff who can provide at-home and community care. This shift is already occurring in some jurisdictions, made increasingly possible by technology necessitated during the COVID-19 pandemic. Moreover, the call for online and home-based services is likely to expand into the future. This means that, in addition to the need for more doctors, nurses, and surgeons in the hospital system, there will be a greater need for more home-based and community service support provided by personal carers, allied health workers, paramedics, specialized technicians who analyze and support diagnosis, and pharmacists who prescribe prevention and treatment options. In addition, the pandemic has caused an increase in mental health issues resulting from the psychological strain of living in a restrictive environment during lockdowns and the fear of possible short- and long-term health effects of the virus. There is already an increasing need for psychologists, social workers, and others who can support patient mental health and life decisions into the future.

A greater focus on preventive care will lead to innovation, disruptive technology, wearable technology, and data and information systems, all of which will have substantial impacts on the care delivered by healthcare organizations in the future. Disruptive technology is continuing to transform the healthcare industry through the emergence of new technologies such as virtual reality, artificial intelligence, and robotics. Until integrated into existing systems and procedures, the use of these technologies may increase the number of intersections and potential failure points of healthcare delivery. Having an awareness of new technologies and what they can do to keep patients safe will reduce the occurrence of healthcare errors and near misses.

Healthcare forecasters are predicting that the future of healthcare will be characterized by a shift toward personalized care. Personalized medicine is an emerging field that tailors medical treatment to an individual's unique genetic makeup, lifestyle, and environment. This approach is based on the understanding that while physiology is largely universal, every individual is unique and medical treatment should be tailored to meet the specific needs of each patient. Personalized medicine has the potential to revolutionize healthcare by enabling targeted treatments for specific conditions and by reducing the likelihood of adverse reactions to medications.

Health futurists are also predicting that patients will play a more active role in managing their own health. Wearable technologies such as smartwatches, fitness trackers, and health monitoring devices are transforming healthcare delivery. These devices track vital signs, physical activity, sleep, and other health-related data. They can transmit these data to healthcare providers in real time, enabling remote monitoring and diagnosis of conditions. Wearable technology is enabling patients to take an active role in managing their health and is helping healthcare providers deliver more personalized care. The opportunities for wearable technology include increased access and affordability, and the enablement of remote monitoring for more proactive management of conditions.

2.2 A Proactive Healthcare System

In the past, the emphasis on patient safety has been on compliance with policies and procedures, investigations to discover the root cause of adverse events, and identification of who to blame. Procedures that focus solely on root causes are retrospective rather than preventative, based on reductionist thinking, and unfortunately are likely to lead to solutions that resolve only one component of the error pathway. This approach is what Hollnagel et al. [6] call the Safey-1 approach to risk management.

2.2.1 Safety-1

The reductionist view of safety can be traced back to the mid-late 1900s when the world was less complex and uncertain, and life was much simpler than it is today. This historical approach to patient safety originated from a "find-and-fix" model of care following a critical event. The event was analyzed not only to determine what happened but also to identify who to blame. There may have been a number of people involved in the pathway process, e.g., the delivery of medication involves a doctor, pharmacist, and nurse. The typical response was to blame the last person in the delivery chain [2, 7, 8]. That person would be punished as a result and may even lose their job. Using Safety-1 thinking, the nurse would be blamed and reprimanded for the error. However, the initiating error may have been caused by a system failure such as undifferentiated labeling of medications which, once blame has been attributed, may not be detected and may even lead to future errors.

Root cause analysis is often proposed as the gold standard in Safety-1 investigations. However, due to staff reluctance to provide information that could indicate their own or others' personal failure, and organizational time pressures to finish the investigation, the outcome of a root cause analysis may not lead to real causal insights. Additionally, the process is often too linear and reductive to result in larger-scale recommendations that would be effective in preventing future incidents from occurring.

Part of the problem is that when an incident occurs, it is usually investigated as a single incident, whereas near misses of a similar trajectory are often not reported. However, near misses are an indicator that harm is likely to occur. The Safety-1 view in relation to patient safety presumes that incidents occur because of identifiable factors such as human error, lack of training or supervision, unclear procedures, or technology failure. When something goes wrong, there is a reaction to try to "fix" it by identifying and eliminating the cause based on the view that the observable factors can be manipulated so that adverse events don't happen again—but they do! Therefore, this way of thinking and approach to adverse events is insufficient to keep patients safe in the increasingly complex and uncertain healthcare environment of the future.

Systemic factors may have played a significant part in creating the event, but because they were not reported or investigated and there is often insufficient visibility across the entire organization, incidents can occur in one department that may have also occurred in other departments, but no one is aware of them. In such instances, clinical specialists and consultants with content knowledge in the area of concern, who are independent of the work team in which the incident occurred, are of great value in bringing the occurrence of such incidents to the attention of relevant decision-makers.

Investigating what happened when an adverse event occurred, identifying the cause, and finding solutions to learn from the event, is currently the role of a patient safety officer or administrator who has been specifically trained to undertake the review process and make recommendations for improvement. Better outcomes result when an investigative patient safety *team* reviews groups of incident reports and aggregates the findings, producing a broader understanding of causation. In these instances, aggregate data assist in providing the basis for change at a larger scale, e.g., developing training programs aimed at proactively recognizing and responding to clinical errors. Even better is when all staff are part of the patient safety *team*, each responsible for keeping each other and all patients safe.

2.2.2 *Safety-11*

Recent thinking has changed in an effort to understand how individuals adapt and respond in complex system environments to ensure that "things go *right*" [9]. That is, clinicians and researchers are now trying to understand how staff can learn from what has already (or nearly) happened and then how they can produce positive outcomes time and time again from what they have learned. This is a Safety-11 [6] approach to the prevention of adverse events.

When healthcare organizations take a proactive approach to patient safety, they preempt possible risks by focusing on the organizational factors that may have allowed adverse events to occur, such as when multiple latent errors align and result in harm to patients [2, 8]. A proactive approach to healthcare takes into account the increasing complexity in healthcare settings, which makes humans and systems vulnerable to error. To counter the possibility of human error and shield healthcare staff from making mistakes, organizational systems, tasks, and processes need to be well-designed from the beginning and modified as necessary as a result of clinical practice [10]. The Safety-II system recognizes that humans, while fallible, are also adaptable and that effective interactions based on human decision-making "in the moment" promote resilience and high performance, which keeps patients safe.

Focusing on system factors that promote effective care marks the start of a proactive journey to identify key success factors for patient safety rather than just the causes of adverse events. It is the beginning of improvements that can only occur in a psychologically safe environment, open to discussion and resolution, and free from blame. This is a culture in which safety is *valued*; staff share the same values, attitudes, and beliefs about safety; and safety is a key lens through which decisions are made [11]. Errors, incidents, and accidents in complex systems are seen to result from more than one antecedent—usually multiple. These factors interact in a complex way and develop over time, and it is not always possible to be certain how they came together at the precise moment that the incident occurred [12]. The future of safe healthcare relies on supporting leadership and staff to identify the triggers as they occur and then communicating effectively so they don't become an adverse event.

Safety-II shifts the focus from merely preventing errors, to understanding and enhancing the everyday work of individuals and teams to drive excellence. Safety-II acknowledges that in complex systems, unexpected events, variations, and adaptations are inevitable. It recognizes that individuals and teams have expertise and the ability to adjust to varying conditions and demands. In a Safety-II culture, the emphasis is on understanding how work is actually done, promoting learning, and creating environments that enable individuals and teams to continuously improve clinical practices and patient safety. Rather than relying solely on reactive measures, Safety-11 seeks to identify and leverage positive outcomes and practices, known as "successes," to enhance patient safety.

To prevent adverse events, a complex, globalized healthcare environment must recognize and leverage the adaptive capacity of their staff. Johnson et al. [13] proposed a *Framework for Better Care* (Fig. 2.1), which was adopted by the Royal

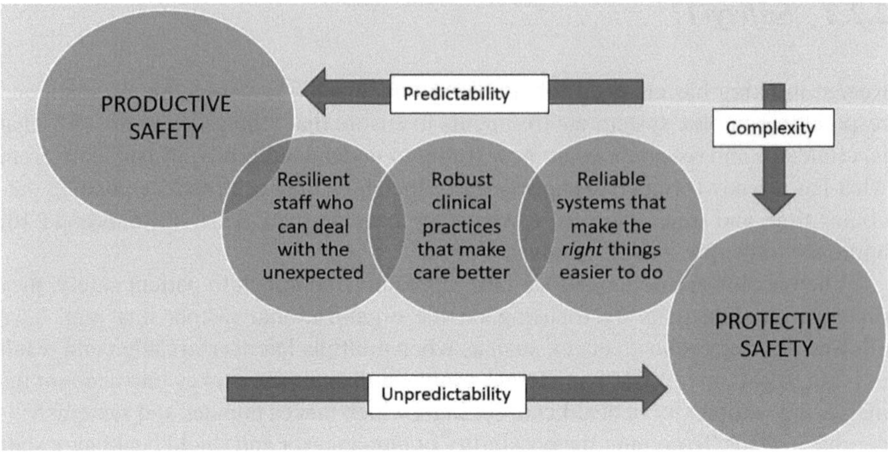

Fig. 2.1 Framework for better care. (Adapted from Johnson et al. [13])

Australasian College of Medical Administrators in 2017. It is a clinical governance framework that recognizes healthcare as a complex, adaptive system. It describes the conditions, principles, and processes by which systems can enhance the resilience, robustness, and reliability of staff working in highly complex and unpredictable environments. Productive safety is goal-oriented and iterative. Protective safety is process-oriented and sequential.

What proponents of the Safety-1 approach fail to recognize is that most things go *right* in the healthcare environment. Hence, rather than spending so much time identifying what has gone *wrong*, why not spend more time on the workplace practices that staff do *right*—the things that keep patients safe? believe that:

> *Safety management should therefore move from ensuring that 'as few things as possible go wrong' to ensuring that 'as many things as possible go right'. We call this perspective Safety-II; it relates to the system's ability to succeed under varying conditions. A Safety-II approach assumes that everyday performance variability provides the adaptations that are needed to respond to varying conditions and hence is the reason why things go right. (Insert reference here rather than above).* Hollnagel et al. [6]

According to Safety-11, "things do not go right because people behave as they are supposed to, but because people can and do adjust what they do to match the conditions of work" [6]. When systems fail, staff need to be able to make adjustments to account for such failures, thereby maintaining safety and performance. With the increasing complexity required in healthcare service delivery, staff need to be able to adjust to uncertainty and not be constrained by the rigidity of systems or procedures. While there are safety protocols and procedures that staff generally adhere to, in an emergency situation or a more complex case, they must be able to do whatever it takes to keep patients safe. Hence, they need to be able to adapt and use their discretion and expertise to make changes to formal procedures if necessary to preserve life.

Hence, the role of staff in a Safety-11 environment is also as a resource to ensure that systems remain resilient and flexible. Debriefs serve to highlight what is going *right* rather than what went *wrong*. They focus on what can be learned from the event to prevent similar occurrences and on what staff need to do to ensure their capacity to respond pre-emptively in the future.

This is not to say that a Safety-1 approach doesn't matter—it does! The protocols and procedures need to be followed. However, when there is a likelihood of system failure, a Safety-11 approach must be incorporated into everyday clinical practice as well, to maintain the surety of healthcare systems and patient safety. Therefore, contemporary healthcare practices need to combine Safety-1 and Safety-11 approaches to patient care so that staff follow procedures but can vary them if necessary. New practices must also be developed to identify the *positive* factors that lead to exceptional patient care (*leading* key performance indicators) while maintaining performance, quality, and safety standards. This book is about providing clinical leaders with the additional knowledge and skills they need to assist staff identify positive patient practices which ensure patient safety.

2.2.3 Differences Between Safety-1 and Safety-11

In the Safety-11 approach to patient safety, healthcare leaders focus on what is going well or *right* in their practices rather than on what went *wrong* when an incident occurred. They do this by using techniques that examine success factors and measure safety attributes associated with a positive approach to learning from excellence. The following are six Safety-11 techniques that leaders can use to improve patient safety in a healthcare organization:

1. *Positive deviance analysis:* This process involves identifying individuals, teams, or departments within the healthcare organization that are consistently achieving better than average or excellent outcomes. These "positive deviants" [14] can be studied to understand the context, structure, practices, strategies, and behaviors that contribute to their success. Positive deviation analysis aims to identify and spread effective practices throughout an organization.
2. *Learning from near misses and good catches*: This strategy involves encouraging healthcare staff to report and analyze near miss events or incidents that were caught before causing harm. While these are often difficult to isolate because harm is the indicator that staff members usually respond to, near misses and good catches provide valuable insights into the system's ability to detect and prevent errors. Analyzing these events can help identify and reinforce the strength of existing systems, leading to changes that cause improvements in the system, processes, and clinical practices.
3. *Safety culture surveys*: Leaders may conduct safety culture surveys to assess the perceptions and attitudes of healthcare staff regarding safety-related practices and behaviors. These surveys provide a snapshot of the organization's safety

culture, allowing leaders to identify strengths and areas for improvement. Safety culture surveys include questions related to communication, teamwork, adaptability, learning, and the organization's response to incidents.
4. *Observational rounds*: This strategy involves leaders and executives conducting observational walk rounds where they directly observe frontline staff members' work and engage in conversations with them. This approach helps leaders gain firsthand insights into the work environment, daily processes, and staff behaviors that contribute to safe and effective care. It also provides an opportunity for leaders to recognize and reinforce positive practices and role model the importance of safety and quality in an organization [15–17].
5. *Performance metrics and key performance indicators (KPIs):* This strategy involves leaders developing and tracking performance metrics and KPIs that capture Safety-II attributes. Metrics may include measures related to proactive safety activities, near miss reporting rates, staff engagement in safety initiatives, and the implementation of improvement suggestions from frontline staff. By measuring and monitoring these indicators, leaders can assess an organization's progress toward developing a Safety-II culture.
6. *Continuous improvement processes*: Processes such as the Lean or Six Sigma methodologies emphasize identifying and eliminating waste, improving workflows, and engaging staff in problem-solving. These processes encourage staff to examine their work processes, enhance safety and efficiency, and identify areas for improvement. When Safety-II principles are integrated into these approaches, opportunities for learning are identified and can be enacted.

In a Safety-11 environment, healthcare leaders use these techniques to support learning from *excellence*. Staff are encouraged to share successes, lessons learned, and suggestions for improvement. Regular feedback, recognition, and celebration of successes also play a crucial role in reinforcing positive behaviors and fostering a Safety-II culture.

2.3 Person-Centered Care

One of the key principles guiding the operation of healthcare organizations is person-centered care, which was first described by Edith Balint in 1969 as "understanding the patient as a unique human being" [18]. However, it was only with the publication of the Institute of Medicine's 2001 seminal report *Crossing the Quality Chasm* [19] that person-centered care became recognized as an essential foundational element for healthcare quality and patient safety and a high priority for the delivery of healthcare services in contemporary healthcare jurisdictions [20]. Person-centered care is an approach in which healthcare organizations partner with patients to co-design and deliver to them the personalized care and services they need. Such an approach understandably takes a toll on established systems, as it requires services and roles to be redesigned and restructured to be more conducive to the implementation of this high-quality model of service provision. But the reward is a higher level of patient safety and care.

Healthcare organizations that implement a patient safety culture have a person-centered approach to patient care. Santana et al. [20] developed a conceptual model of person-centered care to guide practical improvements in healthcare system performance. They used the Donabedian model for healthcare improvement [21] to classify person-centered domains into the categories of structure, process, and outcome. Among these three domains, each component is influenced by the previous component, and each component is interdependent on the other.

Santana et al.'s [20] conceptual framework for person-centered care is organized like a roadmap, depicting the order in which practical person-centered care should be implemented, starting with structural domains that are required as prerequisites, and proceeding to facilitating processes that impact the achievement of person-centered care outcomes. The structural domains refer to the healthcare system or context in which care is delivered. The seven structural foundation elements included in the model are considered essential for the implementation of person-centered care. These are the necessary materials, healthcare resources, and organizational characteristics for healthcare processes to be performed so that patient outcomes can be achieved.

An overview of the structural domains is as follows:

S1: creating a person-centered care culture across the continuum of care
S2: co-designing the development and implementation of educational programs for staff
S3: co-designing the development and implementation of health promotion and prevention programs with patients
S4: supporting a workforce committed to person-centered care
S5: providing a supportive and accommodating person-centered care environment
S6: developing and integrating structures to support health information technology
S7: creating structures to measure and monitor person-centered care performance

An overview of the process domains is as follows:

P1: cultivating communication
P2: respectful and compassionate care
P3: engaging patients in managing their care
P4: integration of care

The higher-level outcomes sought as a result of structural and process improvements include the following:

O1: access to care
O2: patient-reported outcomes (PROs)

2.3.1 Structural Domains

Santana et al.'s [20] model suggests that the structural elements of a person-centered care culture are foundational and need to be embedded into a healthcare organization's strategic vision of how it cares for patients, respecting their human rights as well as the diversity of race, ethnicity, gender, sexual identity, religion, age, socioeconomic status, and disability. These structural elements are underpinned by a core set of common beliefs and principles as to what constitutes quality care in clinical practice.

Patient involvement in their own care is a cornerstone of person-centered care. Patients are provided with sufficient and appropriate information to make decisions about their care and level of engagement [22, 23]. Treatment regimens are co-designed *with* patients rather than *for* them. Dialog is adjusted so that medical language and terminology are understandable to patients and their families. Patient records are shared with the relevant care providers to achieve the best possible outcomes for the patient. Secure e-health technologies and private platforms support access, coordination, and safety in care delivery; they integrate and update across existing healthcare facilities to effectively connect patients and caregivers with practitioners throughout the continuum of care [22, 24].

Another characteristic of person-centered care is that healthcare organizations can establish structures to measure and monitor patient performance based on patient feedback from patient experience surveys, patient-reported outcome measures (PROMs), patient complaints, and patient complements. Public sector reporting mechanisms keep healthcare providers accountable for their use of public funds [24]. Healthcare organizations can build the capacity of healthcare communities by establishing patient advisory groups that enhance the integration, coordination, and continuity of care. These groups identify general issues that present barriers to accessing treatment and care such as finances, accommodation, nutrition, and education [25]. They can support specific patient populations and play a key role in co-designing the development and implementation of health promotion and prevention programs.

Implementing these structural components, having a clear vision of how person-centered care strategies fit within the overall healthcare system goals and priorities, and being vigilant to identify opportunities for systemic quality improvement are crucial in the provision of quality patient care and the achievement of safety outcomes.

2.3.2 Process Domains

Four process domains were identified in Santana et al.'s [20] research, each of which builds upon previous patient-healthcare provider interactions. Communication with patients is enhanced when patients are active participants in their own care [26]. Correlations between physician communication skills and positive patient outcomes have been associated with increased patient satisfaction, recall, understanding, and adherence to therapy [27]. The use of coaching skills such as active and reflective listening communicates to patients that staff care about them and their situation. Through open and curious questioning, staff gather information about the patient which they are able to share with other professionals and care providers, who then feel more comfortable discussing care plans with the patient. Staff invite patients to reflect on their condition, pain, symptoms, and other areas of life that may be linked to their care and elicit the patient's reactions to treatment plans as they continue to engage in active dialog with them.

Respectful and compassionate care acknowledges patients as experts in their own health and as partners in their healthcare. It is about being mindful of, and sensitive and responsive to, patient preferences, needs, and values [28]. This level of care acknowledges patient's personal, cultural, religious, and spiritual values. Patient-centered staff are able to respond to patients' emotional and psychological needs and express appropriate levels of empathy, sympathy, and reassurance. Providing respectful care fosters relationships and has been shown to promote healing and better outcomes [28].

Engaging patients in managing their own care enhances their overall healthcare experience and improves healthcare provision. Research has shown that when doctors and nurses are engaged with their patients, they feel respected and acknowledged as clinical experts and are less likely to make mistakes [29]. Co-designing care plans with patients engages them in shared decision-making, goal-setting, and support, all of which assist clinical management and contribute to better health outcomes, improved quality of care, and improved patient safety [30].

The integration of care is important for streamlining health services between acute and community healthcare providers and the private sector. Linked systems talk to each other and reduce the fragmentation that can occur when there is insufficient or incomplete communication of patient information. Emerging e-health technologies such as EMR portals and the use of email communications between patients and healthcare providers better enable interactions between professionals and facilitate continuity of care [31].

2.3.3 *Outcome Domains*

Access to care has been defined as the system's capacity to provide care efficiently after a need is recognized, as well as meet the costs associated with receiving care [32]. A person-centered access model has been found to promote improved health outcomes while also reducing costs to the healthcare system [33]. Timely access to care includes not only the wait time for a consultation, or to receive test results, or for an operation or referral, but also the availability of healthcare providers outside of working hours [20]. Improving timely access to care has the potential to reduce hospital admissions and decrease the utilization of healthcare services (e.g., emergency department visits and hospital length of stay) and may also help reduce morbidity and mortality for both acute and chronic diseases [34].

The lack of affordability of healthcare services can have a negative impact on patients and families, such as when the costs associated with ambulance and pharmaceutical services hinder access to care. Supporting patients in making their own decisions about their care establishes better value for money, as evidenced in the UK Health Foundation report *Person-Centered Care made Simple* [35], which provides evidence about cost savings and reductions in healthcare service utilization when patients are involved in decision-making. This evidence suggests that when people are better informed, they may choose different treatments—often those that are less invasive and less expensive [30, 36].

The impact of person-centered care on outcomes can be informed through the use of PROs [20], which are patient-centric measures that capture information from patients about their health condition and its management [37]. For example, research has shown that patients who perceive clinical practice to be person-centered experience better recovery and emotional health and need fewer diagnostic tests and referrals two months later [38]. Santana et al. [20] suggested that patient outcomes may be recorded using any or all of the following: PROMs, which measure patient health status, quality of life and symptoms, functionality, and physical, mental, or social health; patient-reported experience measures (PREMs), which measure patient experiences with the healthcare system; and patient-reported adverse outcomes (PRAOs), which record the occurrence of adverse outcomes. Integrating these measures into clinical practice has been shown to improve outcomes as well as quality of care [39, 40].

Santana et al.'s [20] person-centered care framework provides a roadmap for healthcare organizations striving to implement an integrated model of patient care. The adoption of patient-centered care comes with challenges and entails critical changes, particularly with regard to how care is delivered and how patients and their providers interact. However, despite these challenges, the benefits of this approach present a major opportunity for improving patient outcomes.[1]

2.4 Patient Partnerships

With the growth of the Internet, information on medical conditions, symptoms, and treatments has become more accessible to the general public; information that once may have been found only in a medical textbook is now readily available. The public has welcomed the opportunity to learn more about their condition and become more involved in their care and treatment; however, self-diagnosis via the Internet can lead to misdiagnosis and cause even greater problems. Globally, healthcare

[1] Appendix 2.1. Readers may like to ask an executive in your healthcare organization to use this template to evaluate the degree to which their organization delivers person-centered care.

organizations have responded to patients' desires for more information and involvement in their treatment options with great variability. Some organizations have embraced care collaborations with patients, while others have been unable to shift from a hierarchical model in which the patient has healthcare "done to them."

Research has shown that patients can play an important role in the design of healthcare systems that are safer and reduce the risk of harm to them [12]. In its 2016 document *Patient Engagement* [41], the WHO recognized that active patient involvement in all aspects of their diagnosis, treatment, and care is an integral part of healthcare and a critical component of safe people-centered services. Engaged patients are better able to make informed decisions about their care options and agree with recommended care management plans. They are more likely to feel confident in reporting both positive and negative care experiences. A goal of contemporary healthcare systems is to empower patients and their families to a greater extent so that they will be alert to potential sources of risk or harm. For example, the literature reveals that increasing the level of patient involvement in decision-making results in greater patient satisfaction in as many as 93% of patients, with approximately 70% of them wanting to adopt at least a collaborative role regarding the choice of anesthesia [42].

Researchers have distinguished between two broad categories of measures of patient-centered care: patient experience and patient satisfaction [43]. They have proposed the following questions to guide the generation of clear, actionable evidence in future research projects: (i) How will the results of this measure be used? (ii) How will patient subjectivity be accounted for? and (iii) Is this measure validated or tested? By addressing these issues during the design phase, researchers argue that the usability of their findings can be increased.

2.4.1 Patient Experience

Patient experience is the sum of all the interactions that influence a patient's perception across the continuum of care [44]. Patients are increasingly seeking more open and transparent healthcare systems that are responsive to their needs. They expect practitioners to inform them of their test results and diagnosis and discuss treatment options with them so they can be more engaged in the decision-making process. Some developed countries have begun to give patients access to their own EMRs. Engaging patients in monitoring and updating their medication or treatment plans has the potential to increase treatment concordance, as well as enabling healthcare organizations to review and intervene if needed. Patient engagement promotes joint and mutual accountability for the achievement of satisfactory patient care outcomes. From a systemic point of view, resources may be better used if they are aligned with patients' priorities, which is critical for the sustainability of healthcare systems.

Researchers at the Vancouver Centre for Health Services and Policy Research developed a self-reported patient questionnaire to investigate patients' experiences in relation to lifestyle services in a team-based primary care environment [45].

Thirty-eight healthcare providers were recruited to prioritize the variables to be included in the survey. The modified patient questionnaire was then pilot-tested with 164 recipients of a nutrition and physical activity intervention program. The top variables that were found to improve the patient experience were *trust* (including confidence in the healthcare system and patient safety), *general communication*, *whole-person care*, *respectfulness* (including interpersonal communication and shared decision-making), and *first-contact accessibility* (including access, accommodation, and economic accessibility).

2.4.2 Patient Outcomes

In addition to measuring the patient experience and satisfaction with their care, there is increasing research interest in measuring the outcomes of the patient care received [46]. A study by Kilpatrick et al. [47] distinguished between PREMs based on episodic events of how things unfolded during their healthcare visit and PROMs that examined the impact of health conditions and the effectiveness of care from the patient's perspective [48]. They conducted a cross-sectional survey of nurse practitioners across six sites as part of a multiple-case study. From their findings, they concluded that the team processes of decision-making, communication, care coordination, and problem-solving, together with trust, team cohesion, and a focus on the needs of patients and families, are the key components that patients and families appreciate, and that these factors ultimately ensure a higher level of patient and family engagement. Patients and families reported positive outcomes associated with timely care, dealing promptly with complications, and team knowledge and skills. The presence of nurse practitioners was particularly valued.

In 2020, after extensive research, the WHO summarized the measurable elements of patient experience, care, and outcomes in their revised *Patient Safety Assessment Manual* [49]. The measurable elements they identified as significant to the patient partnership included the following:

- Access to care in the hospital
- Respect for patients' cultural and spiritual beliefs and personal preferences
- Access to information and involvement in all medical decisions during care
- Knowledge of how to compliment or complain
- Ability to refuse treatment
- Security, privacy, and confidentiality
- Effectiveness of pain management
- Access to information about hospital services and outcomes

2.4.3 *Measuring Patient Satisfaction with Care*

The measurement of person-centered care is considered to be a key step toward ensuring accountability and quality of care improvement [50]. However, measures of patient quality and care need to be precise so that survey results or research findings can be replicated and achieve the same, reliable results. Then, findings based on precise measurements can be compared with those of other research studies using the same precise measures. When measures do not have a clear purpose or are incorrectly specified or interpreted, they risk conveying an inaccurate and unreliable assessment of the quality of care, making the survey or study a complete waste of time and resources both in the initial collection of data and in the subsequent development of policies and procedures based on those poor measurement outcomes.

Specific outcomes in relation to patient care were noted by Hendricks et al. [51], who conducted an action-research project based on an interprofessional academic-practice, collaborative partnership (IPCP) model in four inpatient acute care units in Australia. They found a significant decrease in readmissions and an overall decrease in catheter-associated urinary tract infections over time as a result of staff engagement and support for education and the use of individual empowerment strategies including coaching. They concluded that an academic-practice partnership can strengthen and support an IPCP environment by allowing clinicians to be directly involved in the selection and implementation of IPCP strategies. They believe that it will also contribute to improved professional, healthcare, and student outcomes.

2.5 Patient Safety Coaching to Improve Patient Engagement

Coaching[2] has been identified as an important developmental approach to assist individuals and teams gain valuable self-awareness and insight into themselves and their behaviors. In a high-risk, complex healthcare environment, staff must often make split-second decisions relating to patient care. On such occasions, and especially when working in an interdisciplinary team, three factors may determine the difference between a successful outcome or an adverse event: communication, engagement, and enablement (Fig. 2.2).

[2] Education and training in patient safety coaching is delivered by the Australian Institute of Professional Coaches. www.professionalcoachtraining.com.au

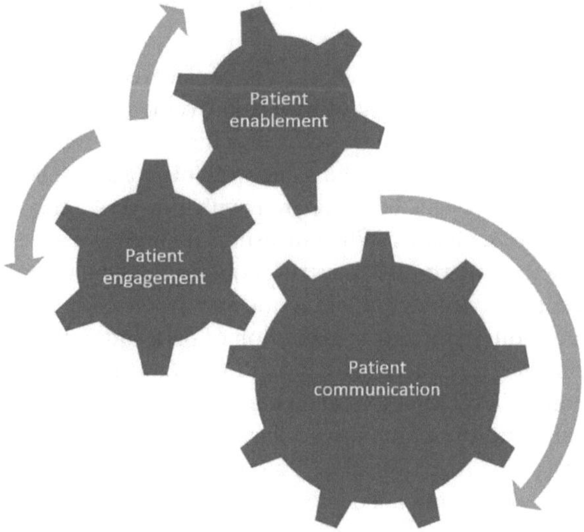

Fig. 2.2 Coaching to improve patient engagement

2.5.1 Patient Communication

The first way that coaching can support patient partnerships is by improving communication between and among invested parties. Communication, partnership, and teamwork have been identified as core domain competencies by a number of regulatory authorities in Europe as well as by the American Medical Association, Medical Council of Canada, and Medical Board of Australia [7]. The Victorian Department of Health's 2008–2009 *Report on Sentinel Events* [52] revealed that 20% of adverse events were due to communication issues. Hence, healthcare organizations need to have an explicit process for how patients can make a complaint and how the complaint will be managed. Best practice suggests that (i) the process needs to be well publicized, making it easier for patients to voice their concerns; (ii) there should be a nominated person responsible for communicating with the complainant, acknowledging, and acting on it; and (iii) all complaints should be logged together with the actions that have been taken to resolve the issue [49].

In a qualitative study conducted across 5600 acute care US hospitals to determine the competencies that senior healthcare leaders need to promote positive patient experiences, patients reported that communication and collaboration inside and outside the organization are key to the provision of quality patient care [44]. Patients believe that leaders need to: demonstrate self-confidence; have compassion and care for patients; have a reputation for providing quality, safe, and effective care; and be culturally aware so that they respect all patients and their values. In addition, to improve the patient experience, what's required is that the patient has a better understanding of the organization and how it operates, processes and procedures are transparent, and the organization takes responsibility for its actions—all necessary components of quality patient care. Coaching can help patients formulate questions they may have in relation to these matters.

2.5.2 Patient Engagement

The second way that coaching can support patient partnerships is by assisting patients in understanding their own care needs and treatment options. Areas in which patients may become actively involved include the following:

Patient education. Contemporary healthcare practice involves providing patients with any educational material and/or written/verbal information that may empower them to play a more active role in their own care. For example, when specific diseases have been diagnosed, staff may inform patients of established networks or groups that offer additional support to those provided through hospital treatment plans; consequently, patients may decide to avail themselves of these education services. Research has shown that when people are supported in managing their own care more effectively, they are less likely to use emergency hospital services [53].

Research participants. Patients may give consent for their samples to be used in research studies that aim to discover more information about their specific disease or condition and develop alternate treatment options. Their data may be included in research studies.

Advisory Committee. Healthcare organizations typically seek feedback from patients in advisory groups to inform them of the veracity of current and anticipated changes to systems and procedures. For example, patients may become actively involved in the design and development of more patient-centered treatment processes and systems.

Staff training. The training of healthcare professionals may be augmented by real patients speaking of their experiences during care and treatment. Their viewpoints help those undertaking training appreciate the patient perspective and the importance of preserving trust between clinicians and patients. Exposure to patient stories during training may also motivate practitioners to improve safety.

Policy development. Increasingly, patients and families are given voice in the development of policy and legislation in relation to specific areas of concern that emerge and are not fully covered by current policies and procedures. Thereafter, patients may be engaged in the development and dissemination of tools, information, and educational materials.

Coaching can assist patients understand the information, processes and groups available to them, and how to access these additional services to enhance their own care.

2.5.3 Patient Enablement

The third way that coaching can support patient partnerships is by assisting leaders to remove barriers to patient care and promoting a positive patient experience. In a qualitative study by Powell et al. [54], three domains that characterize barriers to patient care were revealed: social determinants, health system factors, and patient trust in the health system. Social determinants included insurance and financial shortcomings, mental health and substance abuse issues, housing and transportation-related limitations, and unpredictability associated with living in poverty. Suggestions for addressing these barriers included increasing financial assistance from the healthcare system, and building a workforce to address specific domain-related determinants directly. The healthcare system factors identified in the study as causing patient disablement included poor care coordination, inadequate communication of hospital discharge instructions, and difficulty navigating complex systems. Suggestions for addressing these barriers included enhanced communication between care sites, patient-centered scheduling, and improved patient education especially in discharge planning. Finally, factors related to patient trust in the health system emerged from the study findings; participants reported that patients are often intimidated by the healthcare system, mistrust physicians, and are fearful of receiving a serious diagnosis or prognosis. A suggestion for mitigating these issues was to increase the visibility of the healthcare system within communities to foster trust and help healthcare leaders gain a better understanding of unique community needs.

In the same year, in their review of the factors that present as barriers to patient care, the WHO noted five categories of factors that either support or deter patients from being willing and active participants in their primary care [41]. These include:

- Patient factors (e.g., demographic characteristics, health literacy)
- Health conditions (e.g., the severity of the illness or condition)
- Healthcare professionals (e.g., their knowledge of the condition and attitude toward it)
- Healthcare competence—the care tasks required are within staff clinical abilities
- Healthcare setting (e.g., primary or secondary care)

Moreover, a key factor in this research that was found to hinder patient engagement was patients' perceptions of their role and status (as a subordinate to clinicians).

Other research has shown that patients fear being labeled "difficult" and, consequently, they may take a passive role to protect their personal safety [55]. Such challenges can be overcome by improved communication and breaking down hierarchical systems within the healthcare industry.

The Agency for Healthcare Research and Quality (AHRQ) in the USA makes available a number of patient-related resources for healthcare workers – whether they see patients at a hospital, primary care office or other setting. AHRQ offers free resources that clinical leaders, especially those conducting patient safety coaching, may use to inform and support patient outcomes.

Enabling patient engagement in their own care and within the healthcare organization is a key issue that patients can discuss with their patient safety coach, who will guild them to a solution that fits their circumstances and condition.

These three areas for patient safety coaching—patient communication, patient engagement, and patient enablement—serve to strengthen the patient partnership with staff and increase the level of person-centered care delivered by the healthcare organization.

Key Takeaways

- The context for healthcare is changing. In the future, fixed facilities will treat only the most serious of patients, with the majority receiving in-home or community-based care via personalized treatment regimens delivered by specialist support staff.
- The healthcare workforce is aging and shrinking due to remuneration, cost of living expenses and housing issues, and organizational factors such as inadequate resources and equipment.
- The patient population is changing. People are living longer, often with comorbidities and polypharmacy concerns.
- Person-centered care is a specialized approach that acknowledges the uniqueness of each patient's treatment plan.
- Patient partnerships respect and value the part that patients play in their own care and choice of treatment options.
- Coaching is a key developmental process that healthcare leaders can use to support improved patient communication, engagement, and enablement.

2.6 Case Study 2: Patient Partnerships and Person-Centered Care

The Royal Meridian Hospital is a statewide referral hospital located in the heart of a bustling city, known for its heroic and cutting-edge medical excellence in organ transplantation and burns services. Recently remodeled with philanthropic donation, its state-of-the-art facilities attract world-renowned specialists. It serves as the referral destination for one half of the nation for transplantation and complex trauma with burns requiring reconstruction.

The Transplant unit performs a wide range of transplants including heart, lung, liver, kidney, and multi-organ transplants. It is recognized for its lifesaving therapies and frequent high-profile media presence and celebrity patient recommendations.

The Reconstructive Trauma unit is dedicated to the treatment of complex trauma involving severe burns and complex reconstructive surgeries, utilizing the latest techniques in skin grafting, regenerative medicine, and cutting-edge research. This unit also experiences significant media attention, often receiving mass casualty patients, and patients repatriated after combat-related injuries.

The hospital's illustrious reputation and media presence has, unfortunately, contributed to a dissonance between its general units and the subspecialty units. Over time, an elitist subculture fostering prestige and exclusivity has grown in the subspecialty units. This subculture impacts their approach to person-centered care, since these units are very hierarchical and the consultant medical staff seem to hold all the power. Patients (often having experienced catastrophic injuries and needing major surgery) take a passive role in their care, discouraged from asking questions or challenging their treatment.

In contrast, the general units, while providing essential and high-quality care, have struggled with fewer resources and less recognition. The healthcare professionals in these units, despite their dedication and expertise, feel overshadowed at times by their subspecialty counterparts. This disparity creates tension and a sense of inequality among staff, impacting overall morale, collaboration, and culture. Person-centered care is much more on the minds of these general clinicians; however, they struggle against the bureaucracy to sustain sufficient resources to implement initiatives that would significantly progress their patients' care.

For Discussion

1. What is the difference between Safety-I and Safety-II approaches to managing risk in healthcare?
    - How is risk managed differently in an emergency department as opposed to a ward?
2. How do healthcare organizations implement person-centered care?
    - What happened in this case study, and what could have been done differently?
3. What methods can be used to build patient partnerships?
    - What happened in this case study, and what could have been done differently?
4. How can coaching assist the development of patient partnerships and person-entered care?

Appendix 2.1 Evaluation of Person-Centered Care

Answer the following questions to evaluate the degree to which your organization delivers person-centered care. What can be done to improve current operations and clinical practices? [20]

Structure	*What's currently working*	*How can we improve on what's currently working?*
S1: Creating a person-centered care culture across the continuum of care		
S2: Co-designing the development and implementation of educational programs for staff		
S3: Co-designing the development and implementation of health promotion and prevention programs with patients		
S4: Supporting a workforce committed to person-centered care		
S5: Providing a supportive and accommodating person-centered care environment		
S6: Developing and integrating structures to support health information technology		
S7: Creating structures to measure and monitor person-centered care performance		
Process	*What's currently working*	*How can we improve on what's currently working?*
P1: Cultivating communication		
P2: Respectful and compassionate care		
P3: Engaging patients in managing their care		
P4: Integration of care		
Outcomes	*What's currently working*	*How can we improve on what's currently working?*
O1: Access to care		
O2: Patient-reported outcomes (PROs)		

References

1. WHO. (2005). Draft guidelines for adverse event reporting and learning systems: From information to action. In *World Alliance for Patient Safety*. World Health Organization.
2. Manley, K., & Jackson, C. (2019). Microsystems culture change: A refined theory for developing person-centered, safe and effective workplaces based on strategies that embed a safety culture. *International Practice Development Journal, 9*(2), 1–21.
3. Alwan, A. (2015). *Patient Safety Tool Kit*. World Health Organization, Regional Office for the Eastern Mediterranean.
4. WHO. (2014). *Guide for developing national patient safety policy and strategic plan*. World Health Organization: Regional Office for Africa.
5. Radick, L. E. (2022). Ready for what's next: Future-proofing the healthcare workforce. *Healthcare Executive, 37*(3), 16–24.
6. Hollnagel, E., Wears, R., & Braithwaite, J. (2015). *From safety-I to safety-II: A white paper*. University of Southern Denmark, University of Florida, USA, and Macquarie University.

7. Davis, E., & Beale, N. (2015). It is time: The poor culture regarding safety and quality in Australian hospitals must be addressed! Asia Pacific. *Journal of Health Management, 10*(3), GS36–GS41.
8. Chegini, Z., et al. (2020). The impact of patient safety culture and the leader coaching behavior of nurses on the intention to report errors: A cross-sectional survey. *BMC Nursing, 19*(1).
9. Thompson, L., et al. (2021). Clinical coaches and patient safety—Just in time: A descriptive exploratory study. *Nurse Education in Practice, 54*, 103134.
10. Leape, L., et al. (2012). A culture of respect, Part 2: Creating a culture of respect. *Academic Medicine, 87*, 853–858.
11. Workplace Health and Safety. (2013). *Understanding safety culture*. The State of Queensland.
12. WHO. (2020). *Patient Safety Incident Reporting and Learning Systems: Technical report and guidance*. World Health Organization: License: CC BY-NC-SA 3.0 IGO.
13. Johnson, A., Clay-Williams, R., & Lane, P. (2019). Framework for better care: Reconciling approaches to patient safety and quality. *Australian Health Review, 43*(6), 633–655.
14. WHO. (2021). *Global Patient Safety Action Plan 2021–2030: Toward eliminating avoidable harm in health care*. World Health Organization, License: CC BY-NC-SA 3.0 IGO.
15. de Lima Garcia, C., et al. (2019). Association between culture of patient safety and burnout in pediatric hospitals. *PLoS One, 14*(6), 1–14.
16. AHRQ. (2019). Culture of safety. In *Patient Safety Network*. Agency for Healthcare Research and Quality.
17. WHO. (2016). *Patient safety assessment manual* (2nd ed.). Regional Office for the Eastern Mediterranean.
18. Balint, E. (1969). The possibilities of patient-centered medicine. *Journal of the Royal College of General Practitioners, 17*, 269–276.
19. IOM. (2001). *Crossing the quality chasm: A new health system for the 21st century*. Institute of Medicine Committee on Quality of Health Care in America.
20. Santana, M. J., et al. (2018). How to practice person-centered care: A conceptual framework. *Health Expectations, 21*(2), 429–440.
21. Donabedian, A. (1988). The quality of care: How can it be assessed? *JAMA, 260*, 1743–1748.
22. Pelzang, R. (2010). Time to learn: Understanding patient-centered care. *British Journal of Nursing, 19*, 912–917.
23. Scherger, J. E. (2009). Future vision: Is family medicine ready for patient-directed care? *Family Medicine, 41*, 285–288.
24. Shaller, D. (2007). *Patient-centered care: What does it take?* Commonwealth Fund.
25. WHO. (2007). *People-centered health care: A policy framework* (ISBN 9789290613176). World Health Organization.
26. Laidsaar-Powell, R. C., et al. (2013). Physician–patient–companion communication and decision-making: A systematic review of triadic medical consultations. *Patient Education and Counseling, 91*, 3–13.
27. King, A., & Hoppe, R. B. (2013). "Best practice" for patient-centered communication: A narrative review. *Journal of Graduate Medical Education, 5*, 385–393.
28. Mead, N., & Bower, P. (2002). Patient-centered consultations and outcomes in primary care: A review of the literature. *Patient Education and Counseling, 48*, 51–61.
29. Leiter, M. P., & Laschinger, H. K. (2006). Relationships of work and practice environment to professional burnout: Testing a causal model. *Nursing Research, 55*, 137–146.
30. Coulter, A. (2007). Effectiveness of strategies for informing, educating, and involving patients. *BMJ, 335*, 24.
31. Wu, W. A., et al. (2016). Improving an electronic system for measuring PROs in routine oncology practice. *Journal of Cancer Survivorship, 10*, 573–582.
32. Levesque, J. F., Harris, M. F., & Russel, G. (2013). Patient-centered access to healthcare: Conceptualizing access at the interface of health systems and populations. *International Journal of Equity in Health, 12*, 12–18.

33. Andersen, R. M., Davidson, P. L., & Baumeister, S. E. (2013). Improving access to care. In *Changing the US health care system: Key issues in health services policy and management* (pp. 33–69).
34. Lasser, K. E., Himmelstein, D. U., & Woolhandler, S. (2006). Access to care, health status, and health disparities in the United States and Canada: Results of a cross-national population-based survey. *American Journal of Public Health, 96*, 96(1300-1307).
35. Foundation, T. H. (2014). *Person-centered care made simple. What everyone should know about person-centered care*. Available from: http://www.health.org.uk/sites/health/files/PersonCentredCareMadeSimple.pdf
36. Mulley, A. G., Trimble, C., & Elwyn, G. (2012). Stop the silent misdiagnosis: Patients' preferences matter. *BMJ, 345*, e6572.
37. Lohr, K. N., & Zebrack, B. J. (2009). Using patient-reported outcomes in clinical practice: Challenges and opportunities. *Quality of Life Research, 18*, 99–107.
38. Stewart, M., et al. (2000). The impact of patient-centered care on outcomes. *Family Practice, 49*, 796–804.
39. Snyder, C. F., et al. (2012). Implementing patient-reported outcomes assessment in clinical practice: A review of the options and considerations. *Quality of Life Research, 21*, 1305–1314.
40. Santana, M. J., et al. (2010). Assessing the use of health-related quality of life measures in the routine clinical care of lung-transplant patients. *Quality of Life Research, 19*, 371–379.
41. WHO. (2016). *Patient engagement, in Technical Series on Safer Primary Care*. World Health Organization: License: CC BY-NC-SA 3.0 IGO.
42. Gangakhedkar, G. (2021). Learning as we grow, growing as we learn. *Journal of Anesthesiology Clinical Pharmacology, 37*(2), 297–298.
43. Larson, E., et al. (2019). When the Patient is the Expert: Measuring patient experience and satisfaction with care. *Bulletin of the World Health Organization, 97*, 563–569.
44. Latvis, L., Fick, J., & Dishman, L. (2021). What senior healthcare leadership competencies matter most to affect positive patient experiences in United States inpatient acute care hospitals? *Michigan Academician, 48*(1), 51–52.
45. Brauer, P., et al. (2018). Development of a patient experience questionnaire to improve lifestyle services in primary care. *Primary Health Care Research & Development, 19*(6), 542–552.
46. Bull, C., et al. (2019). A systematic review of the validity and reliability of patient-reported experience measures. *Health Services Research, 54*, 1023.
47. Kilpatrick, K., et al. (2021). Patient and family views of team functioning in primary healthcare teams with nurse practitioners: A survey of patient-reported experience and outcomes. *BMC Family Practice, 22*(1), 1–14.
48. Murphy, M., Hollinghurst, S., & Salisbury, C. (2018). Identification, description and appraisal of generic PROMs for primary care: A systematic review. *BMC Family Practice, 19*, 41.
49. WHO. (2020). *Patient safety assessment manual* (3rd ed.). World Health Organization. Regional Office for the Eastern Mediterranean. License: CC BY-NC-SA 3.0 IGO.
50. Kruk, M. E., et al. (2018). High-quality health systems in the Sustainable Development Goals era: Time for a revolution. *Lancet Global Health, 6*(11), 196–252.
51. Hendricks, S., et al. (2018). Fostering interprofessional collaborative practice in acute care through an academic-practice partnership. *Journal of Interprofessional Care, 32*(5), 613–620.
52. Report. (2008–2009). Report on Sentinel Events. Available from: docs.health.vic.gov.au/docs/doc/.../sentinel_event_program_0809. Victorian Department of Health.
53. De Silva, D. (2011). *Helping people help themselves*. The Health Foundation.
54. Powell, R. E., et al. (2016). A qualitative analysis of interprofessional healthcare team members' perceptions of patient barriers to healthcare engagement. *BMC Health Services Research, 16*, 1–10.
55. Doherty, C., & Stavropoulou, C. (2012). Patients' willingness and ability to participate actively in the reduction of clinical errors: A systematic literature review. *Social Science & Medicine Journal, 75*(2), 257–263.

Chapter 3
Adverse Events in Healthcare

Finding ways to avoid adverse events presents a significant challenge to healthcare organizations and a compelling rationale for the deployment of extensive, resource-intensive initiatives to improve patient safety. Adverse events in healthcare can occur due to a number of causes that may relate to clinical factors, human factors, or systemic/cultural factors. Traditionally, adverse events have been addressed using a Safety-1 [1] investigative approach to discover what happened and who was to blame. More recently, a shift in thinking has caused clinical leaders, healthcare administrators, and executives to operationalize their efforts and direct their budgets to prevent adverse events from occurring in the first place, i.e., toward using a Safety-11 approach to patient care [1]. Safety-11 clinical practices focus on doing more of what is going *right* to identify excellence rather than looking backward at what could have or should have been done to prevent the incident from occurring. Of course, investigations into major incidents must still occur, but could these adverse events have been prevented by learning from contemporary procedures that showcase the very latest and best in clinical practice and healthcare technology?

Contemporary clinical leaders and governance executives are now attempting to eliminate the causes of adverse events by taking a broader view of care quality, with a focus on *leading* safety and quality markers such as preventable admissions, hospital-acquired complications, and length of stay. Skilling leaders in the nontechnical coaching process, which enhances communication, relationships, and interdisciplinary teamwork, has been found to be highly effective in reducing the occurrence of adverse events in frontline care.

Adverse events have been defined as unintended, negative consequences of healthcare [2]. They increase the chances of patients being admitted to intensive care units and dying in the hospital. From a systems perspective, adverse events result in longer hospital stays and increased use of healthcare resources; they also contribute to access issues for the broader population. Hence, from both patient and systemic perspectives, finding ways to avoid adverse events presents a significant challenge to healthcare organizations.

© The Author(s), under exclusive license to Springer Nature Switzerland AG 2024
S. Knowles, *Patient Safety Coaching*,
https://doi.org/10.1007/978-3-031-68722-8_3

Hospital-level factors that may be relevant to patient safety can be conceptually grouped into four broad domains: patient safety culture; patient safety strategies; staffing; and hospital volume and capacity [3]. This book aims to provide healthcare leaders and governance executives with the strategies they can use to develop a patient safety culture within teams and organizations. It does not address staffing and resourcing issues that are dictated by budget allocations. Instead, it informs leaders of the benefits of delivering patient safety coaching[1] to team members who witness or have been involved in an adverse event and may have been traumatized by it. Coaching is a developmental process that can support staff through trauma to restore balance, promote resilience, and foster overall wellbeing.

3.1 The Statistics

The World Health Organization (WHO) has reported that millions of patients unnecessarily suffer injury or die every year because of unsafe and poor-quality healthcare [4]. Patients may be injured or disabled when infections are acquired, mistakes are made in medication use, or procedures are performed badly. They may be injured in falls, their condition may be undiagnosed or misdiagnosed, or they may experience poor clinical management of their acute illnesses. Many of these harmful events are avoidable. Unfortunately, although the scale of each type of harm varies, the overall burden of care has not dramatically decreased over the past two decades, despite the unprecedented priority and resources that have been given to patient safety within healthcare systems during this period.

In 2000, the Institute of Medicine in the USA published its seminal paper, *To Err is Human: Building a Safer Health System* [5]. The report estimated that between 44,000 and 98,000 patients die in American hospitals every year as a result of medical errors. The authors concluded that the majority of medical errors were not the fault of any individual or team, but rather were due to poor systems and processes related to the provision of patient care.

A similar analysis in the United Kingdom (UK) in that same year revealed that medical errors in patients admitted to the National Health Service (NHS) caused an estimated 850,000 adverse events annually—representing 10% of all patient admissions [6]. The authors suggested that the lack of organizational learning from previous incidents was responsible for these errors and associated this deficiency with the organization's culture. They recommended that a patient safety culture is the preferred way to address medical errors.

In Australia, the need for a national approach to patient safety was first raised in 1995 as a result of the increasing number of adverse events in hospitals [7]. The definition of an adverse event that researchers adopted back then consisted of three

[1]Education and training in patient safety coaching is delivered by the Australian Institute of Professional Coaches. www.professionalcoachtraining.com.au

components: (i) an unintended injury or complication, which (ii) resulted in disability, death, or prolongation of hospital stay, and (iii) was caused by healthcare management issues rather than the patient's disease [8, 9]. In the past, the Australian Institute of Health and Welfare published the incidence of adverse events for all public and private hospitals annually. The incidence of recorded adverse events in 2013/14 exceeded 500,000 for the second time, which was 47.6% greater than the figures recorded in 2006/07 [10]. Sadly, even with extensive encouragement and demands from accreditation bodies, State Departments of Health, insurers, and authorities such as the Australian Commission on Safety and Quality in Healthcare (ACSQHC), the occurrence of adverse events has continued to increase each year.

Hence, the thinking in relation to patient safety is shifting to a broader view of quality care with a focus on safety and quality markers such as preventable admissions, hospital-acquired complications, and length of stay. This shift in thinking has caused administrators and executives to operationalize their efforts and direct their budgets to implement a Safety-11 [1] approach to patient care and safety. Meanwhile, there continues to be a focus on those Safety-1 patient safety indicators necessary for governance functions such as the number of Severity Assessment Code 1 (SAC1) incidents, incident reports of investigations, and the use of risk management plans and assessments.[2]

3.2 Causes of Patient Harm

Adverse events in healthcare are classified as occurring due to three main causes [11]:

- *Clinical factors* such as poor hand hygiene, unsafe use of injections, blood products, or medication, unsafe use of medical devices, and unsafe practices during surgery.
- *Human factors* including poor leadership, communication failure, ineffective teamwork, poor patient handovers, misdiagnosis, and poor test follow-up.
- *Cultural factors* which, combined with ineffective systems and processes, ineffective regulation or accountability mechanisms, poor training and education, and a lack of organizational knowledge transfer and learning from adverse events, create a culture of blame.

3.2.1 Human Error

The most common patient safety issues caused by human errors are described below:

[2] Chapter 9 addresses governance issues in healthcare.

- *Medication errors* are a leading cause of injury and avoidable harm in healthcare systems. Globally, the cost associated with medication errors is estimated to be US$42 billion annually [12]. For example, a patient in a hospital might receive the wrong medication because of a mix-up that occurs due to similar packaging; perhaps two similar medications that perform opposite functions have similar labels or names. The prescription passes through different levels of care starting with the doctor in the ward, then to the pharmacy for dispensing, and finally, to the nurse who administers medication to the patient. At each step in this process, there is the potential for error. In this example, a lack of standard procedures for the storage of medications that look alike, poor communication between the different providers, lack of verification before medication administration, and lack of patient involvement in their own care, might all be underlying factors that led to medication errors.
- *Healthcare-associated infections* occur in 7 out of every 100 hospitalized patients in high-income countries and 10 out of every 100 in low- and middle-income countries [13].
- *Unsafe surgical care procedures* cause complications in up to 25% of patients. Almost seven million surgical patients suffer significant complications annually, one million of whom die during or immediately following surgery [14].
- *Unsafe injection practices* in healthcare settings can transmit infections and pose direct danger to patients and healthcare workers. They account for a burden of harm, estimated at 9.2 million years of life lost to disability and death globally [15].
- *Diagnostic errors* occur in approximately 5% of adults in outpatient care settings at any time, more than half of which have the potential to cause severe harm. Alarmingly, it has been suggested that most people will suffer a diagnostic error in their lifetime [16].
- *Unsafe transfusion practices* expose patients to the risk of adverse transfusion reactions and the transmission of infections [17]. Data on adverse transfusion reactions from a group of 21 countries show an average incidence of 8.7 serious reactions per 100,000 distributed blood components [18].
- *Radiation errors* involve overexposure to radiation and cases of incorrect-patient and incorrect-site identification [19]. A review of 30 years of published data on safety in radiotherapy estimates that the overall incidence of errors is approximately 15 per 10,000 treatment courses [20].
- *Sepsis* is frequently not diagnosed early enough to save a patient's life. Under-recognition and delay of definitive treatment can lead to rapid deterioration and death, affecting an estimated 31 million people globally and causing more than five million deaths per year [21].
- *Venous thromboembolism* is one of the most common and preventable causes of patient harm, contributing to one-third of the complications attributed to hospitalization. Annually, there are an estimated 3.9 million cases in high-income countries and six million cases in low- and middle-income countries [22].

3.2.2 *Systemic Error*

In addition to the human factors that may cause patient harm, several systemic factors have been identified in the literature as potential causes of patient harm within healthcare organizations. These include [23]:

- Inadequate communication
- Prevailing punitive and blaming culture with inadequate reporting
- Limited leadership and management capacity
- Inadequate training or supervision of clinical staff
- Weak healthcare systems
- Suboptimal infrastructure and limited supplies of essential equipment for safety
- Absence of protocols or policies
- Failure to implement protocols and policies
- Delays in providing, or failure to provide, a reliable service

Many of these systemic failures are significant factors in incidents that occur in healthcare, whether they result in harm or not. James Reason is famously known for his Swiss cheese model that illustrates how weaknesses in defenses, latent failures, or unseen deficiencies within complex systems can result in an adverse event [24]. Reason advocated the importance of adopting a systemic approach to causation of patient harm: "When an adverse event occurs, the important issue is not who blundered but how and why the defenses failed" [25].

3.3 Factors Contributing to Adverse Events

The WHO 2010 document, *Learning from Error* [26], identified a number of pressure areas that may contribute to the occurrence of adverse events in healthcare organizations. These factors are related to individual and organizational factors that may distract attention from patient care, leading to patient harm. In their training package, the authors focused on five ways in which error could be reduced:

- Instigating standard operating procedures and guidelines
- Ensuring valid and up-to-date training
- Effective communication
- Medication safety
- Patient engagement

Root cause analysis (a Safety-1 approach) focuses on a number of individual factors that may have contributed to that one-time adverse event. However, since organizational factors are often the precursors of adverse events, staff need to be flexible and resilient enough to navigate systemic factors to manage the whole system so that adverse events do not occur and quality care can be delivered (a Safety-11 approach). Figure 3.1 represents the complex environment in which healthcare staff

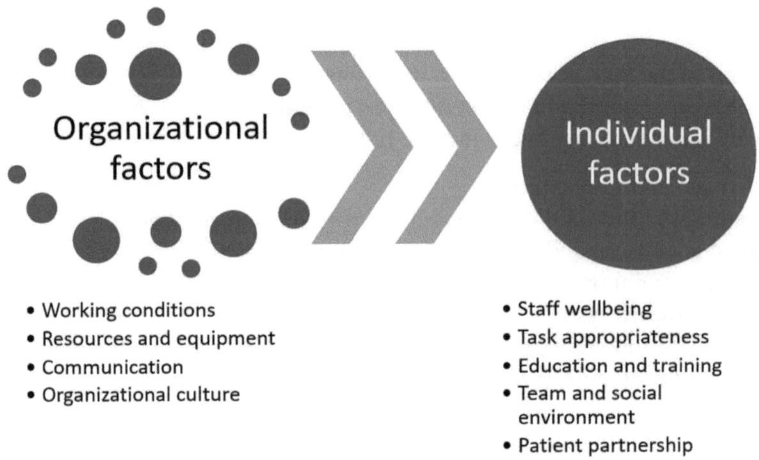
Organizational factors
Individual factors
• Working conditions
• Resources and equipment
• Communication
• Organizational culture
• Staff wellbeing
• Task appropriateness
• Education and training
• Team and social environment
• Patient partnership

Fig. 3.1 Organizational and individual factors that contribute to adverse events

work and the systemic factors that may, at times, either constrain care outcomes or facilitate quality patient care. In the following sections, the effect of systemic issues on patient care are addressed first, followed by the consideration of individual factors.

3.3.1 Organizational Factors

Historically, the causes of staff distress used to center on physical working conditions such as lighting and heating—the physical working environment. Currently, it centers on both the working conditions and the mental/emotional working environment that either supports staff to perform effectively and feel satisfied that they have done a good job or not. Workplace issues prevail in every organization and must be addressed to ensure that a psychologically safe work environment exists, particularly those relating to bullying and harassment which can lead to poor mental health, stress, and burnout.[3]

According to the WHO [26], there are four organizational factors that cause distress to workers in relation to the healthcare system, each of which is discussed in the following sections:

(1) Working conditions
(2) Resources and equipment

[3] Issues of bullying and harassment are addressed in Chap. 9.

(3) Communication
(4) Organizational culture

3.3.1.1 Working Conditions

The first organizational factor that may contribute to adverse events is working conditions. Article 23 of the *Universal Declaration of Human Rights* affirms that the right to work includes "just and favorable conditions of work" [27] as a fundamental human right. Other international conventions, resolutions, and instruments, including the WHO's 2030 *Agenda for Sustainable Development* and its *Sustainable Development Goals*, have heralded the need for governments and other stakeholders to provide safe, secure, and supportive working environments for all staff, particularly for women who make up approximately 70% of the health workforce globally [27]. The health, safety, and well-being of health workers are legal and moral responsibilities of governments and prerequisites for the provision of essential health services.

Every workplace must provide the requisite working conditions for effective clinical care to be performed such as adequate lighting, ventilation, and temperature control. In addition, staff must be given adequate time to rest in-between shifts, before returning to work. Once these basic working conditions are met, staff can feel assured that their physical welfare needs are being addressed. In exceptional circumstances, additional safeguards are put in place such as for staff working in COVID-19 wards with infected patients. However, even in normal circumstances, these basic workplace conditions are not sufficient to ensure that staff are satisfied with their job and the work that they do. What also needs to happen is that they find the work meaningful and important because if they don't do it well, patients may suffer.

Recognizing health worker safety as a priority for patient safety, in 2020 the WHO Member States and all relevant stakeholders urged healthcare organizations to take urgent and sustainable action to rectify any staff-related work issues by undertaking the following, as relevant and applicable to context and responsibilities [27]:

(1) Establish synergistic relationships between health worker safety and patient safety policies and strategies
(2) Develop and implement national programs for occupational health and safety of health workers
(3) Protect health workers from violence in the workplace
(4) Improve the mental health and psychological well-being of health workers
(5) Protect health workers from physical and biological hazards

3.3.1.2 Resources and Equipment

The second organizational factor that may contribute to adverse events is resources and equipment. The *Job Demands Resources (JD-R) model* [28, 29] proposes that without sufficient resources to perform a job, there is an increased risk that high levels of job demands will lead to staff burnout. Studies have associated high job demands and low job resources with reduced patient safety outcomes [29–31]. Seljemo et al. [32] reported that job demands and job resources explained 7.8% of patient safety culture and 4.7% of the overall perception of patient safety ($p < 0.001$). More importantly, transformational leadership explained 47.2% of the variance in patient safety culture and 25.4% of the overall perception of patient safety, controlling for age and gender ($p < 0.001$).

Technological resourcing in healthcare is becoming increasingly important. It involves the following:

- Information technology required to run business systems (e.g., computers, phones, Wi-Fi, email, accounting software)
- Patient-related information systems (e.g., booking systems, medical records, radiology, pathology, operating theatre software)
- Specialized medical equipment (e.g., patient monitors, telemetry, ventilators, intravenous infusion pumps, CT scanners)

If any component of business-related systems is nonfunctional or poorly integrated, it risks business continuity and disruption to the provision of business services—in this case, healthcare. If any component of clinical-related systems is nonfunctional, patient lives may be at risk. As technology advances, specialized medical equipment becomes increasingly safe, with built-in safeguards to prevent errors and harm. Examples of this include IV infusion pump software designed to ensure that medication errors do not occur. Even so, most of these error prevention safeguards still require human input, at the very least to respond to alerts or issues and not dismiss them. Leaders are key in advocating for the resolution of technology integration issues and supporting their staff in managing issues safely until their resolution.

3.3.1.3 Communication

The third organizational factor that may contribute to adverse events is communication. Effective communication needs to occur at a number of levels within the workspace. Interpersonal communication needs to be respectful of the opinions of others; staff concerns need to be heard. Communication within the team must center on cooperation and collaboration so that tasks can be performed effectively and efficiently. Misunderstandings or misinterpretations in communication can lead to mistakes being made, sometimes with dire consequences. Within multiprofessional teams, the same courtesy should be given to all individuals regardless of their discipline—respect, listening, and concern for care. When there are discrepancies in

Table 3.1 An unconditionally constructive strategy

Principle	Actions required of the leader
Rationality	Use reason to balance emotion.
Understanding	Even if they do not understand you, seek to understand them and how they see things.
Communication	Always consult and listen before making a decision, on any matters that affect them.
Reliability	Be able to be relied upon, such that others can trust you, even if others are not reliable.
Persuasion (not coercion)	Negotiate side by side, be open to being persuaded, and try to persuade others. Do not use coercion or yield to it.
Acceptance	Take on treating others from whom you differ seriously. Treat others as worthy of being considered even if they reject you as unworthy of their consideration.

Adapted from Fisher et al. (1989) [33]

disciplinary approaches to treatment, a number of strategies can be employed to negotiate differences so that the most effective treatment plan for maintaining patient safety can be determined.

Fisher et al. [33] developed a number of key principles that are useful strategies when communicating with others, whether they are intact team members or interdisciplinary team members. Adopting these actions will smooth communication and ensure that, if differences occur, they can be resolved in the most meaningful way (Table 3.1).

3.3.1.4 Organizational Culture

The fourth organizational factor that may contribute to adverse events is organizational culture. A culture of individual blame is still found in traditional healthcare organizations [34]. This kind of culture creates fear in staff who then become reluctant to report errors. Since some errors may be due to individual staff members' lack of expertise or poor work performance, the WHO is calling for not a "no blame" culture but a "just" culture [35], which places responsibility and accountability where the error originated so that the individual can improve. A just culture recognizes the complexity of situations and events and acknowledges that, while most patient safety failures are the result of weak systems, there is a minority of situations where an individual should be held accountable. For example, in situations of reckless behavior or willful misconduct, the relevant professional authority's guidelines for managing poor performance should be followed.

A "no blame" culture [35] focuses on identifying and addressing systemic issues that lead individuals to engage in unsafe behaviors, while maintaining individual accountability by establishing zero tolerance for reckless behavior. It distinguishes between human error (e.g., slips), at-risk behavior (e.g., taking shortcuts), and reckless behavior (e.g., ignoring required safety steps). Bullying and harassment are increasingly causes of concern for staff in healthcare settings [36]. If a culture of blame and fear is dominant in a healthcare organization, it is often impossible to implement a successful program of patient safety.[4]

3.3.2 *Individual Factors*

The WHO document, *Learning from Error* [26], identified a number of individual factors that may contribute to the occurrence of adverse events in healthcare organizations, including the following:

(1) Staff well-being
(2) Task appropriateness
(3) Education and training
(4) Team and social environment
(5) Patient partnership (see Chapter 2)

The COVID-19 pandemic highlighted the fragility of the healthcare system and exposed the vulnerability of the healthcare workforce. During the pandemic, the usual stresses on individuals were set aside by the need to work extraordinary hours in the care of COVID-19 patients. Nevertheless, even in everyday health systems under better circumstances, staff well-being may be tested.

3.3.2.1 Staff Well-Being

The first individual factor that may contribute to adverse events is staff well-being. Preserving the physical and mental health of staff is essential to ensure the delivery of safe patient care and avoid adverse events. Physically and psychologically sound health staff are less prone to make errors, contributing to safer care. The safety of health staff therefore directly impacts the safety of patients [27]. For example, a heavy physical workload may lead to musculoskeletal disorders that impact staff quality of life. At times, staff may be subjected to violent behavior from patients and relatives. Burnout may occur if issues such as these are not addressed.

Staff well-being was especially important during the COVID-19 pandemic which exposed and exacerbated the underlying challenges facing current healthcare systems. At times, staff were required to work extra shifts to cover staff shortages due to staff illness. When staff absenteeism and attrition aggravate the physical and mental well-being of those staff who remain, the possibility of suboptimal care increases. During the pandemic, factors that may have been ignored in the past took on increased significance. These factors have been identified as related to either

[4] More information of how to develop a patient safety culture is discussed in Chap. 7.

human factors such as disrespectful behaviors, or systemic issues such as a blame culture, working conditions, bullying, and harassment.

Disrespectful behavior has been identified in the literature as one of the main causes of stress in the healthcare workplace [37]. Although the impact of the disrespectful behavior of doctors has been researched the most [38, 39], there is no suggestion that this category of healthcare profession is alone in exhibiting this type of behavior. Davis and Beale [40] believe that, to a greater or lesser extent, disrespectful behavior occurs in all professional and nonprofessional groups in hospitals. They concluded that this behavior is an underlying cause of many of the problems in relation to safety and quality care within healthcare organizations.

Personal issues may also affect an individual's ability to be fully present in the clinical setting. These issues may relate to family concerns such as childcare arrangements, the care of aged parents, economic/financial issues, separation/divorce, or major illness. In some cases, the effects of a stressed, disrupted household may impact children who exhibit difficult behaviors at home or at school. These distressors can cause staff to be less focused than normal on the clinical care of patients.

3.3.2.2 Task Appropriateness

The second factor that may contribute to adverse events is task appropriateness. For individuals to perform successfully, there must be clear and achievable objectives aligned with the clinical goals for the patient. Any vagueness or ambiguity can lead to confusion. Individuals must be able to identify what they are supposed to do and to what standard. There must be realistic timelines for them to achieve the task that has been set in relation to a particular patient. Too much time and laziness or disinterest may set in. Too little time and stress may become too great and interfere with performance. In addition, individuals must be able to make decisions within their area of expertise and according to their qualifications and experience. If they cannot, they will always be running back to their clinical supervisor for permission. This can create a dependent situation in which the individual becomes demoralized and stressed and questions why they have been given the job in the first place. Why cannot they be trusted to make decisions within their authority limits? Bakker and Demerouti [28, 29] specifically note the supervisory nature of the leadership relationship in providing supportive feedback to individuals and teams as they perform their tasks.

When task factors cause individuals distress, coaching helps them restructure their work and/or workload to the degree that they are able to make changes on their own. If not, the coach can assist coachees in structuring a future conversation with their clinical supervisor in relation to their situation and their desired task/role changes so that they find increased satisfaction at work. To do this, the coach may use the Job Characteristics Model [41], which is based on how jobs are designed, to help them identify the elements with which they are satisfied and those elements about which they need to speak with their supervisor to bring about changes in their

Table 3.2 Job characteristics model

Job characteristics model
● *Skill variety*—The degree to which the job requires a variety of different activities
● *Task identity*—The degree to which the job requires completion of a whole and identifiable piece of work
● *Task significance*—The degree to which the job has a substantial impact on the lives or work of other people
● *Autonomy*—The degree to which the job provides substantial freedom and discretion to the individual in scheduling the work and in determining the procedures to be used in carrying it out
● *Feedback*—The degree to which the individual obtains direct and clear information about the effectiveness of their performance

Adapted from Hackman & Oldham (1980) [41]

role. The model proposes five job characteristics that can be adjusted to increase satisfaction at work (Table 3.2).

Role Clarity

A major impediment to task completion and performance, that may contribute to adverse events, is role clarity. The need for role clarity among team members has long been recognized as an imperative to optimize team functioning and outcomes [42]. It has been identified as one of the most important factors causing confusion and uncertainty in clinical settings. Who is responsible for what? What actions need to be taken by whom? Interdependency among team members is likely to be high in clinical teams. With the important team goal of quality patient care and safety, good leadership has been particularly evidenced in research as enabling effective team huddles with clarity of purpose and co-constructed expectations of patient care [43]. However, unless all individuals are committed to achieving their clinical goals, they will let down the team and colleagues. When only one or two individuals shoulder responsibility in a particular area, this may be acceptable for a time provided that their responsibility is later shared with other team members. However, if the one or two continue to shoulder the extra burden, this situation does not generate the kind of commitment that is needed from each team member. In relation to patient safety, the attitude of "I'll do whatever it takes" is what the leader is looking for from every team member.

Given the many challenges identified in healthcare and how staff work in interdisciplinary teams, it is essential that the various roles played by each team member are clarified prior to the commencement of patient care. Evidence-informed strategies, such as structured communications, speaking up, and debriefing, show promise for improving team functioning [44]. The utilization of nontechnical skills such as coaching has been identified as crucial for issue resolution. In addition, the co-development of a *Patient Implementation Plan* with key stakeholders, including patients, families, care providers, and decision-makers, can support role clarification in teams [45].

A study by Kilpatrick et al. [46] revealed the critical role of nurse practitioners in patient care. It measured the influence of role clarity on care outcomes and identified the mediating role that team processes play. Patient characteristics, such as type of respondent, location, being employed, and attendance at a routine health visit, were also identified as significant predictors of perceived outcome success.

3.3.2.3 Education and Training

The third individual factor that may contribute to adverse events is education and training. Being adequately educated and trained can alleviate any professional competence issues that may cause individuals stress and ensure that all team members are fully capable of performing in their role. The *World Health Assembly Resolution WHA72.6,2* on *Global Action on Patient Safety* recognized the importance of "education, training and continuous professional development to build and maintain a competent, compassionate and committed healthcare workforce operating within a supportive environment to make health care safe" [27].

In interdisciplinary teams, the primary concern is to identify team members' skills and capabilities as they perform the task. However, the traditional hierarchical nature of healthcare organizations is not conducive to developing systems and processes that support interdisciplinary collaboration and teamwork and equalize the status of clinicians on the care team. Status equalization greatly assists the achievement of the *WHO Strategy 2.1*: *Develop and sustain a culture of respect, openness and transparency* [35] that promotes learning rather than blame and retribution and fosters the display of attitudes and behaviors that reduce hierarchical structures and support a "speak-up" culture.

Nontechnical skills such as communicating more effectively and building more robust relationships are particularly important during a team response to a medical emergency. In 2011, the WHO issued the *Patient Safety Curriculum Guide: Multi-Professional Edition* [47], a document that stressed the need for clinicians to learn how to function more collaboratively in a multidisciplinary team environment. This implies that training in nontechnical skills should be provided not only for leaders but also for current and future workers so that everyone can contribute to positive and effective interdisciplinary teamwork. The nontechnical (human) skills critical to effective teamwork are communication, cooperation, and collaboration. The challenge is that the presence of these skills is difficult to measure and hence can only be evidenced by observation of the results in domain-specific clinical areas. The development of these and other nontechnical skills can be enhanced when individuals receive coaching and/or are trained in coaching skills.

Recognition that the nontechnical skills of individual team members are just as important as their technical skills is an important step in the evolution of cultural improvement in healthcare safety and quality [48–51]. However, as the education of developing healthcare professionals continues to be delivered in silos, the task of integrating interdependent professionals into a cohesive working team is difficult unless nontechnical skills are utilized by the team leader to smooth the process.

Moreover, researchers note that, while the education of younger doctors now includes training in interpersonal skills, senior clinicians may not have received this training; hence, they may not know how to work effectively with other disciplines [40]. They recommend initial and ongoing training for clinicians to develop the knowledge, behaviors, and attitudes necessary for highly reliable and effective team performance to occur. Moreover, they suggest that periodic mandatory reviews of these skills should be incorporated into continuing professional development activities.

3.3.2.4 Team and Social Environment

The fourth individual factor that may contribute to adverse events is the team and social environment. Using nontechnical skills such as coaching, the team leader is able to develop high-quality patient care as an outcome of the coordinated, cooperative efforts of multiple technically competent healthcare clinicians working in concert over time, spanning disciplinary and professional boundaries [40]. Teamwork skills that pay attention to group dynamics are vital to the delivery of safe patient care. The team should be well-informed of the situation and goals to be achieved so that they can support each other knowing that, if one component of the care fails, the outcome may be disastrous for the patient. Hence, it is in everyone's interest to assist and support each other. The shared social experience of participating in a multidisciplinary team assists in advancing team learning about how members relate to each other, truthfully communicate, and trust that their colleagues will support them.

Working toward a common goal is a highly motivating factor that keeps everyone on track and engenders a feeling of comradery within the team. If there are hidden agendas, cliques, or groups, these may have a disruptive influence on the overall harmony of the team. The leader's role is to ensure that these cliques/groups support each other so that everyone feels part of the larger team. Otherwise, a sense of isolation and separation from the team may result in some individuals leaving the team because of these factors.

In a recent US research project aimed at nurturing the academic-practice partnership between nursing and medical practitioners [52], researchers used team-based, collaborative approaches to interdisciplinary care which are known to have had a positive influence on healthcare organizations [53, 54]. These interventions included distributive interdisciplinary unit-level leadership, daily huddles, and data-driven care including information sharing and collaborative problem-solving. Results from academic-practice partnership studies confirm that they nurture a culture that fosters shared practice and create the conditions to meet mutual goals [55].[5]

---

[5]Appendix 3.1. Readers may like to assess the extent to which you believe these organizational and human factors are affecting the likelihood of adverse events occurring in the team or department in which you predominantly work.

3.4 How Adverse Events Occur

Investigations into how adverse events occur have analyzed major safety catastrophes around the world since the 1970s [56, 57]. Turner [58] was the first to conceptualize accidents as processes rather than as sudden events. His theoretical model identified an incubation period of communication and information difficulties long before the actual event occurred, e.g., repeated violations of procedures. He stated that any failure to heed these signals was the result of "rigidities of perception and beliefs" [59], which constitute the frames of reference through which organizational members interpret information about the organization's activities and environment. Chernobyl (1986) was the first recorded catastrophic event to illustrate Turner's man-made disaster theory. Turner's investigative approach spawned a plethora of methods to discover the underlying cause of catastrophic events based on a "What went wrong?" scenario and led Rasmussen [60] to examine the trajectory of processes that led to an adverse event impacting safety.

3.4.1 Boundary of Acceptable Performance

In 1997, Rasmussen proposed a dynamic model of risk and safety to rectify the risks plaguing high-risk industries at that time [60]. He noted that "a major problem appeared to be management's commitment to safety and the related efforts of society to control management incentives by safety regulation" [60]. The traditional way to manage risk at that time was "to constrain … behavior by rules and equipment design, to increase … performance" [60]. Rasmussen observed that research findings and safety models at that time focused on a "bottom-up" approach to managing risk driven by rigid management controls and procedures that proved insufficient to prevent harm since these safety practices were being "compensated by people adapting to … change in an unprecedented way" [60] to keep people safe. He concluded that work processes could not be slavishly followed when there was danger of accidental side effects that may cause harm to people. He proposed that a "top-down" system-oriented approach based on control concepts needed to be embedded within an adaptive social-technical system to acknowledge the social and interactional nature of doing work. This was a shift in thinking—identifying what staff were actually doing to keep each other safe—rather than just taking a remedial approach to prevention or rectification. Rasmussen believed that controlling activities and people's safety via the prescriptive *command-and-control* approach may be effective in a stable society where instruction and work tools at all levels can be based on task analysis; however, in a dynamic situation, this approach was insufficient for managing risk in a complex, high-risk environment.

Rasmussen noted that "risk management at the upper levels is usually studied with a 'horizontal' orientation of research across the technological hazard sources" [60]. Therefore, because the "profession" of management believes that managers can manage across any area of expertise, the result of this "horizontal orientation" is that managers tend to have no detailed knowledge of, or experience in, the "actual processes found at the productive bottom level" [60]. Moreover, because a "rule or instruction is often designed separately for a particular task in isolation whereas in the actual situation, several tasks are active in a time sharing mode … rules, laws and instructions practically speaking are never followed to the letter" [60].

He also noted that any variations to procedures often appear to be quite rational given the "actual workload and timing constraints" [60]. Moreover, because people who violated the rules could easily be identified in the Safety-1 environment at that time [1], they were typically blamed, and accidents were considered to be the result of human error. However, with further investigation, court reports of failures such as Chernobyl showed that human error was not the cause of these accidents. Instead, the cause was "a systemic migration of organizational behavior toward accident under the influence of pressure toward cost-effectiveness in an aggressive, competitive environment (Rasmussen, 1993b, 1994b)" [60], resulting from a sequence of decisions made by many operatives over a period of time, which suggests "a natural migration of activities toward the boundary of acceptable performance" [60].

Rasmussen concluded that "a new approach to representation of system behavior was necessary, not focused on human errors and violations but on the mechanisms *generating* behavior in the actual, dynamic work environment" [60]. He advocated for the identification of "the boundary conditions of the work space and the process criteria guiding drift across this space" [60] and recommended that "rather than attempting to control behavior by *fighting deviations* from a particular pre-planned path, the focus should be on the control of behavior by *making the boundaries explicit and known* and by giving opportunities to develop *coping skills at boundaries*" [60].

3.4.2 Acceptable Performance in Healthcare

Later, in 2005, Rasmussen teamed up with Cook [61] and they applied Rasmussen's dynamic model of risk and safety [60] to the healthcare sector. As a dynamic environment that is fraught with risk, healthcare systems struggle to balance *tight coupling* to ensure compliance and *loose coupling* to ensure patient safety. Hospitals and other healthcare facilities often operate on short timeframes. Decisions regarding patient diagnosis and treatment need to be made "in the moment," often amidst the presence of other complicating factors both internal to the patient (e.g., allergic reactions to medicines, comorbidity concerns) and external interferences (e.g., blocked access to beds, conflicting patient demands).

Drawing on Rasmussen's original model [60], Cook and Rasmussen [61] formulated a dynamic model of risk and safety in the healthcare sector that addressed the patient safety dynamics associated with tight coupling, which they referred to as "going solid." "Going solid" [61] means that the organization has reached the

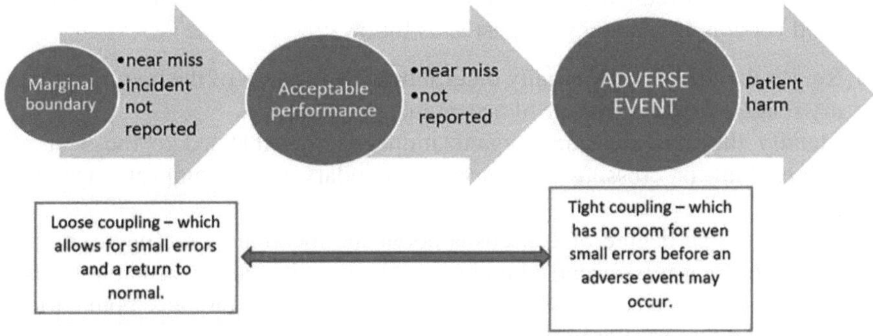

Fig. 3.2 From marginal boundary to adverse event (Adapted from Cook & Rasmussen (2005) [61])

"boundary of acceptable performance" [60], which implies that incidents are likely to occur if that boundary is crossed, causing patient harm (Fig. 3.2).

In the past, healthcare systems were loosely coupled, i.e., activities and conditions in one part of the system had only limited effects on other parts of the system. This arrangement allowed the system to cope with conditions such as short-term surges in demand. However, in today's increasingly complex environment, tight coupling must be observed in specific areas to ensure that legal and regulatory requirements are met. Tight coupling occurs when activities in one area of the healthcare organization are interdependent on those occurring in other areas of the system. No longer is there a buffer to soak up the compression between activities, which light coupling affords. Tight coupling is most easily observed as a financial pressure to do more with less, ensure cost-efficiencies, and optimize resources, including new technologies.

In healthcare settings, daily operations take place amidst a number of events that occur simultaneously. Variations in processes or procedures (near misses) due to pressures in the environment (e.g., staff shortages, resource constraints, bed inaccessibility) shift the "normal" boundary of acceptable performance further toward the margin and may even establish a new margin further toward the "boundary of acceptable performance" [61], putting pressure on this outer marker. When a new near miss occurs, it may shift the new margin over the acceptable performance boundary into unacceptable territory, causing an adverse event to occur. Cook and Rasmussen recommended looser coupling, which allows for a greater margin of error. This is accomplished by addressing the first near miss when it occurs to learn from it and reduces the pressure gradient on staff, resources, and hospital capacity so that another near miss does not occur and tip the system over the edge. So, even though from a resourcing and financial point of view, healthcare organizations would like to "go solid" [61] with tight coupling, it is imperative that executives and staff heed the warnings of near misses so that situations do not escalate into adverse events that may cause patient harm or even death.

Cook and Rasmussen [61] provided guidance for how healthcare executives can proceed once a near miss has been reported, to move the marginal boundary back to where it was, thus reducing pressure on the acceptable performance boundary. A modified version of what they suggest is as follows:

(1) Revisit the factors that initially determined the location of the marginal boundary relative to the boundary of acceptable performance.
(2) Identify the individual and organizational factors that led to the near miss approaching or crossing the marginal boundary and its impact—actual and possible.
(3) Determine the degree of consensus about the location of the operating point where the near miss occurred relative to the marginal and acceptable boundaries, and what needs to be done to release the pressure on these boundaries so that they return to "normal."

3.4.3 *Shifting Thinking to Safety-11*

Hollnagel et al. [1] expanded on the concept of the "boundary of acceptable performance" [61] when they developed their Safety-11 approach to risk management and safety. They added another dimension when their research reinforced that operatives work in a sociotechnical system in which the work that is performed is composed of design and work principles from various research disciplines that impact significant actors in the system (e.g., government legislators and regulators, managers implementing company policies, and staff doing the work) under various environmental conditions (e.g., political climate, market conditions, financial pressure, technological change). However, because designers do not often work at coalfaces, the processes they put in place do not always work exactly as planned. They need to be modified "on-the-run" by workers to ensure that the work gets done to specifications while also keeping them and patients safe. However, when near misses have not been reported, the next occurrence may cross the boundary of acceptable performance and become an adverse event, possibly with tragic consequences. If staff had felt psychologically safe to speak up and if management had listened, the event may not have occurred.

3.5 Adverse Event Reporting

Adverse event reporting is regarded as a significant indicator when assessing patient safety culture in the healthcare system. It serves as an indispensable tool for monitoring and promoting the quality and safety of patient care. Adverse events accounted for 55.6% of the complaints made during admissions, or approximately 1 out of every 3 [62]. According to Schwendimann et al. [63] and Hibbert et al. [64], the most acknowledged inpatient adverse events are medication errors, falls, surgical site infections, and bed sores. These complaints are all challenges to the quality and safety of care administered in the healthcare environment. Abuosi et al. [65] believe that adverse events identified through staff observation and patient/relationship complaints are a particularly underutilized source of information for improvement in most healthcare settings.

The study by Abuosi et al. [65] investigated the frequency of adverse event reporting, the determinants of adverse event reporting, and the implications for patient safety culture in healthcare facilities. They used the *Hospital Survey of Patient Safety Culture* (HSOPSC)[6] to survey 1651 health professionals in 13 healthcare facilities in Ghana. The results showed that "Teamwork" and "Response to errors" were the main determinants of a satisfactory patient safety culture. They noted that the ability of health professionals to voluntarily report adverse events can be improved through factors such as managers' responsiveness to errors, open communication about errors, adequate handovers and information exchange among staff, and adequate staffing. To increase the adverse event reporting rate, they advised hospital managers to put in place a nonpunitive reporting system while rewarding staff who reported adverse events. Promoting an effective patient safety culture is the ultimate way to overcome the challenges of adverse event reporting, and this can be effectively addressed by developing policies to regulate the incidence and reporting of adverse events. The quality of healthcare and patient safety can also be enhanced when healthcare managers dedicate adequate resources to support teamwork, effective communication, and a blame-free culture. The researchers listed several implications of their research for healthcare management in relation to leadership, teamwork, the work environment, and communication. Moreover, they stated the obvious issue for management—that adequate healthcare financing can address human and material resource issues associated with patient safety.

Also researching in Ghana, Tenza et al. [34] found that behaviors such as open communication, organizational learning, and strong teamwork within units contributed to a positive patient safety culture in selected facilities. These findings are consistent with those of previous studies indicating a positive relationship between organizational learning, good teamwork, and communication about errors, as factors for improving patient safety culture [66, 67]. Moreover, they also identified a number of other factors that inhibited patient safety culture: lack of teamwork across units, fear of reporting adverse events, the existence of a blame culture, inconsistent response to errors, extreme shortage of staff, substandard handover, and lack of management support and resources. The lack of standardized policies for reporting adverse events and responding to errors allowed managers to use various approaches, some of which resulted in a culture of blame. Staff shortages contributed to poor quality safety practices, including poor handover, which was also influenced by lateness to duty. They concluded that there is a need to normalize a just culture [35] in the hospitals they surveyed and to train managers in the effective reporting of errors.

[6] Read more about the HSOPSC in Chap. 8.

Binkheder et al. [68] explored the relationship between patient safety culture and nationally reported sentinel (adverse) events in Saudi hospitals over one year. They found that the domains most highly correlated with patient safety culture were "Teamwork within units" (80.65%) and "Organizational learning" (80.33%). In addition, the correlation analysis showed that three domains were significantly associated with lower rates of reported sentinel events, namely, "Teamwork within units," "Communication openness," and "Handovers and transitions." Conversely, multivariate analyses showed that the "Handovers and transitions," "Nonpunitive response to error," and "Teamwork within units" domains were significant predictors of the number of sentinel events. Their study confirmed that a more positive patient safety culture is associated with a lower occurrence of sentinel events. They concluded that to minimize the fear of sentinel event reporting, thereby improving overall patient safety, a cultural change is needed and can be achieved by promoting a blame-free culture and improving teamwork, handovers, and communication openness.

Similarly, Beyene et al. [69] reported that poor handovers and transitions had the most detrimental effect on a positive patient safety culture and most frequently impacted the lack of event reporting. Participants working in surgical wards were more likely to record the presence of a patient safety culture than those working in medical wards. They concluded that ensuring a blame-free working environment increased the likelihood of there being a patient safety culture within the unit.

3.5.1 Incident Reporting Systems

Although originating in a Safety-1 environment, incident reporting systems are also a vital part of a proactive Safety-11 patient safety approach. To promote error reporting, incident reporting systems were first established in the USA and Australia in 2000, in the UK in 2003, and in France in 2006 [70]. These systems vary in relation to the actual data recorded, the extent of patient involvement, and the depth of the investigation undertaken when an incident occurs. Typically, the more significant the harm from the event is, the more detailed the investigation is. Implementing an incident reporting system requires the presence of a number of factors: training and education on the importance of reporting and how to use the system; financial resources to conduct an investigation; technology, data analysis, and storage facilities; data security policies; and protocols for dealing with and reporting confidential information [4] as well as investigative processes to understand the incidents and their causation.

Reporting and learning systems around the world have developed the content of their reports either by deciding from first principles what information they want to collect or by adopting one of the commercially available or open source-based tools/software for incident reporting. Generally, whichever approach is used, incident reporting systems seek to capture and assemble information in three main domains [4]:

- *Description* (what happened), including patient characteristics, incident characteristics, and location
- *Explanation* (why it happened), including perceived causes of the event, contributing factors, and mitigating factors
- *Remedial measures* (what happened then)—the actions that were taken as a result, including reviewing and redesigning processes and procedures, preventative educational measures, and organizational changes

The value of a reporting system is that the stored data can be used to identify risk and harm, assess differences by place and over time, serve as the starting point for investigations into causation, prevent repetition of similar incidents, promote a culture of patient safety, and engage staff curiosity and commitment so they can learn from these events. However, this value may or may not be realized depending on the quality and veracity of the data collected on each incident and how it is recorded.

In a healthcare environment, reporting errors and near misses is essential because they provide the opportunity for staff to review the practices that contributed to the event, and act to correct it so this does not happen again [71]. However, unfortunately, not all medical errors and near misses are reported by staff for a number of reasons, including the following:

- Fear of being blamed for an adverse event, particularly if they are the end users of the process [43, 72]
- Fear that a record of their mistakes will be stored in their personal file and may be used against them at some time in the future [72]
- Fear that there may be repercussions or punishment inflicted [73]
- Other staff members developing a negative impression of them and a lack of adequate support from their colleagues [74]
- Administrative factors such as time to report and ease of the reporting system[7]
- Social and cultural barriers
- Organizational factors such as rigid systems and protocols, cost-cutting imperatives, and lack of or cumbersome policy and standard operating procedures [75]

These findings are consistent with those from international studies suggesting that a major barrier to error reporting is the risk of punitive response [76–78]. When nonpunitive measures are taken, errors are detected and reported early, and further occurrences are prevented [79].

[7] Appendix 3.2 contains a simple tool that you can use to rate your current patient safety incident reporting system to assess its strengths against key points.

3.5.2 Patient Safety Indicators

Following the WHO initiative, health jurisdictions have developed their own versions of patient safety reporting systems. For example, the Agency for Healthcare Research and Quality (AHRQ) in the USA developed *Patient Safety Indicators* (PSIs), which use the hospital's administrative data as quality measures of patient safety. PSIs reflect the quality of inpatient care but also focus on preventable complications and iatrogenic events. PSIs have been found to be useful for understanding adverse events and identifying possible areas for improvement within healthcare delivery systems. For example, PSIs have been shown to accurately identify certain accidental inpatient injuries. In addition, the AHRQ has developed a *Patient Safety Incident Response Framework*, which is a comprehensive, systemic, and process-focused incident examination approach to ensuring organizational learning. This framework replaces the current method used by the UK NHS to support overarching patient safety strategic aims for their agency.

3.5.3 Data Quality

Data on incidents are collected not only to discover new information but also to act upon it, i.e., to bring about behavioral and organizational change. While the reporting system acts as a way to document and track the management of an individual adverse event, at a systemic level, it allows for aggregate data to be collated that can guide the organization to broader trends in its care that need to be addressed. Adverse events provide "information-rich" data for learning and system improvement to proactively strengthen a patient safety culture [80]. Patient safety culture is significantly impacted by education and coaching when leaders follow-up on reports [81]. However, studies have repeatedly shown that insights into patient safety may be hampered by a number of factors such as the volume of data (overload), poor specification of what is to be reported, over-interpretation of incident analyses to judge safety performance, selectivity and incompleteness of data, taxonomies and classifications that do not enable aggregation of reports into categories that reliably highlight systemic weaknesses, and lack of investment in analysis compared with reporting [4].

In addition to collecting data on *lagging* PSIs, a Safety 11 ([1]) approach recommends that consideration be given to collecting data on *leading* indicators of adverse events such as the number of hospital admissions, bed access and congestion rate, and staffing ratios.

At a systemic level, large quantities of automated data are not yet widely available in healthcare, nor has the opportunity been taken on any large scale, to adapt existing electronic monitoring in patient care for safety purposes. This may be because in healthcare, more decisions and procedures are carried out by people than by machines. There is more emphasis on the observation of clinical practices and procedures than on data collection and analysis, although it is only through such analysis that insights can be gleaned for improvement and learning purposes—to assess risk, identify poor safety performance, and expose the potential occurrences of harm.

3.6 Coaching to Prevent Adverse Events

One important area of clinical care that *coaching* has been reported to significantly influence is that of error reporting [82]. The reporting of adverse events is a necessary first step in identifying and addressing lapses of patient safety. However, adverse events are underreported, especially by frontline leaders such as resident physicians [83]. Leaders trained in patient safety coaching are better able to encourage their staff to speak up and report errors even though they recognize the potential barriers to doing so, such as the following:

- Fear of how others will respond
- Concerns over appearing incompetent
- Not being able to collect the facts and accurately report them with positive intent
- Not knowing the most appropriate person to be spoken to
- Feeling a lack of personal control and impact

Research has shown that a number of individual factors, such as job satisfaction, responsibility toward patients, professional standing, confidence based on experience, communication skills, and educational background influence whether a person feels able to speak up [82]. Contextual factors such as hospital administrative support, interdisciplinary policy-making, teamwork and relationships between other team members, and the attitudes of leaders/superiors, were also found to be significant. These inhibitors of speaking up to report errors have been associated in the literature with other factors occurring in the workplace such as ineffective leadership and lack of individual and team psychological safety. Ways that leaders can support speaking up to prevent the occurrence of adverse events include assisting coachees in communicating more effectively with their leader and within interdisciplinary teams, becoming more mindful and observant as they deliver patient care, and providing constructive feedback to individuals and teams so they can learn and grow professionally (Fig. 3.3).

3.6.1 Communicating Effectively

The first way that leaders can prevent adverse events from occurring is by communicating more effectively with individual team members and their team as a whole and with members of interdisciplinary teams. They can do this by fostering daily dialog within their team; supporting effective communication within

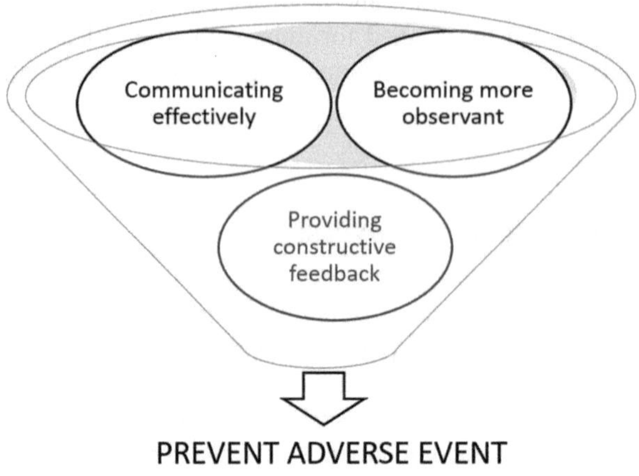

Fig. 3.3 How leaders can prevent adverse events

interdisciplinary teams, e.g., during clinical rounds; and utilizing the beneficial relationships that exist within staff networks and disciplines.

3.6.1.1 Daily Dialog within a Team

Dialog optimizes safe clinical decision-making for patients and promotes staff well-being based on respectful communication and relationships. Dissonance between espoused values and values-in-action is identified as potential areas for individual and team improvement [84, 85]. Lee et al. [86] studied the everyday language used by healthcare professionals as they described their daily duties of providing quality healthcare. Following Wetherell and Potter's premise that social and psychological realities are "constructed, defined and articulated through discourse" [87], they identified the actions taking place within a period of talk during interdisciplinary team meetings. Thereafter, they examined the realities that these discursive actions constructed (e.g., in relation to the patient as a malfunctioning body) to explicate patterns of communication that impact team decision-making. They found that individual, lifeworld, and interpretative language repertoires assisted health professionals within the same discipline in assessing, articulating, and practicing care provision and describing patients' clinical and social conditions efficiently. However, they were insufficient to promote collaborative discourse within multidisciplinary teams.

In other studies, researchers concluded that healthcare professionals could enrich their representations of patients by using the discursive strategy of perspective-taking more often to recognize patients as people with preferences and constraints [88]. The perspective-taking strategy can be used to gain knowledge of the patients' historical and personal situation so that what is shared at the meeting table is included in collaborative decision-making regarding care and discharge planning.

In a study investigating patient safety culture in Austria, Draganović and Offermanns [37] reported that the most highly rated factors contributing to patient safety culture were communication openness, supervisor/manager expectations, and actions promoting safety. They noted that evidence-based tools and approaches exist to improve communication—such as *SBAR* (situation, background, assessment, and recommendation), *Checkback*, *Call out*, and *Ask Me* 31—and that leaders can encourage improved communication and foster a supportive team culture by making themselves approachable and inviting everyone into the conversation. However, the study noted that there are significant differences in the perceptions of patient safety culture among nurses, doctors, and other groups.

3.6.1.2 Interdisciplinary Teams

Healthcare teams consist of individuals communicating with one another during patient care delivery. The coordination of multiple specialties is critical for patients with complex health conditions and requires interdisciplinary and intraprofessional communication [89]. This is especially true when multidisciplinary healthcare teams are tasked with creating new, individual, patient-centered solutions to improve a patient's long-term healthcare situation such as when assessing the needs and care options for patients with rare diseases [90].

Managing the communication flow within teams is essential so that all team members are "on the same page," i.e., they understand the clinical goals for the patient and the part they are responsible for delivering. In a psychologically safe environment, team members can speak openly and candidly about their concerns and ask the "silly questions." They do not feel that they will be punished for speaking up about errors or omissions. When communication is clear, there is no room for misunderstanding or misinterpretation. Clear communication is free from assumptions and innuendos, is evidence-based, and supports learning. There is no opportunity for individuals to deny responsibility or attribute blame. There is a collaborative approach with a focus on ensuring quality and safe patient care.

If difficulties arise in interdisciplinary team communications, a strategy by which clinical leaders can better manage the situation is either to change the situation (by avoiding or altering the stressor) or change their reaction to the situation (by adapting to or accepting the stressor). The latter strategy is particularly useful in situations in which they have very little, or no, control over the situation or the likely outcome. The Thomas–Kilmann negotiation style of accommodating, avoiding, collaborating, competing, or compromising [91] provides further options for resolution. The style chosen will depend on whether the relationship with others involved in the situation is more important than the desired outcome or vice versa.

3.6.1.3 Respecting Social and Cultural Differences

Primary care teams increasingly depend on the contributions of multiple professionals. Hence, the interdisciplinary team composition consists of a variety of job roles and different staff members, which has been described as "functional heterogeneity" [92]. Based on the premise that a broader range of knowledge and skills enhances problem-solving and work efficiency, functional heterogeneity is expected to improve team performance [93]. Patient care is enhanced by increased efficiency, improved continuity of service, reduced errors, and a culture of shared resources [94].

Leaders need to be alert to how social and cultural factors can distort communication within an interdisciplinary team. For example, a study by Fernando et al. [95] explored the enablers and barriers to interdisciplinary communication between surgical trainees and ward nurses, and how power is deployed and experienced, which they believed may negatively impact interdisciplinary communication. Findings from observations and semi-structured interviews revealed issues derived from contested meanings of space and time. Trainees experienced the contested spatial boundaries of the surgical ward when they perceived nurses to project a sense of territoriality. Nurses expressed difficulty getting trainees to respond and attend to pages from the ward and believed them to have a poor understanding of the nurses' role. Trainees perceived seasoned nurses to devalue their clinical knowledge. Nurses viewed the limited time that trainees spent in clinical rotation in the ward as adversely affecting communication. The researchers proposed that challenges to interdisciplinary communication are rooted in team and professional cultures and suggested that interventions to improve communication should therefore identify and target the social and cultural dimensions of healthcare team member relations. They also encouraged interdisciplinary team members to develop an enhanced understanding and appreciation of the temporal and spatial dimensions of communication, as these dimensions apply to their daily work with staff members of different social groups or cultures.

3.6.1.4 Clinical Rounds

The need to communicate effectively is particularly important during clinical rounds when patient details are shared and treatment options discussed. Clinical rounds are an essential organizational process within the hospital setting. They play an important role in the flow of clinical information and coordination of care. Key clinicians involved in the patient's care come together on a daily basis to check their medical records, appraise their progress, inform and consult with the patient, and allow for collaborative planning in relation to their immediate and longer-term care needs [96]. Goals and expectations are made clear so that team members do not feel that they are "left in the dark," which can cause resentment and negative feelings.

In interdisciplinary teams, nurses and physicians develop short- and long-term patient goals that incorporate up-to-date information and address potential issues. The structure of such teams is important to their effectiveness because improved communication during interdisciplinary rounds may lead to earlier order entry, laboratory collection, and diagnostic scheduling, resulting in early intervention and resolution of current medical issues [97] which can improve patient outcomes [98]. However, for interdisciplinary care teams to be successful, team members must be willing to overcome hierarchies, blur professional boundaries, respect one another's contributions, learn from each other, share skills, and understand that many patient care needs are not discipline specific [94].

There are many benefits of interdisciplinary clinical rounds including improved communication and a reduction in adverse events, morbidity and mortality rates [99]. Interdisciplinary rounds build supportive care teams, improve patient care outcomes, and increase patient satisfaction [100]. They provide an opportunity to create a therapeutic alliance among members of the interdisciplinary care team by virtue of their in-person accessibility [98]. Additionally, standardized interdisciplinary rounds serve to increase productivity among healthcare teams and build better connections with patients [101]. They are forums to address concerns, engage in collaborative information sharing, and better conduct discharge planning [102].

A study by Verhaegh et al. [97] explored the perceptions of healthcare professionals about the effectiveness of interdisciplinary communication and collaboration during clinical rounds. Nurses, physicians, and other staff members identified a number of barriers that they believe impede communication and collaboration, such as the social and spatial structures between the healthcare team and patient. Specific ways to generate more effective interdisciplinary communication and collaboration during clinical rounds were reported as pre-round briefing to prepare the team for patient interaction; scheduling rounds at times other than mornings, which are usually quite hectic in terms of patient care and activity; and using a communication tool such as that developed by Adams [102] to structure communication or a safety checklist, which has been found to reduce adverse events, morbidity and mortality [99].

Standardizing the focus and communication channels of the interdisciplinary care team is an effective method for achieving quality patient outcomes because it can streamline workflow and provide a forum for open discussion of patient care issues. Other ways that the interdisciplinary team can improve communication with patients include summarizing a daily care plan for them, setting goals with them for the next 24 h or until discharge, and involving them in decision-making and discharge planning. Strong leadership is required to strengthen communication between physicians, nurses, and other staff members. It ensures that all members of the team are involved in decision-making and leads to the development of a strong team culture [97]. A clear division of roles and responsibilities supports the organization and effectiveness of clinical rounds.

3.6.1.5 Communication Networks

Networking is a favored approach for expanding knowledge, understanding, and relationships into other areas of clinical expertise. Shoham et al. [89] examined a communication network of 71 health professionals in four professional roles—physician, nurse, health management, and support personnel (dietitian, pharmacist, or social worker)—compared with other health professionals (including physical, respiratory, and occupational therapists and medical students) working in a burn unit. The data for this cross-sectional study were collected by surveying members of a healthcare team. "Ties" were defined by asking team members whom they discussed patient care matters with on the shift. Researchers built an exponential random graph model to determine whether professional roles influence the likelihood of a tie and whether ties are more likely between team members from different professions than between team members from the same profession. They also investigated which professions were more likely to form interdisciplinary ties. They found that health management and support personnel ties were interdisciplinary in 94% of nurses, while ties among nurses were interdisciplinary in 60% of cases. Nurses and other health professionals were significantly less likely than physicians to form ties. Nurses were 1.64 times more likely to communicate with nurses than with non-nurses; however, there was no significant role homophily for physicians, other health professionals, or health management and support personnel. They concluded that understanding communication networks in healthcare teams is an early step in understanding how teams work together to provide care.

3.6.2 Observation of Incidents, "Near Misses," and "Good Catches"

The second way that leaders can prevent adverse events from occurring is by enhancing team members' ability to become more observant. Observation of clinical practices is a powerful means of highlighting where improvements can be made in individual and team approaches to patient care. The discussion of observations generates staff ownership for change and celebrates collective learning [43]. Team members grow professionally as they learn to preempt the occurrence of possible harm to patients. Contributing to cultural change, team members also learn from observations of *excellent* clinical practices of those who do things *well* in their daily clinical duties.

Staff become more observant when they are mindful of the situation and remain fully "present" during clinical activities. Mindfulness is the degree to which individuals notice what is happening around them, pay attention to others and things in their environment, and fully "experience life "in the moment" [103].

The mind has a tendency to wander and lose focus, traveling in the past and future to ignore or escape the present [104]. In this process, the mind constructs its own reality that is not necessarily consistent with the actual present situation [105]. Being mindful brings the wandering mind back to the present. It allows individuals to develop nonjudgmental and nonbiased awareness as they experience and come to accept the present. Consequently, thoughts and cognitive processes are formed based on the experience itself and not on prior judgments and biases [106].

The process of mindfulness involves focusing attention on an object or activity (such as a clinical activity) and noticing the visual stimuli and physical sensations in the body while also distancing the mind from distracting thoughts and emotions [107]. During this focused-attention process, individuals meta-cognitively observe their psychological experience as well, focusing on the quality of their self-awareness instead of on any particular content of which they are aware [108]. Mindfulness practice activates the cognitive functions of attentional vigilance, attentional reorientation, executive monitoring of working memory, response inhibition, and emotion regulation, into a combined whole [109].

Training in patient safety coaching hones leaders' observational skills of what went *well* and improves their ability to demonstrate to team members the specific ways in which they can improve their daily patient care. Initially, the leader may identify an individual who would benefit from learning how to become more observant. Thereafter, all team members may benefit from becoming more observant of patient conditions, environmental situations, and potential risk areas.[8]

Typically, the most common way in which clinical practice is observed is through job-embedded training. In a Safety-11 environment [1], coaching is coupled with this approach to expeditiously transfer the learning and maximize the benefits.[9] Feedback on observed practices that are immediate, honest, constructive, and focused on learning enhances its effectiveness (Table 3.3).

Table 3.3 Learning from observations and excellence

Observation	Feedback
● Job-embedded training	● Immediate
● Coaching	● Honest
	● Constructive
	● Focused on learning

[8] Appendix 3.3. The reader may like to observe the interactions of a leader with their team during a clinical activity. The activity may be a regular daily occurrence, a pre-emptive attempt to avoid an incident, a debrief post-incident, or an examination of something that went well.

[9] Coaching for patient safety is discussed in Chap. 4.

3.6.2.1 Job-Embedded Training

A type of professional development that is frequently used in technical skill-based occupations is competency-based instruction, especially in occupations where outcomes matter such as medicine [110]. Competency-based professional development activities focus on the acquisition of defined occupational competencies specific to the field of endeavor. Skills are acquired via observation, feedback, and monitoring of progress. When this form of professional development is embedded in workplace learning, it is called job-embedded training and is intended to increase the work-related knowledge and skills required in the performance of a job. It is specifically focused on ongoing learning in the workplace and uses real data observations, conversations, and evaluations to foster the application of knowledge and skills to job-related practices [111]. It is usually followed by expert supervision.

This method of improvement may involve the observation of single or multiple work episodes by single or multisource supervisors. Observation assists individuals and teams in applying the learning from critical self-reflection back into the workplace to improve performance and professional effectiveness. Team members are encouraged to reflect, plan, and create experiences as part of their daily routine to further their own professional development [112]. They identify a discreet issue or propose a well-defined question about their practice and then systematically gather, analyze, and interpret data to discover an improvement solution.

However, instructional and training professional development activities alone are inadequate for meeting the characteristics of high-quality professional development activities. Coaching has been found to significantly facilitate the transfer of learning back into the workplace following attendance at structured professional development events [113, 114]. Multiple researchers have suggested that ongoing support in the form of coaching following the training is required to sustain long-term gains from the event [115–117].

Contemporary research places increased emphasis on evidence-based coaching approaches to achieve improved learning and expected outcomes [118]. Researchers have differentiated between supervisory and side-by-side coaching [119]. Supervisory coaching refers to job-embedded practice and competency-based instruction. This type of coaching occurs when the individual's performance is observed and monitored to gauge progress and when strengths and opportunities for improvement are recorded. Side-by-side coaching occurs when the coach provides immediate feedback regarding the accuracy of the implementation of the job-related competency [119]. Following observation and feedback, coaches help coachees develop strategies, and change their actions, with immediate impact back into the workplace; this also increases their confidence and helps them improve their performance into the future [120]. The impact of side-by-side coaching is considerably improved when a systemic, multitiered approach is used to transfer learning back into the workplace [121], as it more readily bridges the gap from knowing to doing [122].

3.6.3 Feedback That Is Constructive

The third way that leaders can prevent adverse events from occurring is by improving their ability to provide immediate and constructive feedback to team members on what went *well* and what they can do differently to make improvements. Feedback conversations are an opportunity for an open, honest conversation without justification or blame, to help team members improve their clinical practice from debriefs of incidents or near misses, and especially from observations of clinical excellence.

First, the leader "unpacks" what was happening in the team when an incident occurred or when a team member reported a near miss or good catch. How did they and team members respond or react? Did they judge? blame? justify? Was the leader dispassionate enough to provide objective initial comments? Or did everyone need time to process their thoughts and feelings? The insights generated by the debriefing allow the leader and team members to reorient, start over, and move in the right direction. They now have the information they need to guide new behaviors and performance improvements.

As a guideline when conducting a debrief after an adverse event has occurred, a near miss been reported, or a good catch been observed, leaders may use the following approach:

(1) The adverse event is debriefed as soon as possible after its occurrence but when all emotions have subsided. Rational thought and learning are possible only when emotions are contained. Using a coaching approach, questions such as the following promote learning:

   - What happened? With what outcome?
   - Who was involved?
   - What could have prevented the incident from occurring?
   - What can we learn from this incident?
   - What systems need to be changed?

(2) The near miss is debriefed as soon as possible after its occurrence but when all emotions have subsided. Questions such as the above are asked.

(3) The good catch is debriefed as soon as possible after its occurrence so that recall is not diminished over time, using the above questions (except c). Instead, the leader asks the following:

   - How can these excellent outcomes be replicated within our team?

Throughout, the leader applauds the positive behaviors observed and highlights new behaviors to be practiced in future events. As improvements are made based on this feedback, they continue to debrief future events with their team in a similar way. Team members are encouraged to reflect on their own actions, take responsibility for them, and make suggestions for learning and improvement so that positive behaviors can be reinforced.

While the best feedback is delivered in person, on occasions, feedback may be delivered in written form such as by displays that compare performance or via audio or video formats. The use of interactive technology enables real-time performance to be observed and debriefed, providing immediate feedback. Although online tools and resources are emerging that assist individuals in giving and receiving feedback (such as simulations through virtual reality, augmented reality, and extended reality) [123], there is no substitute for the personal approach to such interactions that can be provided by in-person coaching by the leader during a debrief with the individual or team.

3.6.3.1 How to Deliver Feedback

In addition to arranging debriefs when adverse events, near misses, and good catches have occurred, the contemporary leader will also be engaging in daily conversations with their direct reports and providing feedback on their performance. In a feedback conversation, the leader gives immediate feedback that is specific and descriptive. What needs improvement is conveyed in objective terms so that the individual understands what they need to do differently. Feedback is always constructive and positively focused on how individuals can change their clinical practice and/or standards. The leader acknowledges excellent clinical practices and recognizes excellent skills and positive abilities and attitudes when they occur (a Safety-11 approach) [1] rather than focusing on poor performance (a Safety-1 approach). With constructive feedback, leaders actively seek opportunities to notice and reward good performance on a daily basis.

Following the debriefing of an incident, near miss, or good catch, leaders can seek feedback from their coach on factors such as how "present" they were during the debriefing, whether they paid attention and showed that they were listening to team members' ideas/suggestions, deferred judgment, and responded appropriately. Specifically, the feedback focuses on observations of how the leader demonstrated the following behaviors during the debriefing:

Remaining "present"

- Did they focus on the team member and their story?
- Were they fully present—"in the moment"—reflecting on both the content and the team member's feelings?
- Were they completely aware of the task at hand?

Paying attention

- Did they give team members their undivided attention and acknowledge their messages?
- Did they look at team members directly?
- Did they seem to put aside distracting thoughts and avoid mentally preparing a rebuttal?
- Did they avoid being distracted by environmental factors?
- Did they "listen" to team members' body language and take note of their own?
- Did they refrain from side conversations when listening during the debriefing?

Showing that they were listening

- Did they use their body language and gestures to convey their attention?
- Did they nod occasionally?
- Did they smile and use other facial expressions?
- Did they note their posture and make sure that it was open and inviting?
- Did they encourage team members to continue talking by making small verbal comments such as "yes," "uh huh," and "go on"?

Deferring judgment

- Did they allow team members to finish what they had to say without interrupting with counterarguments?
- Did they seem to "park" their own thoughts so that they were fully present with the team member who was speaking?

Responding appropriately

- Were they candid, open, and honest in their responses to team members?
- Did they assert their opinions respectfully?
- Did they treat team members as they would want to be treated?[10]

In an atmosphere of openness, commitment, and reflective learning based on mutual respect and freedom of expression, the beginnings of a patient safety culture start to emerge.

Key Takeaways

- Adverse events are frequently the result of system failure rather than human error.
- When a near miss occurs, it should be reported so that action can be taken to make the system more robust.
- If the near miss is not reported, learning cannot occur.
- If learning doesn't occur, the next incident may push the system over the "boundary of acceptable performance" [60] which could result in dire consequences for the patient such as disablement or death.
- Clinical practices are enhanced and adverse events prevented when staff learn from observations of excellent clinical practices and leaders provide constructive feedback for performance improvement.
- Coaching is a developmental process that supports improved communication and daily dialog in teams, cooperation and collaboration in interdisciplinary teams, and respect for others and their social and cultural differences.

---

[10] Appendix 3.4. The reader may like to provide feedback to the leader on how 'present' they were during a debrief, whether they paid attention and showed that they were listening to team members' ideas/suggestions for improvement, deferred judgment and responded appropriately.

3.7 Case Study 3: Detailed Adverse Event

Rupika is a registrar working in a regional, emergency department in a low socio-economic area. Her night shift has been busy and a surge of patients arrive around 7 pm. The department is full. At this time of night, it is difficult to get the wards to take their admissions and processes can grind to a halt, making flow difficult in the emergency department. Jerry, a senior shift nurse, asks Rupika to order and sign an X-ray form for an older male who has presented with breathlessness. Rupika hasn't seen the man or assigned herself to his case. Jerry puts Rupika's name next to the patient on the system, so no one else picks up his case. The X-ray is carried out but Rupika is busy and doesn't realize that it has been performed. The nursing staff handover and change shifts, and around 10 pm the medical staff change shifts. At the medical handover, Rupika indicates that the man is still awaiting his X-ray, uncertain about his care and glosses over the case. A cardiac arrest comes in and takes all the night shift staff to resuscitate. The older man dies later that night, never being treated for his pneumonia or having his X-ray reviewed.

His death was recorded on a death certificate but the event (delay in treatment) was not recorded. Eventually, at the monthly morbidity and mortality meeting, the death review process picks up a significant delay in the man's treatment. It is discussed internally as an issue with handover in the emergency data, but the event is not recorded in the incident reporting system and the factors beyond handover are not considered.

This scenario highlights several critical issues in emergency department workflow, communication, and patient safety. Here are some points to consider for a detailed analysis:

(1) Breakdown in Processes:

- Responsibility for patients: Jerry assigned the patient to Rupika without her knowledge or consent, leading to a lack of clarity in patient responsibility.

(2) Communication Failures:

- Jerry did not effectively communicate the urgency or details of the patient's condition to Rupika.
- During the medical handover, Rupika did not provide complete and accurate information about the patient's status and care plan.
- The handover between shifts failed to adequately address and communicate the patient's needs and the status of his care.

(3) Systemic Issues:

- The emergency department was already under strain due to the surge in patients, making it difficult to manage workflow and patient care safely.
- There was no follow-up mechanism to ensure that critical diagnostics, such as the X-ray, were reviewed promptly.

For Discussion

(1) Discuss your understanding of the concept of the "boundary of acceptable performance."
   - What were the system failures in this case study?
(2) This study brings communication between colleagues and within teams into the spotlight.
   - What are the various methods by which communication can be enhanced between colleagues and within teams?
   - What happened in this case study, and what could have been done differently?
(3) How can clinical staff become more observant in their daily practices?
(4) What is the best way for leaders to provide feedback so that staff can learn?
(5) In what other ways can coaching support leaders and their teams to keep patients safe?

Appendices

Appendix 3.1: Survey of Factors Contributing to Adverse Events

To what extent do you believe that the following factors affect the likelihood of adverse events occurring in the team or department in which you predominantly work? Put an X in the relevant box and then make notes for improvement.

(1) Considerable improvement is needed.
(2) Needs some improvement.
(3) Average.
(4) Working well enough.
(5) Working very well.

#		1	2	3	4	5	Notes for improvement
1	Staff well-being						
2	Task appropriateness						
3	Education and training						
4	Team and social environment						
5	Patient partnerships						
6	Psychological safety						
7	Communication—dialog (within team)						
8	Relationships (within interdisciplinary teams)						
9	Social and cultural awareness						
10	Using strengths and appreciating diversity						

Appendix 3.2 Incident Reporting Form

The table below is adapted from the first portion of Table 2 in the WHO report, *Patient Safety Incidence Reporting System: a self-assessment* [4].

You can use this form to rate your current patient safety incident reporting system to assess its strengths against key points in the WHO report guidelines.

Section	Details	Rating				
		Strongly disagree	Disagree	Neither agree nor disagree	Agree	Strongly agree
Environment for reporting	It is easy for me to report an incident.					
	I have time to make a report.					
	I absolutely understand what needs to be reported.					
	I receive personalized feedback on the progress and action taken after I make a report.					
	I am motivated to report an incident.					
	Staff are encouraged to report incidents. It is rare that we are blamed. Disciplinary action is only taken if there has been serious misconduct.					
	Our leaders are committed to policies that establish a patient safety culture and their commitment is visible.					

(continued)

Section	Details	Rating				
		Strongly disagree	Disagree	Neither agree nor disagree	Agree	Strongly agree
Reporting rules and content	The criteria and definition for what constitutes a patient safety incident is clear.					
	The rules for what kinds of incident should be reported are clear.					
	Training on the purpose of reporting is provided.					
	We are trained in how to complete an incident report and what information to include.					
	We understood what kind of incident is voluntarily reported and which is mandatory (and the circumstances to report both).					
	As a minimum, the content of incident reports covers the elements of the MIM PS.					
	Incident reports capture both structured information and free text narrative commentary.					
	You can go back to the reporter to gather further information.					
	It is clear what types of incident can be analyzed by the hospital and what types nationally.					
	A rigorously constructed telephone hotline is in place for staff to report serious incidents that require immediate escalation and investigation, and actions to protect other patients.					
	There is a specific mechanism for patients and families to make reports.					

Appendix 3.3: Learning from Observations

Observe and record the interactions of a leader with their team during a clinical activity. The activity may be a regular daily occurrence, a preemptive attempt to avoid an incident, a debrief post-incident, or an examination of something that went *well.* Record your observations in relation to the following factors for feedback to the leader in a later coaching session.

#	Identify the factors involved in the clinical activity	Record your observations of the leader's interaction with their team during the activity
1	What's the context? Where did the activity take place (e.g., theatre, ward, office)?	
2	What's the content (type of activity, topic of discussion, e.g., review of patient obs)?	
3	Who was involved?	
4	What was the clinician doing? With what outcome?	
5	What happened then?	
6	What were the general feelings of the clinician and others as the activity unfolded and afterward?	
7	What was the impact of this activity on the clinician and others involved? (personal/professional, pre and post activity)	
8	What did team members learn from debriefing this activity?	
9	What improvements were noted for the future?	

Appendix 3.4: Feedback on Being "Present"

Observe a leader and how "present" they were during a debrief of a recent incident—whether they paid attention and showed that they were listening to team members' ideas/suggestions for improvement, deferred judgment, and responded appropriately. Tick the behaviors you observed and make comments as evidence to guide a later coaching session with the leader.

Behavior	Tick if observed	What did the leader do to demonstrate this behavior?
Remain "present"		
Did the leader focus on the team member and their story by being: ● Fully present—"in the moment"—reflecting on the content and their feelings ● Completely aware of the task at hand		

(continued)

Behavior	Tick if observed	What did the leader do to demonstrate this behavior?
Pay attention		
Did the leader give the team member their undivided attention and acknowledge their message? (Remember that nonverbal communication also "speaks" loudly). Did they: ● Look at the individual directly ● Put aside distracting thoughts and not mentally prepare a rebuttal ● Avoid being distracted by environmental factors ● "Listen" to the individual's body language ● Refrain from side conversations when listening in a group setting		
Show that you are listening		
Did the leader use their own body language and gestures to convey their attention? Did they: ● Nod occasionally ● Smile and use other facial expressions ● Note their posture and make sure it was open and inviting ● Encourage the individual to continue by making small verbal comments such as "yes" and "uh huh"		
Defer judgment		
Interrupting is a waste of time. It frustrates the individual and limits full understanding of the message. Did the leader: ● Allow the individual to finish speaking ● Not interrupt with counterarguments ● "Park" their own thoughts so they were fully "present" with the individual team member		
Respond appropriately		
Active listening is a model for respect and understanding. You are gaining information and perspective. You add nothing by attacking the individual or otherwise putting them down. Did the leader ● Provide feedback candidly, openly, and honestly in their responses ● Assert their opinions respectfully ● Treat the individual as they would want to be treated		

References

1. Hollnagel, E., Wears, R., & Braithwaite, J. (2015). *From safety-I to safety-II: A white paper*. University of Southern Denmark, University of Florida, Macquarie University.
2. de Vries, E. N., et al. (2008). The incidence and nature of in-hospital adverse events: A systematic review. *Quality & Safety in Health Care, 17*, 216–223.

3. Sauro, K. M., et al. (2021). The role of hospital characteristics in patient safety: A protocol for a national cohort study. *CMAJ Open, 9*(4), E1041–E1047.
4. WHO. (2020). *Patient safety incident reporting and learning systems: Technical report and guidance*. World Health Organization: Geneva: Licence: CC BY-NC-SA 3.0 IGO.
5. Ehsani, S. R., et al. (2013). Medication errors of nurses in the emergency department. *Journal of Medical Ethics, 6*(11).
6. Pham, J. C., et al. (2011). National study on the frequency, types, causes, and consequences of voluntarily reported emergency department medication errors. *Journal of Emergency Medicine, 40*(5), 485–492.
7. Wilson, R. M., et al. (1995). The quality in Australian health care study. *Medical Journal of Australia, 163*(9), 458–471.
8. Wilson, R. M., et al. (1995). The quality in Australian healthcare study. *Medical Journal of Australia, 163*, 458–471.
9. Wilson, R. M., et al. (1999). An analysis of the causes of adverse events from the quality in Australian healthcare study. *Medical Journal Australia, 170*, 411–415.
10. Vazin, A., Zamani, Z., & Hatam, N. (2014). Frequency of medication errors in an emergency department of a large teaching hospital in southern Iran. *Drug Health Patient Safety, 6*, 179–184.
11. WHO. (2014). *Regional Strategy on Patient Safety*. World Health Organization: Geneva SEA-HSD-371.
12. Aitken, M., & Gorokhovich, L. (2012). *Advancing the responsible use of medicines: Applying levers for change*. IMS Institute for Healthcare Informatics.
13. WHO. (2011). *Report on the burden of endemic health care-associated infection worldwide*. World Health Organization.
14. WHO. (2009). *Guidelines for safe surgery*. World Health Organization.
15. Jha, A. K., et al. (2013). The global burden of unsafe medical care: Analytic modelling of observational studies. *British Medical Journal of Quality and Safety, 22*, 809–815.
16. Singh, H., Meyer, A. N., & Thomas J, E. (2014). The frequency of diagnostic errors in outpatient care: Estimations from three large observational studies involving US adult populations. *British Medical Journal of Quality and Safety, 23*(9), 727–731.
17. WHO. (2010). *Clinical transfusion process and patient safety: Aide-mémoire for national health authorities and hospital management*. World Health Organization.
18. Janssen, M. P., & Rautmann, G. (2014). The collection, testing and use of blood and blood components in Europe. In *European Directorate for the Quality of Medicines and HealthCare (EDQM) of the Council of Europe*. Strasbourg.
19. Boadu, M., & Rehani, M. M. (2009). Unintended exposure in radiotherapy: Identification of prominent causes. *Radiotherapy and Oncology, 93*(3), 609–617.
20. Shafiq, J., et al. An international review of patient safety measures in radiotherapy practice. *Radiotherapy and Oncology, 92*, 15–21.
21. Fleischmann, C., et al. (2016). Assessment of global incidence and mortality of hospital-treated sepsis: Current estimates and limitations. *American Journal of Respiratory Critical Care Medicine, 193*(3), 259–272.
22. Raskob, E., et al. (2014). Thrombosis: A major contributor to global disease burden. *Thrombosis Research, 134*(5), 931–938.
23. WHO. (2020). *Patient safety assessment manual, Third Edition*. World Health Organization. Regional Office for the Eastern Mediterranean. License: CC BY-NC-SA 3.0 IGO.
24. Reason, J. (1997). *Managing the risks of organisational accidents*. Ashgate.
25. Reason, J. (2000). Human error: Models and management. *Education and Debate, 320*(7237), 768–770.
26. WHO. (2010). *Learning from error: Patient safety workshop*. World Health Organization.
27. WHO. (2020). *Health worker safety: A priority for patient safety*. World Health Organization.
28. Bakker, A. B., & Demerouti, E. (2001). The job demands-resources model of burnout. *Journal of Applied Psychology*.

29. Bakker, A. B., & Demerouti, E. (2007). The job demands-resources model: State of the art. *Journal of Managerial Psychology*.
30. Sturm, H., et al. (2019). *Do perceived working conditions and patient safety culture correlate with objective workload and patient outcomes: A cross-sectional explorative study from a German university hospital*. PLoS. OneWorkSafeMed Consortium.
31. Nahrgang, J. D., Morgeson, F. P., & Hofmann, D. A. (2011). Safety at work: A meta-analytic investigation of the link between job demands, job resources, burnout, engagement, and safety outcomes. *Journal of Applied Psychology*.
32. Seljemo, C., Viksveen, P., & Ree, E. (2020). The role of transformational leadership, job demands and job resources for patient safety culture in Norwegian nursing homes: A cross-sectional study. *BMC Health Services Research, 20*(1), 1–12.
33. Fisher, R., Brown, S., & Payne, R. (1989). *Getting together*. Business books.
34. Tenza, I. S., et al. (2022). Hospital managers' views on the state of patient safety culture across three regions in Ghana. *BMC Health Services Research, 22*(1), 1–14.
35. WHO. (2021). *Global Patient Safety Action Plan 2021–2030:Towards eliminating avoidable harm in health care*. World Health Organization, Licence: CC BY-NC-SA 3.0 IGO.
36. Arnetz, J. E., et al. (2019). Organizational determinants of bullying and work disengagement among hospital nurses. *Journal of Advanced Nursing, 75*(6), 1229–1238.
37. Draganović, Š., & Offermanns, G. (2022). Patient safety culture in Austria and recommendations of evidence-based instruments for improving patient safety. *PLoS One, 17*(10), 1–17.
38. Leape, L., et al. (2012). A culture of respect, part 1: The nature and causes of disrespectful behaviour by physicians. *Academic Medicine, 87*, 1–8.
39. Leape, L., et al. (2012). A culture of respect, part 2: Creating a culture of respect. *Academic Medicine, 87*, 853–858.
40. Davis, E., & Beale, N. (2015). It's time: The poor culture regarding safety and quality in Australian hospitals must be addressed! *Asia Pacific Journal of Health Management, 10*(3), GS36-GS41.
41. Hackman, J., & Oldham, G. (1980). *Work redesign*. Addison-Wesley Publ. Co.
42. Rosen, M., et al. (2018). *Teamwork in healthcare: Key discoveries enabling safer, high-quality care*. American Psychologist.
43. Manley, K., & Jackson, C. (2019). Microsystems culture change: A refined theory for developing person-centred, safe and effective workplaces based on strategies that embed a safety culture. *International Practice Development Journal, 9*(2), 1–21.
44. Kilpatrick, K., et al. (2020). Systematic review of the characteristics of brief team interventions to clarify roles and improve functioning in healthcare teams. *PLoS One, 15*(6), 1–28.
45. Pomey, M., et al. (2018). Development of patient-inclusive teams: Toward a structured methodology. *Healthcare Quarterly*.
46. Kilpatrick, K., et al. (2021). Patient and family views of team functioning in primary healthcare teams with nurse practitioners: A survey of patient-reported experience and outcomes. *BMC Family Practice, 22*(1), 1–14.
47. WHO. (2011). *Patient safety curriculum guide—Multi-professional Edition*. World Health Organization.
48. Mitchell, L., & Flin, R. (2008). Non-technical skills of the operating theatre scrub nurse: Literature review. *Journal of Advanced Nursing, 63*(1), 15–24.
49. Flin, R., & Maran, N. (2004). Identifying and training non-technical skills for teams in acute medicine. *Quality Safety Healthcare, 13*(suppl 1), i80–i84.
50. Yule, S., et al. (2006). Development of a rating system for surgeons' non-technical skills. *Medical Education, 40*, 1098–1104.
51. Yule, S., et al. (2015). Coaching non-technical skills improves surgical residents' performance in a simulated operating room. *Journal of Surgical Education, 72*(6), 1124–1130.
52. Hendricks, S., et al. (2018). Fostering interprofessional collaborative practice in acute care through an academic-practice partnership. *Journal of Interprofessional Care, 32*(5), 613–620.

53. Kara, A., et al. (2015). Redesigning inpatient care: Testing the effectiveness of an accountable care team model. *Journal of Hospital Medicine, 10*(12), 773–779.
54. Kim, C. S., et al. (2014). Unit-based interprofessional leadership models in six US hospitals. *Journal of Hospital Medicine, 9*(8), 545–550.
55. Broome, M. E., Everett, L. Q., & Wocial, L. (2014). Innovation through partnership: Building leadership capacity in academe and practice. *Nurse Leader, 12*(6), 91–94.
56. Turner, B. (1989). Accidents and nonrandom error propagation. *Risk Analysis, 9*(4), 437–444.
57. Roberts, K. (2015). Organizational errors: Catastrophic. In J. D. Wright (Ed.), *International encyclopedia of the social & behavioral sciences* (2nd ed., pp. 370–374). Elsevier.
58. Turner, B. (1978). *Man-made disasters*. Wykeham Press.
59. Turner, B., & Pidgeon, N. (1997). *Man-made disasters* (2nd ed.). Butterworth Heinemann.
60. Rasmussen, J. (1997). Risk management in a dynamic society: A modelling problem. *Safety Science, 27*(2/3), 183–213.
61. Cook, R., & Rasmussen, J. (2005). Going solid: A model of system dynamics and consequences for patient safety. *Quality Safety Health Care, 14*, 130–134.
62. de Vos, M. S., et al. (2019). Connecting perspectives on quality and safety: Patient-level linkage of incident, adverse event and complaint data. *BMJ Quality Safety, 28*(3), 180–189.
63. Schwendimann, R., et al. (2018). The occurrence, types, consequences and preventability of in-hospital adverse events—A scoping review. *BMC Health Services Research, 18*(1), 1–13.
64. Hibbert, P. D., et al. (2016). The application of the global trigger tool: A systematic review. *International Journal of Quality Health Care, 28*(6), 640–649.
65. Abuosi, A. A., et al. (2022). Safety culture and adverse event reporting in Ghanaian healthcare facilities: Implications for patient safety. *PLoS One, 17*(10), 1–18.
66. Aljaffary, A., et al. (2021). Patient safety culture in a teaching hospital in eastern province of Saudi Arabia: Assessment and opportunities for improvement. *Risk Management Healthcare Policy, 14*, 3783–3795.
67. Zabin, L. M., Zaitoun, R. S. A., & Abdullah, A. A. (2022). Patient safety culture in Palestine: University hospital nurses' perspectives. *BMC Nursing, 21*(1), 204.
68. Binkheder, S., et al. (2023). The relationships between patient safety culture and sentinel events among hospitals in Saudi Arabia: A national descriptive study. *BMC Health Services Research, 23*(1), 1–15.
69. Beyene Shashamo, B., et al. (2023). Patient safety culture and associated factors among nurses working at public hospitals in Gamo zone, Southern Ethiopia. *BMC Health Services Research, 23*(1), 1–12.
70. Garrouste-Orgeas, M., et al. (2012). Overview of medical errors and adverse events. *Annals of Intensive Care, 2*(1), 2.
71. Sinclair, J. E., et al. (2018). Barriers to self-reporting patient safety incidents by paramedics: A mixed methods study. *Prehospital Emergency Care, 22*(6), 762–772.
72. Chegini, Z., et al. (2020). The impact of patient safety culture and the leader coaching behaviour of nurses on the intention to report errors: A cross-sectional survey. *BMC Nursing, 19*(1).
73. Kim, M. Y., et al. (2014). Nurses' willingness to report near misses: A multilevel analysis of contributing factors. *Social Behavior Personal International Journal, 42*(7), 133–146.
74. Ali, H., et al. (2018). Baseline assessment of patient safety culture in public hospitals in Kuwait. *BMC Health Services Research, 18*(1), 158.
75. Ko, Y., & Yu, S. (2017). The relationships among perceived patients' safety culture, intention to report errors, and leader coaching behavior of nurses in Korea: A pilot study. *Journal of Patient Safety, 13*(3), 175–183.
76. Alahmadi, H. (2010). Assessment of patient safety culture in Saudi Arabian hospitals. *Quality Safety Health Care, 19*(5), e17.
77. El-Jardali, F., et al. (2010). The current state of patient safety culture in Lebanese hospitals: A study at baseline. *International Journal of Quality Health Care, 22*(5), 386–395.
78. Habibi, M., et al. (2017). Patient safety culture and factors that impact that culture in Tehran hospitals in 2013. *Iran Red Crescent Medical Journal, 19*(1), e30874.

79. Sarac, C., et al. (2011). Hospital survey on patient safety culture: Psychometric analysis on a Scottish sample. *BMJ Quality & Safety, 20*(10), 842–848.
80. Parand, A., Dopson, S., & Vincent, C. (2013). The role of chief executive officers in a quality improvement initiative: A qualitative study. *BMJ Open, 3*(1), e001731.
81. DuPree, E., et al. (2011). Professionalism: A necessary ingredient in a culture of safety. *Journal of Quality Patient Safety, 37*(10), 447–455.
82. Okuyama, A., Wagner, C., & Bijnen, B. (2014). Speaking up for patient safety by hospital-based health care professionals: A literature review. *BMC Health Services Research, 14*(1), 61.
83. Appelbaum, N. P., et al. (2016). The effects of power, leadership and psychological safety on resident event reporting. *Medical Education, 50*(3), 343–350.
84. Schön, D. (1994). *The Reflective Practitioner: How professionals think in action*. Routledge.
85. Argyris, C., & Schon, D. (1974). *Theory in practice: Increasing professional effectiveness*. Jossey-Bass.
86. Lee, M., Ong, Y. H., & Martimianakis, M. A. (2021). Understanding decision-making in interprofessional team meetings through interpretative repertoires and discursive devices. *Journal of Interprofessional Care, 35*(2), 164–174.
87. Wetherell, M., & Potter, J. (1992). *Mapping the language of racism: Discourse and the legitimation of exploitation*. Harvester Wheatsheaf and Columbia University Press.
88. Berger, J., & Mohr, J. (1997). *A fortunate man: The story of a country doctor*. Vintage International.
89. Shoham, D. A., et al. (2016). A network model of communication in an interprofessional team of healthcare professionals: A cross-sectional study of a burn unit. *Journal of Interprofessional Care, 30*(5), 661–667.
90. Hannemann-Weber, H., et al. (2011). Shared communication processes within healthcare teams for rare diseases and their influence on healthcare professionals' innovative behavior and patient satisfaction. *Implementation Science, 6*(1), 40–46.
91. Thomas, K. W., & Kilmann, R. H. (1974). *Thomas-Kilmann conflict mode instrument (TKI)*. [Database Record].
92. Somech, A. (2006). The effects of leadership style and team process on performance and innovation in functionally heterogeneous teams. *Journal of Management, 32*(1), 132–157.
93. van Knippenberg, D., de Dreu, C. K. W., & Homan, A. C. (2004). Work group diversity and group performance: An integrative model and research agenda. *Journal of Applied Psychology, 89*, 1008–1022.
94. Pickering, J. and E. Embry, So long, silos. The ASHA Leader, 2013. 18(6) 38–45.
95. Fernando, O., et al. (2016). Interprofessional communication between surgery trainees and nurses in the inpatient wards: Why time and space matter. *Journal of Interprofessional Care, 30*(5), 567–573.
96. Gurses, A. P., & Xiao, Y. (2006). A systematic review of the literature on multidisciplinary rounds to design information technology. *Journal of the American Medical Informatics Association, 13*(3), 267–276.
97. Verhaegh, K. J., et al. (2017). An exploratory study of healthcare professionals' perceptions of interprofessional communication and collaboration. *Journal of Interprofessional Care, 31*(3), 397–400.
98. Sharma, U., & Klocke, D. (2014). Attitudes of nursing staff toward interprofessional inpatient-centered rounding. *Journal of Interprofessional Care, 28*(5), 475–477.
99. Thomassen, O., et al. (2014). The effects of safety checklists in medicine: A systematic review. *Acta Anaesthesiologica Scandinavica, 58*(1), 5–18.
100. Gonzalo, J. D., et al. (2014). Patient-centered interprofessional collaborative care: Factors associated with bedside interprofessionalrounds. *Journal of General Internal Medicine, 29*(7), 1040–1047.
101. Ashcroft, S., et al. (2016). Interprofessional clinical rounding: Effects on process and outcomes of care. *Journal of Healthcare Quality, 39*(2), 85–94.

102. Adams, H. A. (2018). Implementation of a structured rounding tool for interprofessional care team rounds to improve communication and collaboration in patient care. *Pediatric Nursing, 44*(5), 229–246.
103. Brown, K., & Ryan, R. (2003). The benefits of being present: Mindfulness and its role in psychological well-being. *Journal of Personality and Social Psychology, 84*(4), 822–848.
104. Sheldon, K., & Vansteenkiste, M. (2005). Personal goals and time travel: How are future places visited, and is it worth it? In A. Strathman & J. Joreman (Eds.), *Understanding behavior in the context of time: Theory, research, and application* (pp. 143–163). Lawrence Erlbaum.
105. Hayes, S., Strosahl, K., & Wilson, K. (1999). *Acceptance and commitment therapy: An experiential approach to behavior change*. Guilford Press.
106. Brown, K., Ryan, R., & Creswell, J. (2007). Mindfulness: Theoretical foundations and evidence for its salutary effects. *Psychological Inquiry, 18*(4), 211–237.
107. Lutz, A., Dunne, J., & Davidson, R. (2007). Meditation and the neuroscience of consciousness: An introduction. In P. Zelazo, M. Moscovitch, & E. Thompson (Eds.), *The Cambridge handbook of consciousness* (pp. 497–549). Cambridge University Press.
108. Lutz, A., et al. (2008). Attention regulation and monitoring in meditation. *Trends in Cognitive Science, 12*, 163–169.
109. Vago, D., & Silbersweig, D. (2012). Self-awareness, self-regulation, and self-transcendence (S-ART): A framework for understanding the neurobiological mechanisms of mindfulness. *Front Human Neuroscience, 6*(296), 1–30.
110. Armson, H., et al. (2019). Identifying coaching skills to improve feedback use in postgraduate medical education. *Medical Education, 53*(5), 477–493.
111. Croft, A., et al. (2010). *Job-embedded professional development: What it is, who is responsible, and how to get it done well.* National Comprehensive Center for Teacher Quality.
112. Nolan, J., & Hoover, L. (2008). *Teacher supervision and evaluation: Theory into practice* (2nd ed.). John Wiley.
113. Barkley, S. (2005). *Quality teaching in a culture of coaching*. Scarecrow Education.
114. Costa, A., & Garmston, R. (2002). *Cognitive coaching: A foundation for renaissance schools* (2nd ed.). Christopher-Gordon Publishers, Inc.
115. Hemmeter, M., et al. (2011). Impact of performance feedback delivered via electronic mail on preschool teachers' use of descriptive praise. *Early Childhood Research Quarterly, 26*, 96–109.
116. Garbacz, S., et al. (2015). Strategies for effective classroom coaching. *Preventing School Failure, 59*(4), 263–273.
117. Kretlow, A., Wood, C., & Cooke, N. (2011). Using in-service and coaching to increase kindergarten teachers' accurate delivery of group instructional units. *The Journal of Special Education, 44*(4), 234–246.
118. Hartz-Mandell, K., & Umaschi, S. (2016). Classroom coaching for professional development in early care and education. *Brown University Child & Adolescent Behavior Letter, 32*(4), 1–7.
119. Kretlow, A., & Bartholomew, C. (2010). Using coaching to improve the fidelity of evidence-based practices: A review of studies. *Teacher Education and Special Education, 33*(4), 279–299.
120. Nichols, W., et al. (2006). What affects instructional choice? Profiles of K-2 teachers' use of reading instructional strategies and methods. *Journal of Literacy Research, 37*(4), 437–458.
121. Schnorr, C. (2013). *Effects of multilevel support on first-grade teachers' use of research-based strategies during beginning reading instruction, in unpublished doctoral dissertation.* University of North Carolina.
122. Freeman, J., et al. (2017). MTSS coaching: Bridging knowing to doing. *Theory Into Practice, 56*(1), 29–37.
123. Radick, L. E. (2022). Ready for what's next: Future-proofing the healthcare workforce. *Healthcare Executive, 37*(3), 16–24.

Chapter 4
Patient Safety Coaching in Healthcare

Coaching is a developmental, relational, and social process that motivates and supports coachees to solve their own problems and achieve their goals [1]. The coaching process helps individuals and teams gain greater self-awareness and insight into their current situation and guides them toward behavioral change, which leads to better outcomes. In a healthcare setting, coaching supports the utilization of strengths and learning from excellence, develops staff capability in nontechnical interpersonal skills, reduces stress, and promotes resilience and well-being. When adopted by all leaders and teams as a better way of behaving, communicating with, and relating to others, coaching leads to transformational cultural change [2]. Coaching of teams post-incident results in improved clinical practices that are utilized in the future. Coaching pre-emptively highlights learnings from observations and feedback as a result of exceptional clinical practice.

Traditional professional development activities typically include learning, implementation, feedback, and reflection [3]. However, professional development programs based on this approach are insufficient to ensure sustained learning and practice changes [4]. To better link attendance at professional development events with implementation in practice, *coaching* has been proposed as the necessary additional skillset needed by clinicians and executives to overcome obstacles and eliminate barriers so that improvements in clinical practice can be sustained [5, 6]. Contemporary professional development activities incorporate coaching as an essential component of the learning experience.

4.1 Coaching

Coaching is a bespoke form of development that places the learner at the center of the learning process [7–10]. It was developed from therapeutic approaches that focused on observing human behavior and changing ineffective or inappropriate

© The Author(s), under exclusive license to Springer Nature Switzerland AG 2024
S. Knowles, *Patient Safety Coaching*,
https://doi.org/10.1007/978-3-031-68722-8_4

behavior to condition new responses [11]. Cognitive therapeutic approaches have proposed that interpersonal difficulties are caused by habits and associated thoughts and feelings [12]. Coaching can change disruptive thoughts, beliefs, attitudes, and feelings by focusing on goal-oriented behaviors [13]. During coaching, coachees are encouraged to find their own solutions rather than blaming external forces [14]. When combined with elements of cognitive and rational-emotive behavioral therapy, solution-focused coaching is effective in building a greater depth of self-understanding and self-efficacy in coachees [15–17], reducing negative affect [18–20], and achieving goals [12, 21, 22].

Coaching is a pluralist process grounded in individual learning, personal mindsets, motivations, and self-efficacy. According to implicit person theory [23, 24], coachees with self-efficacy believe in their ability to learn, grow, and change as a result of their own effort and persistence [25, 26]. The coaching process integrates mindset theory, social learning theory, and work motivation theory with principles of self-efficacy to effect change and enhance an individual's ability to grow [23, 27, 28].

4.1.1 Coaching Process

As a dynamic, interactive, developmental process that promotes self-improvement [29], coaching focuses on assisting coachees achieve their life and work goals [30]. It is a particularly effective process for stimulating learning, creating new meanings, and changing behavior [31–35]. As coachees build trust in their own values, motives, thoughts, and feelings, they develop personally and professionally [36]. When the coach aligns the process to the coachees' targeted needs and situation [37–39], they reach their full potential and achieve meaningful, important goals [40]. The effectiveness of the coaching experience depends on a range of factors including the personality match between the coach and coachee [41, 42], the coach's empathic understanding and the quality of the coaching relationship [42, 43], and the coachee's self-efficacy and positive expectations [44–46]. The coachee is responsible for taking action, but both parties are accountable for obtaining results [47].

As a relational process aimed at supporting coachee growth and development [48, 49], coaching nonjudgmentally holds the coachee as the expert in their life with the necessary resources to address their own challenges [50, 51]. The working relationship that develops between coach and coachee is an equal partnership [52] with clear, mutually defined expectations [53]. A strong working relationship allows coaches to reveal candid and honest feedback on the coachee's performance and behavior [54]. A meta-analysis conducted by Graßmann, Schölmerich, and Schermuly [55] revealed a moderate and consistent correlation between a high-quality coach–coachee working relationship and cognitive and affective coaching outcomes such as staff well-being, self-efficacy, motivation, and work satisfaction. Self-awareness increases as the coaching relationship deepens [56–59], allowing the coachee to bring "tacit understandings to a level of conscious awareness" [60]. However, to create change, coaches may first need to challenge the coachee's mental model "through inquiry and an outside or etic perspective" [61] which shifts their thinking, thus allowing them to achieve a different outcome [23].

As a social process, coaching reshapes the coachee's social context by influencing power structures and individual agency [62]. Hence, coaching is either an "enabler of conformity or change ... [or] a process of control or resistance" [63]. Individuals learn through social interactions with other individuals, groups, and communities in their environment [64]. Sharing can have a profound impact on individuals and their relationships, leading to new perspectives and transformation [65].

Coaches use a variety of skills during coaching, such as active and reflective listening, powerful questioning, summarizing, and critical reflection, to build a trusting coach–coachee relationship that enhances responsibility and accountability [66]. At times, they may demonstrate a particular concept or skill [67]. The skill of the coach is to facilitate rather than prescribe outcomes [68]. Using coaching skills not only builds trust and alignment but also engages individuals both cognitively and emotionally. Coaching behaviors that "ask the right questions and model behaviors [that] workers can replicate are more productive than traditional 'tell me' feedback approaches" [69] because they establish expectations of the coachee's active involvement in, and responsibility for, achieving their desired outcomes from the coaching. Sustained change is achieved when coaching satisfies the coachee's needs for autonomy, relatedness, and competence [70].

During coaching, coaches invite critical self-reflection by the following means: focusing on a "disorienting dilemma" [47] for the coachee; recognizing the resulting discontent; exploring options for new roles, relationships, and actions; and supporting action. Transformative learning occurs when coaching brings about significant changes in coachees' fundamental beliefs about themselves [71], producing paradigm shifts that affect their subsequent thought processes and actions [72]—changes that are often more profound than the learning achieved by using single- or double-loop learning processes [73, 74].

Coachees who have not been coached before or who are reluctant participants in the coaching process may decide to start slowly and address a small issue first. Once resolved and trust is established, even a reluctant coachee usually decides to become fully involved in the coaching process thereafter. Actions that coachees take following the coaching session are reviewed at the beginning of each subsequent session until all their goals are achieved and the coaching program is completed.

4.1.2 *Differences Between Coaching and Mentoring*

Several factors distinguish coaching from other types of personal, developmental interventions: its dynamic and interactive qualities, its relational and social nature, and the coach's ability to first identify deep-seated issues and subsequently assist coachees' goal-set and action plan solutions. *Coaching* is often confused with *mentoring*, and research has shown that the two terms are frequently used interchangeably [75–80]. Both processes deepen the coachee's understanding of themselves and improve their personal and professional effectiveness [7, 81–83], but there are key differences in a number of areas. Principally, coaching is an "asking" process focused on promoting the coachee's agenda. The coach partners with the coachee as an equal and helps them achieve their desired outcomes. Mentoring is mainly a "telling" process in which the mentee seeks to extract wisdom and ideas for action from an often more-qualified, content expert. This definitional confusion between coaching and mentoring was noted in a literature review of the virtues of coaching for doctors and medical students [84]. The researchers found that the strongest evidence for coaching lies in the teaching of technical medical skills pertinent to a doctor's practice expertise but concluded that there is great scope for further studies to investigate the power of coaching as an important tool to enhance doctor/student well-being and nontechnical skills.

There is increasing consensus in the literature that the nontechnical aspects of healthcare delivery are responsible for a majority of adverse events in healthcare organizations rather than issues related to technical competence [85]. This finding has generated increased interest in the provision of nontechnical education and training for clinical and healthcare professionals alike. Within healthcare, where there is an imperative to get things *right* lest patients are harmed or die, coaching skills can be categorized as either process-oriented or content-oriented. Process-oriented coaching skills support communication, cooperation, and collaboration between individuals and within teams—the nontechnical skills. Content-oriented coaching skills support the development of clinical skills that enhance professional expertise—the technical skills. Contemporary solutions to professional development activities are most effective when technical skills training is coupled with process-oriented coaching—a Safety-11 approach [86].

4.1.3 Process-Oriented Coaching

Process-oriented coaching has been described as intangible in content or technical knowledge and difficult to assess [87]. Also known as nontechnical or "soft skills," they are instrumental in the delivery of successful coaching outcomes. Coaches use the skills of active and reflective listening, powerful questioning, and summarizing to assist coachees achieve their goals. Communication, collaboration, and cooperation are also nontechnical skills that individuals use every day in their interactions with others, which coaching can help develop.

The use of nontechnical skills contributes significantly to the creation of a trusting working relationship in which learning occurs and personal change results. Coaches position themselves as co-learners with coachees; they seek resolution based on constructive feedback and collaborative accountability. Coaching conversations are focused on the issue rather than the person; hence, they can be actioned in a dispassionate, realistic way. The coach enhances the coachee's personal growth by first focusing on developing their nontechnical skills before using content-oriented coaching to assist them develop professionally as they goal-set and action plan improvements in their clinical practice.

4.1.4 *Content-Oriented Coaching*

Content-oriented coaching is aligned with a competency-based, performance agenda such as required in a corporate or regulatory environment like healthcare. In occupations or professions where strict adherence to implementation guidelines is required (such as in medicine), content-oriented skills of observation, feedback, and correction are necessary. Researchers have investigated the difference between process- and content-oriented coaching skills in a medical education setting [88]. They discovered that in this workplace, supervisors used process skills in relation to preparation, relationship development, micro-communication skills, reflection, and self-assessment. They used content skills when providing feedback, goal setting, and development planning. The researchers noted the interconnectedness of the process- and content-oriented coaching skills and observed that, in prescriptive environments such as medical practice, there are tensions between encouraging self-direction on the one hand and progressing performance and competence on the other. They also noted difficulties in balancing the use of process versus content skills in the "partnership–teaching" relationship between the coach/supervisor and the medical residents.

4.1.5 *Role of the Coach and Coachee*

The coach and coachee play different roles in the coaching process. The coach challenges coachees' underlying beliefs, assumptions, and meaning perspectives and may question their fundamental value judgments and expectations [47, 73]. They express curiosity in relation to actions that do not serve coachees well and assist them in making more appropriate behavioral choices [1]. The coaching relationship is central to successful outcomes from the coaching experience. Initially, coaches seek to understand coachees' issues and objectives as they help them examine their situation with greater depth and clarity than they could do alone. Next, they stimulate recall from coachees to identify what they know about their situation and uncover what they do not know [32]. Insight is facilitated by improving coachees' "existing skills, competence and performance … personal effectiveness, personal development or personal growth" [78]. They may use role-playing, behavior modeling, and intensive feedback to release individual potential [89, 90]. Coaches believe that coachees have the necessary insights to solve their own problems [55] and discover better solutions [1, 91].

The coachee's role is to engage with the coach in open and honest communication to reveal their innermost thoughts, dreams, and fears for the future in the hope of generating new learning [92]. Using curiosity, encouragement, and joint accountability, coaches promote self-discovery as coachees reflect on and delve beneath the surface of each desire [59]. Coachees begin to acknowledge the part they have played in creating their current situation and start to take responsibility for it [93].

They identify the actions that will achieve their future goals, acknowledging that they may need to revisit these goals if circumstances change [15, 38, 94].

4.1.6 Coachee Readiness for Change

When coachees are ready for change, the coach helps them discover more effective ways of communicating with and relating to others so that they learn, and teams work better together. The principles that guide coaching as an experiential process [47, 73] are those that underpin adult learning interventions and change processes in the workplace [95–98]. Core andragogical principles [99] include the learner's need to know, self-directed learning, prior experiences of the learner, readiness to learn, orientation to learning and problem-solving, and motivation to learn [97, 100]. Coaches acknowledge coachees as independent learners with control of, and responsibility for, their own actions.

Coachees learn best when they relate the relevance of the issue to their life or work and when they feel valued, supported, and involved in the self-evaluation of their own learning [101]. Self-reflection, self-learning, and self-evaluation are particularly important in healthcare since staff frequently work in interdisciplinary teams that need to communicate effectively to achieve the best outcomes for patients. Coaching does not have to be conducted in formal, scheduled sessions; it can be conducted "on the go" as situations emerge that require shifting perspectives and generating alternate solutions.

4.1.7 Organizational Readiness for Change

Healthcare organizations will be at varying stages in their readiness to support the introduction of a coaching program depending on the degree to which executives understand the meaning of coaching. Executives who are unsure of what coaching is may be unwilling to allocate funding and resources, facilitate access to staff and data, and commit to program implementation. Leaders trained in patient safety coaching should expect to explain the benefits of coaching to a healthcare executive when they request to establish a coaching program and outline to them the expected outcomes.

4.2 Patient Safety Coaching

Patient safety coaching is the process of assisting healthcare leaders create a patient safety culture within their team and organization so that staff feel psychologically safe to pre-emptively raise issues or concerns in relation to patient care, learn from excellence and the lessons from adverse events, and ensure that staff well-being is constantly maintained, including after being involved in or witnessing an adverse event. In a clinical setting, coachees are provided with opportunities to be observed, obtain feedback, and reflect on their actions, to identify ways to improve patient safety. Through critical self-reflection based on Borton's [102] "what–so what–now what?" framework, team members are encouraged to become more self-aware and identify the changes they need to make in their clinical practice. When multisource observations and feedback data are available, these provide powerful stimuli to assist staff become more focused in their application of learning to enhance their personal effectiveness and professional performance [103].

In recent years, medical educators who seek to move away from purely competency-based assessment models of clinical performance have turned toward a more holistic, coaching approach to professional growth [104–106]. Medical residents' competence has been shown to increase when "disorienting dilemmas" [47] based on direct observation and feedback surfaced during coaching. Targeted professional development plans are then put in place as a result of learning from facilitated reflection on actions [103]. When opportunities for learning are available through both formal coaching sessions and informal coaching [107, 108], healthcare organizations are moving toward cultural change through coaching [109].

4.2.1 Purposes of Patient Safety Coaching

The coaching of individuals influences the degree to which they feel supported and empowered to grow and flourish. Hence, it is important to support the development of leaders who are willing to embrace all the technical and nontechnical skills required to assist team members improve patient safety. There are three main purposes for patient safety coaching in healthcare. The first is to increase leader capability so that leaders become more personally and professionally effective in guiding teams to improve patient safety (Chap. 5). The second is to maintain staff well-being so that clinical workers can provide the best possible patient care (Chap. 6). The third is to create a patient safety culture within their team and influence its development across the entire organization (Chaps. 7 and 8) (Fig. 4.1).

The first purpose of patient safety coaching is to develop *leader capability* so that leaders can prevent the occurrence of adverse events and keep patients safe from harm. Coaches show leaders how to use process-oriented coaching skills to encourage staff to raise issues or concerns regarding patient safety and to resolve communication and relational issues that are often experienced in workplaces. They show leaders how to use content-oriented coaching skills to become more observant and deliver constructive feedback to team members on their performance so they improve and so that everyone in the team learns from incidents and near misses, as well as from observations of excellent clinical practice. Overall, patient safety coaching supports leaders to: (i) become more self-and-other aware as they develop their emotional intelligence, (ii) adopt a coaching leadership style to lead and

Fig. 4.1 Purposes of patient safety coaching

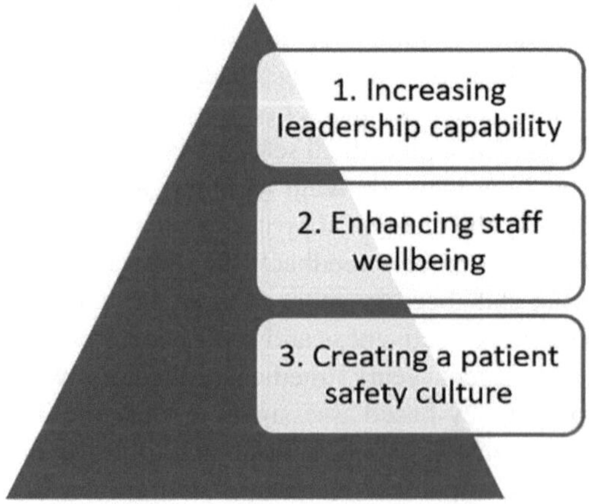

communicate more effectively and build trusting relationships within their team, and (iii) assist team members critically reflect on incidents and near misses so they learn from these mistakes, and (iv) speak up without fear to prevent further occurrences. This is a Safety-11 [86] response to reduce the incidence of adverse events in healthcare.

The second purpose of patient safety coaching is to enhance *staff well-being* and job satisfaction so that staff are fully "present" with patients and alert to their care needs. Patient safety coaching addresses the areas that cause staff stress in the workplace. Coachees determine which area for resolution they would like to work on first, which is usually the area that is most pressing or of most concern to them. Through coaching, coachees identify ways to relieve their stress and develop their ability to cope with future challenges. They gain insight into how to better manage their emotions and behaviors so that they can grow personally and professionally. Coaching helps them better communicate, learn how to prioritize tasks, and identify strategies to manage their workload. It provides a safe space for staff to share their thoughts and feelings without fear of judgment. By creating a supportive environment, leaders who deliver patient safety coaching can help healthcare workers better manage their stress and find more effective ways to cope with workplace issues and trauma.

The third purpose of patient safety coaching is to bring about *cultural change*. Patient safety coaching supports leaders in developing a patient safety culture within their team so that staff feel psychologically safe to bring forward omissions, errors, or potential failure points and learn from them. Leaders in a patient safety culture highlight good clinical practices they have observed and bring them to the team's attention so that everyone learns from these examples. Staff feel able to propose opportunities for their own personal growth and be heard. Team members develop professionally in an environment in which everyone willingly shares feedback in a positive, constructive manner. There is no blame, recrimination, bullying, or harassment in an environment that keeps everyone safe to do their job and improve their work practices. Patient safety coaching for cultural change enables team members to engage in self-reflection and self-evaluation, leading to improved performance and enhanced collaboration. This ensures that team members consistently apply safe care practices in their daily duties and are invested in the team's shared commitment to demonstrating safe behaviors in every setting.

4.2.2 Benefits of Patient Safety Coaching

Research findings have revealed the value of coaching as a major developmental process that promotes alternative perspectives and supports positive change [1, 110]. Patient safety coaching supports leaders in developing their leadership skills in the most appropriate ways to enable the engagement, commitment, and participation of team members in keeping patients safe and in contributing to the creation of a patient safety culture within frontline teams [110].

The first major benefit of coaching is that, when individuals are coached, they develop greater self-awareness and insight into who they are and the situation in which they find themselves. They realize that these circumstances are of their own making and hence, they have the power to change them. They just need the motivation and commitment to do so! This is where the support of a trusted partner coach comes to the fore. The coach is someone to whom they can turn to better understand how their thoughts and actions have created the problem or situation in which they find themselves. The coach helps them reframe their problem into a positively motivating goal to which they commit actions. As a goal-oriented, solution-focused developmental process, coaching provides individuals with the means to better transform their life and work.

A second major benefit of individual coaching, particularly in work settings, is that coachees learn how to better communicate with and relate to members of a team. In a complex working environment, healthcare workers may become stressed, which puts a strain on interpersonal relationships. When coached, individuals learn how to manage their stress so they can perform better as valued members of a clinical team. They re-engage with patients and colleagues and feel able to offer advice and support when requested by others. Consequently, the team performs *well* to keep patients safe since there is less disruption, conflict, absenteeism, and complaints.

In healthcare, individuals may become members of multiple teams depending on their professional expertise and patient needs. Learning to negotiate the compromises that are often necessary in multidisciplinary teams to ensure patient safety, and to remain flexible in responding to others, are skills that can be learned and nurtured through coaching. Coaching helps individuals develop these skills to reduce any negativity within the team, foster cooperation, and build collaboration as necessary. There is no doubt that there are multiple benefits when a number of healthcare professionals work *well* together to administer patient care in its many forms, such as when pharmacists work collaboratively with doctors and nurses in hospital settings [111].

A major organizational benefit of patient safety coaching is that as staff well-being improves, so does staff job satisfaction and staff retention.

4.3 Delivery of Patient Safety Coaching

Within the healthcare sector, patient safety coaching is an important supplementary intervention to the education provided by clinical and health coaches and an enabler of change in team-based care [112, 113]. In healthcare organizations, "coaching" is typically delivered as part of a leader's role or by specialists who are directly responsible for educational activities and professional development. Experienced and highly competent individuals in these positions have clinical expertise in a range of disciplines. They may have titles such as clinical nurse, nurse educator, or nurse practitioner. Individuals in these roles educate and provide practical support to staff who deliver safe, high-quality patient care in their specialist area. At the point of care, they assist staff in anticipating and proactively responding to emerging issues, particularly when complex practice situations change unexpectedly. To estimate the extent to which clinical coaches are accessed, a research study surveyed registered nurses about their experiences intervening in a number of clinical situations involving errors in dispensing medication, clinical procedures, documentation, assessment skills, and clinical handover [114]. The results revealed that clinical coaches intervened with both junior and senior staff with varying skill levels on average of 3–4 h per day in this role, depending on patient acuity. The researchers concluded by affirming the value of the supportive, education services provided by clinical coaches.

In the private sector and community settings, clinical coaches provide primary care and use interpersonal skills to focus patients on managing their disease and preventing health risks [111]. Their role is to ensure that patients are educated about their health, guided toward setting realistic health goals, and expect realistic outcomes [115, 116]. For example, clinical coaches may support patients with chronic conditions such as hypertension, diabetes, and asthma who can be treated in the community, thus considerably reducing the need for hospital infrastructure and resources and for specialist medical staff and services [117]. Research has shown that the education, regular monitoring, and follow-up of patients with chronic health conditions by clinical and health coaches results in a considerable improvement in outcomes for patients who learn to manage their conditions in the long term [118]. Moreover, it has been proposed that the inclusion of multidisciplinary healthcare professionals in the healthcare system improves clinic wait times and reduces unnecessary costs to public health insurance schemes such as Medicare [119].

4.3.1 Patient Safety Coaching Process

When healthcare leaders are formally trained by the *Australian Institute of Professional Coaches*[1] to deliver *coaching* to individuals and teams in an organization, they follow the positive psychology ©AIPC COACH Model to assist coachees discover solutions to their problems and achieve their goals [1] (Fig. 4.2).

The first step in the model is to identify the *Critical issue* that the coachee needs to address. This issue may relate to a problem they are experiencing or a goal they have tried to attain but were unsuccessful in achieving on their own. The second step is to identify the *Opportunities* that are available to them once the problem has been resolved or the goal achieved. The opportunity is often the reverse of the problem and represents the ideal situation that the coachee would like to find themselves in long term into the future. The third step is to identify the *Actionable goals* the coachee wants to achieve and how they will do this. The fourth step is *Commitment.* What is the coachee's level of commitment to taking the actions they have decided to take? While the coachee is responsible for taking action, the final step is to identify how the coach and coachee will *Hold* each other *accountable* for achieving the outcomes of the coaching program. By implementing these five steps in the ©AIPC COACH Model, the coach helps coachees become more self-aware, responsible, and committed to solving their own problems and achieving their goals.

Specifically, during *patient safety coaching*, the coach works with coachees to find ways to:

- Increase their leadership capability
- Enhance staff well-being
- Develop a patient safety culture within their team or organization (Fig. 4.1)

One of the first skills that leaders develop during coaching is the ability to become more observant so that they and team members can prevent adverse events from occurring while also learning from examples of clinical excellence. Coaching

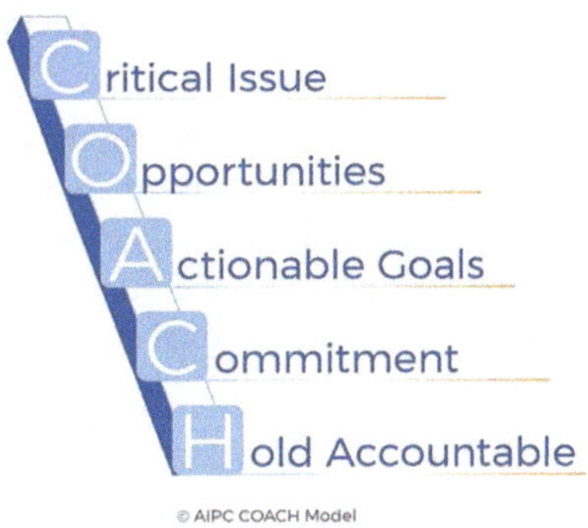

Fig. 4.2 The ©AIPC COACH Model [1]

[1] www.professionalcoachtraining.com.au

also assists leaders provide open, honest, and constructive feedback to staff to improve their clinical performance.

4.3.1.1 "Coachable" Moments

Leaders who deliver patient safety coaching support team members in becoming more observant during a clinical activity. Observations of practice are best conducted routinely as team members go about their daily duties. A "coachable moment" [107] is sought thereafter to provide constructive feedback and extend the individual's learning. When an adverse event occurs, a debrief is undertaken as soon as possible to identify how the leader and team members responded (or reacted) to the event. The debrief may occur immediately or at a later date when emotions have subsided—but in the not-too-distant future. In the debrief, the team critically reflects on the adverse event to identify what they can learn from it. Is formal coaching required to debrief the trauma associated with the event? What improvements in processes, resources, or systems are needed? What barriers need to be overcome? Similarly, when a good catch has been observed, the leader uses coaching skills to facilitate discussion on what occurred to achieve a positive outcome so that team members can repeat the behavior or adapt it to other situations.[2]

Coaching of the individual or team continues as "coachable moments" are identified on a daily basis. Team members are encouraged to continue to be observant, and the leader continues to arrange opportunities for self-reflection and learning for both themselves and team members. If the leader has participated in a formal coaching program, it is recommended that "refresher" coaching sessions be conducted every few months, even if there have been no incidents in the intervening period. This keeps the need for observation, identification of excellent clinical practice, self-reflection and learning, front-of-mind for leaders and reinforces the good work they are doing.

4.3.2 Formal Training in Patient Safety Coaching

Clinical and health coaches in the healthcare industry are often registered nurses or doctors with many years of experience in patient care, but they are not usually trained as professional coaches according to international standards, as regulated by professional associations such as the *International Coaching Federation* (ICF). Training to an international standard is important for supporting individuals who are traumatized or dealing with personal issues, and for teams who struggle with internal, interdisciplinary, or multidisciplinary issues that impact patient safety and

[2] How leaders can become more observant and provide constructive feedback is fully discussed in Chap. 3.

quality care. Similarly, a healthcare executive with a risk management or governance responsibility may not understand the full benefits that coaching can bring to the organization if they have not undertaken formal coach training.

When clinical coaches are formally trained in patient safety coaching, they add to their skillset and are better able to assist leaders work more effectively with their team and learn from excellent clinical practices. They assist leaders in preventing adverse events by instigating preemptive safety practices such as addressing team issues as they arise and creating a patient safety culture (a Safety-11 strategy [86]). Clinical coaches or leaders who deliver patient safety coaching strengthen their leadership capability when they use their nontechnical coaching skills on an ongoing basis to promote excellent clinical practice so that fewer adverse events occur [114].

Individuals and teams benefit from receiving patient safety coaching from a coach who:

- Is formally qualified, experienced, and trained in human behavior or psychology and uses a comprehensive coaching methodology that takes into account more than just a formulaic, goal-setting, and action planning approach.
- Possesses a genuine coaching mindset and a coaching philosophy that respects the individual and what they have done to resolve their situation, aiming to unleash the potential of all workers.
- Displays by their behavior a combination of personal resilience and systems awareness that is underpinned by their relatively advanced level of socioemotional and cognitive maturity.
- Engages in continuous learning and invests in their own personal growth and development, e.g., by being supervised, as they embrace this new aspect of their role.
- Acts as a role model for leaders and team members who learn how to conduct informal coaching conversations with others. In doing so, they contribute to the development of a patient safety culture within teams that can have positive systemic ramifications into other areas of the healthcare organization.

4.3.3 Informal Coaching

In addition to formal coaching sessions being conducted within healthcare organizations by formally qualified coaches to improve patient safety and staff well-being, informal coaching may also be conducted by leaders to assist staff become more effective in their role. Informal coaching approaches include coaching conversations and corridor conversations, which help team members achieve immediate resolution of their issue or concern. The leader models coach-like behaviors and, as time passes, team members start to emulate these informal coaching methods and behaviors and become role models to peers themselves [49, 120, 121].

4.3.3.1 Coaching Conversations

Coaching conversations are a form of coaching in which the person acting as "coach" uses coach-like behavior and coaching language to explore what is happening, often in relation to a problem that is getting in the way of the coachee's performance. Using active listening, the coach elicits their story and helps them pinpoint their concerns with greater clarity. At times, the simple act of listening unconditionally, without interruption, is enough to give the coachee insight into what they need to do next. The conversation may take just 15–20 min—enough time and headspace for the coachee to distance themself from their dilemma and view their situation objectively—because it is only when emotions have subsided that an individual can start to think rationally and problem-solve. The conversation continues as the coach asks the coachee what they think they need to do next and what assistance or support they need. The coachee is motivated to take action now that they can see a way ahead and are energized to achieve a particular goal [122]. Goal-directed activity serves not only to improve individual performance but also to increase the overall outcomes of the team. Coaching conversations can occur at any level of the organization, aimed at driving clinical practice forward toward improved quality patient care and staff well-being.

Leaders who are coached, especially if they are trained in coaching skills, can use their nontechnical coaching ability to engage their direct reports in coaching conversations as and when needed, initiated either by themselves or their team member. The focus of coaching conversations is driven by the coachee and can cover a range of topics—except when the issue is serious and requires a more in-depth, formal coaching session to be conducted by a qualified coach. Coaching conversations aim to assist team members in finding an immediate solution to a problem or providing direction in terms of, say, a particular resource. After each conversation, the team member feels that the leader has heard what is on their mind, asks constructive questions, and helps them discover the solution by themself.

4.3.3.2 Corridor Conversations

Corridor conversations are those conducted "on-the-run" as staff go about their daily duties. They are mostly peer-to-peer conversations that can occur at any time of day or night when a situation arises in which a staff member needs support, advice, or information. The conversation may take just a few minutes—in the hallway, by a patient's bed, at the nurses' station. The most effective corridor conversations are those in which the "coach" uses active listening and powerful questioning to elicit from the "coachee" what they already know and think they should do. These conversations are often confirmatory rather than exploratory. When a situation arises and the staff member is unsure of what to do next—although they think they know—they just want to confirm that next step or gather new information from another who may have a different perspective. Once confirmed, they are confident that they are doing the right thing by the patient and will not cause any harm, or they have another treatment option to consider that may be more effective. Corridor conversations typically occur informally multiple times during a shift, as staff members endeavor to deliver the best possible quality patient care.

Key Takeaways

- Coaching is a developmental, relational, and social process that promotes self-awareness and insight from reflection on clinical practice.
- As a nontechnical skill, coaching supports healthcare staff to communicate more meaningfully with patients and develop better relationships with others.
- Coaching skills are both process-oriented to improve interactions with colleagues and content-oriented to support technical improvements in clinical practice.
- Coaching can be conducted in formal, scheduled sessions by leaders or clinical coaches trained to international standards.
- Informal *coaching conversations* are conducted as the need arises to assist a staff member resolve a patient concern so they know what to do next. "On-the-run" *corridor conversations* can take just a few minutes to get staff members back on track.

4.4 Case Study 4: Learning from Excellence

As the new emergency department registrar, Jean, enters the resuscitation bay, he is immediately struck by the calm and collaborative atmosphere. The team is already in full swing, responding to a triage Category 1 cardiac arrest with precision and focus. Nurses are efficiently preparing medications and equipment according to protocol, while the senior doctors lead the resuscitation efforts with confidence. Everyone seems to have a place and they all look to each other as if they each know what to expect next.

Despite the high-stress situation, there is a sense of unity among the team members. Everyone knows their role and performs it with precision, communicating effectively and respectfully with each other. The registrar, who is used to more chaotic and less organized team environments, is impressed by the level of professionalism and teamwork displayed by his new colleagues. He immediately feels safe and relaxed and is able to notice things he otherwise would not.

He quickly joins in, seamlessly integrating into the team and contributing to the resuscitation efforts. As the minutes tick by, despite the patient's condition not stabilizing, the senior doctor in charge of the resuscitation calls out her overview of the arrest and asks for input from the team. Jean realizes that he has a lot to learn from his new team and looks forward to working with them in the future.

In this scenario, the use of protocols and effective communication techniques such as reflection and repetition play a crucial role in improving the way the case is handled to eliminate all reversible causes of cardiac arrest.

Later that evening, Jean shares his sense of wonder from this experience with his partner at home and describes the following key success factors:

(1) *Protocols:* The team followed their established protocol for managing cardiac arrest, ensuring that no critical steps were missed and that interventions were carried out in a systematic manner. This helped to identify and address reversible causes promptly and kept everything in order, with greater clarity and comfort for the team.
(2) *Effective Communication*: Throughout the resuscitation process, team members engaged in repetitive call-out practices, where they repeated key steps aloud to share with the team what had been completed. This not only aided the scribe in documenting progress but also signaled to the team which part of the protocol they were up to. There was also a built-in pause to review the progress of the resuscitation and consider alternative approaches if needed. This allowed for a more thoughtful and effective response.
(3) *Training and Experience*: Jean wonders how much of the team's ability to handle the case effectively is also influenced by their training and experience. He reflects that regular training sessions and simulations help staff familiarize themselves with protocols and improve their communication skills, leading to better outcomes in real-life scenarios.

For Discussion

(1) What is your understanding of coaching, and how could it be conducted in healthcare?
    - What was done *well* in this case study and what could have been done differently?
(2) When would you use process-oriented coaching with staff? Content-oriented?
    - What conclusions can be drawn from this case study?
(3) Discuss the purpose of patient safety coaching in healthcare. What are the benefits?
    - What was the purpose of this case study, and how can improvements to your clinical practice be made?
(4) Is there a place for informal coaching in healthcare?
    - Provide examples.

References

1. Knowles, S. (2021). *Positive psychology Coaching*. Springer Nature.
2. Knowles, S. (2022). *Coaching culture*. Springer Nature.
3. Snow, C., Griffin, P., & Burns, M. (2005). *Knowledge to support the teaching of reading: Preparing teachers for a changing world*. Jossey-Bass.
4. Fixsen, D., et al. (2005). *Implementation research: A synthesis of the literature*. The National Implementation Research Network.
5. Adelman, H., & Taylor, L. (2007). Systemic change for school improvement. *Journal of Educational and Psychological Consultation, 17*, 55–77.
6. Lewis, T., & Newcomer, L. (2002). Examining the efficacy of school-based consultation: Recommendations for improving outcomes. *Child & Family Behavior Therapy, 24*, 165–181.
7. Bozer, G., & Jones, R. (2018). Understanding the factors that determine workplace coaching effectiveness: A systematic literature review. *European Journal of Work and Organizational Psychology, 27*(3), 342–361.
8. Hunt, J., & Weintraub, J. (2004). Learning developmental coaching. *Journal of Management Education, 28*(1), 39–61.
9. Kim, S., et al. (2013). The impact of managerial coaching behavior on employee work-related reactions. *Journal of Business and Psychology, 28*(3), 315–330.
10. Theeboom, T., Beersma, B., & van Vianen, A. (2014). Does coaching work? A meta-analysis on the effects of coaching on individual level outcomes in an organizational context. *The Journal of Positive Psychology, 9*(1), 1–18.
11. Skinner, B. (1938). *The behaviour of organisms: An experimental analysis*. Appleton-Century.
12. Beck, A. (1976). *Cognitive therapy and the emotional disorders*. International Universities Press.
13. Locke, E., & Latham, G. (2002). Building a practically useful theory of goal setting and task motivation: A 35-year odyssey. *American Psychologist, 57*(9), 705–717.
14. Neenan, M. (2008). From cognitive behaviour therapy (CBT) to cognitive behaviour coaching (CBC). *Journal of Rational-Emotive & Cognitive-Behavior Therapy, 26*(1), 3–15.
15. Ives, Y., & Cox, E. (2012). *Goal-focused coaching: Theory and practice*. Routledge.
16. O'Connell, B., Palmer, S., & Williams, H. (2013). *Solution-focused coaching in practice*. Taylor and Francis.
17. Roeden, J., Maaskant, M., & Curfs, L. (2012). The nominal group technique as an evaluation tool for solution-focused coaching. *Journal of Applied Research in Intellectual Disabilities, 25*(6), 588–593.
18. Nagel, R. (2008). Coaching with a solutions focus—Focusing on the solution not the problem. *Development and Learning in Organizations: An International Journal, 22*(4), 11–14.
19. Grant, A., et al. (2012). Development and validation of the solution-focused inventory. *The Journal of Positive Psychology, 7*(4), 334–348.
20. Wakefield, M. (2006). New views on leadership coaching. *The Journal for Quality and Participation, 29*(2), 9–43.
21. Ellis, A. (1962). *Reason and emotion in psychotherapy*. Lyle Stuart.
22. Grant, A., & O'Connor, S. (2018). Broadening and building solution-focused coaching: Feeling good is not enough. *Coaching: An International Journal of Theory, Research and Practice, 11*(2), 165–185.
23. Dweck, C. (2012). Mindsets and human nature: Promoting change in the Middle East, the schoolyard, the racial divide, and willpower. *American Psychologist, 67*(8), 614–622.
24. Dweck, C. (2014). Teachers' mindsets: "Every student has something to teach me". *Educational Horizons, 93*(2), 10–15.
25. Dweck, C., Chiu, C., & Hong, Y. (1995). Implicit theories: Elaboration and extension of the model. *Psychological Inquiry, 6*(4), 322–333.
26. Molden, D., & Dweck, C. (2006). Finding "meaning" in psychology: A lay theories approach to self-regulation, social perception, and social development. *American Psychologist, 61*(3), 192–203.

27. Bandura, A. (1977). Self-efficacy: Toward a unifying theory of behavioral change. *Psychological Review, 84*, 191–215.
28. Latham, G., & Pinder, C. (2005). Work motivation theory and research at the dawn of the twenty-first century. *Annual Review of Psychology, 56*, 485–516.
29. Kersten-van Dijk, E., et al. (2017). Personal informatics, self-insight, and behavior change: A critical review of current literature. *Human-Computer Interaction, 32*(5/6), 268–296.
30. Megginson, D. (2014). Goal-focused coaching: Theory and practice. *Action Learning: Research and Practice, 11*(2), 243–245.
31. Wilson, C. (2011). Developing a coaching culture. *Industrial and Commercial Training, 43*(7), 407–414.
32. Celoria, D., & Hemphill, D. (2014). Coaching from the coaches' perspective: A process-oriented focus. *International Journal of Mentoring and Coaching in Education, 3*(1), 72–85.
33. de Souza, R., & Brunstein, J. (2018). Critical reflection in the workplace and management competencies: In service of transformation? *Australian Journal of Adult Learning, 58*(2), 266–291.
34. Chatterjee, A., Pereira, A., & Bates, R. (2018). Impact of individual perception of organizational culture on the learning transfer environment. *International Journal of Training & Development, 22*(1), 15–33.
35. Nicolaidou, M., Karagiorgi, Y., & Petridou, A. (2018). Professional learning through reflection promoted by feedback and coaching (PROFLEC) in Cyprus. *International Journal of Leadership in Education, 21*(4), 412–426.
36. Grant, A. (2001). *Towards a psychology of coaching, in department of psychology*. Macqualrie University.
37. McDermott, I., & Jago, W. (2005). *The coaching bible*. Piatkus Books.
38. Stober, D., & Grant, A. (2006). *Evidence based coaching handbook: Putting best practices to work for your clients*. John Wiley & Sons.
39. Downey, M. (2003). *Effective coaching: Lessons from the coaches' couch*. Texere/Thomson.
40. Rosinski, P. (2003). Coaching across cultures. *The International Journal of Coaching in Organizations, 1*(4), 99–106.
41. Bozer, G., Joo, B., & Santora, J. (2015). Executive coaching: Does coach-coachee matching based on similarity really matter? *Consulting Psychology Journal: Practice and Research, 67*(3), 218–233.
42. Boyce, L., Jackson, R., & Neal, L. (2010). Building successful leadership coaching relationships: Examining impact of matching criteria in a leadership coaching program. *Journal of Management Development, 29*(10), 914–931.
43. Kim, S., & Kuo, M.-H. (2015). Examining the relationships among coaching, trustworthiness, and role behaviors: A social exchange perspective. *The Journal of Applied Behavioral Science, 51*(2), 152–176.
44. de Haan, E., Culpin, V., & Curd, J. (2011). Executive coaching in practice: What determines helpfulness for clients of coaching? *Personnel Review, 40*(1), 24–44.
45. de Haan, E., et al. (2013). Executive coaching outcome research: The contribution of common factors such as relationship, personality match, and self efficacy. *Consulting Psychology Journal, 65*(1), 40–57.
46. de Haan, E., et al. (2016). A large-scale study of executive coaching outcome: The relative contributions of relationship, personality match, and self-efficacy. *Consulting Psychology Journal: Practice and Research, 68*(3), 189–207.
47. Gray, D. (2006). Executive coaching: Towards a dynamic alliance of psychotherapy and transformative learning processes. *Management Learning, 37*(4), 475–497.
48. Parker, P., Hall, D., & Kram, K. (2008). Peer coaching: A relational process for accelerating career learning. *Academy of Management Learning & Education, 7*(4), 487–503.
49. Parker, P., et al. (2015). A relational communication approach to peer coaching. *The Journal of Applied Behavioral Science, 51*(2), 231–252.

50. Baron, L., & Morin, L. (2009). The coach-coachee relationship in executive coaching: A field study. *Human Resource Development Quarterly, 20*(1), 85–106.
51. Swift, J., & Parkin, S. (2017). The client as the expert in psychotherapy: What clinicians and researchers can learn about treatment processes and outcomes from psychotherapy clients. *Journal of Clinical Psychology, 73*(11), 1486–1488.
52. Bozer, G., Sarros, J., & Santora, J. (2013). The role of coachee characteristics in executive coaching for effective sustainability. *Journal of Management Development, 32*(3), 277–294.
53. Silsbee, D. (2004). *The mindful coach: Seven roles for helping people grow*. Ivy River Press.
54. Sherman, S., & Freas, A. (2004). The wild west of executive coaching. *Harvard Business Review, 82*(11), 82–90.
55. Graßmann, C., Schölmerich, F., & Schermuly, C. (2019). The relationship between working alliance and client outcomes in coaching: A meta-analysis. *Human Relations, 73*(1), 35–58.
56. Lawrence, E., Dunn, M., & Suri, W.-S. (2018). Developing leadership potential in graduate students with assessment, self-awareness, reflection and coaching. *The Journal of Management Development, 37*(8), 634–651.
57. Orton, T. (2015). *Leadership self-awareness development through the amelioration of fear-based thoughts: An eastern perspective* (p. 312). Gonzaga University.
58. Axelrod, S. (2012). Self-awareness: At the interface of executive development and psychoanalytic therapy. *Psychoanalytic Inquiry, 32*(4), 340–357.
59. Hadin, K., & Steinwedel, J. (2006). Developing global leaders: Executive coaching targets cross-cultural competencies. In *Global business and organizational excellence*. Wiley Periodicals Inc.
60. Bond, C., & Seneque, M. (2012). Conceptualizing coaching as an approach to management and organizational development. *Journal of Management Development, 32*(1), 57–72.
61. Offstein, E., et al. (2013). Rebuilding reliability: Strategy and coaching in a high hazard industry. *Journal of Organizational Change Management, 26*(3), 529–555.
62. Cushion, C., & Partington, M. (2016). A critical analysis of the conceptualisation of 'coaching philosophy'. *Sport, Education and Society, 21*(6), 851–867.
63. Shoukry, H., & Cox, E. (2018). Coaching as a social process. *Management Learning, 49*(4), 413–428.
64. Kurland, H., & Hasson-Gilad, D. (2015). Organizational learning and extra effort: The mediating effect of job satisfaction. *Teaching and Teacher Education, 49*, 56–67.
65. Glăveanu, V. (2011). Children and creativity: A most (un)likely pair? *Thinking Skills and Creativity, 6*(2), 122–131.
66. Bommelje, R. (2015). Managerial coaching. *New Directions for Adult and Continuing Education, 2015*(148), 69–77.
67. Crawford, A., et al. (2017). Integrating professional development content and formative assessment with the coaching process: The Texas school ready model. *Theory Into Practice, 56*(1), 56–65.
68. Lam, P. (2016). Chinese culture and coaching in Hong Kong. *International Journal of Evidence Based Coaching & Mentoring, 14*(1), 57–73.
69. Pulakos, E., et al. (2015). Performance management can be fixed: An on-the-job experiential learning approach for complex behavior change. *Industrial and Organizational Psychology, 8*(1), 51–76.
70. Taylor, S., Passarelli, A., & Van Oosten, E. (2019). Leadership coach effectiveness as fostering self-determined, sustained change. *The Leadership Quarterly*, 1013.
71. Mezirow, J. (1997). Transformative learning: Theory to practice. *New Directions for Adult and Continuing Education, 1997*(74), 5–12.
72. Clark, M. (1993). In S. Merriam (Ed.), *Transformational learning, in new directions for adult and continuing education: No. 57 an update on adult learning theory* (pp. 47–56). Jossey-Bass.
73. Cox, E. (2015). Coaching and adult learning: Theory and practice. *New Directions for Adult and Continuing Education, 148*, 27–38.

74. Argyris, C. (2002). Double-loop learning, teaching, and research. *Academy of Management Learning & Education, 1*(2), 206–218.
75. Cleary, M., & Horsfall, J. (2015). Coaching: Comparisons with mentoring. *Issues in Mental Health Nursing, 36*(3), 243–245.
76. Hackman, J., & Wageman, R. (2005). A theory of team coaching. *The Academy of Management Review, 30*(2), 269–287.
77. Cowan, K. (2013). What are the experiences of external executive coaches working with coaches'assigned goals? *International Journal of Evidence Based Coaching and Mentoring, 7*, 1–14.
78. Hamlin, R., Ellinger, A. D., & Beattie, R. (2008). The emergent 'coaching industry': A wake-up call for HRD professionals. *Human Resource Development International, 11*(3), 287–305.
79. Thompson, R., Wolf, D. M., & Sabatine, J. (2012). Mentoring and coaching: A model guiding professional nurses to executive success. *Journal of Nursing Administration, 42*(11), 536.
80. Werner-Washburne, M. (2018). Principles of intentional mentoring. *CBE Life Sciences Education, 17*(3).
81. Hamlin, R., Ellinger, A. D., & Beattie, R. (2006). Coaching at the heart of managerial effectiveness: A cross-cultural study of managerial behaviours. *Human Resource Development International, 9*(3), 305–331.
82. Kim, S. (2014). Assessing the influence of managerial coaching on employee outcomes. *Human Resource Development Quarterly, 25*(1), 59–85.
83. Egan, T., & Hamlin, R. (2014). Coaching, HRD, and relational richness: Putting the pieces together. *Advances in Developing Human Resources, 16*(2), 242–257.
84. Lovell, B. (2018). What do we know about coaching in medical education? A literature review. *Medical Education, 52*(4), 376–390.
85. Davis, E., & Beale, N. (2015). It's time: The poor culture regarding safety and quality in Australian hospitals must be addressed! *Asia Pacific Journal of Health Management, 10*(3), GS36-GS41.
86. Hollnagel, E., Wears, R., & Braithwaite, J. (2015). *From safety-I to safety-II: A white paper*. University of Southern Denmark, University of Florida, USA, and Macquarie University.
87. Bates, C., & Morgan, D. (2018). Literacy leadership: The importance of soft skills. *Reading Teacher, 72*(3), 412–415.
88. Armson, H., et al. (2019). Identifying coaching skills to improve feedback use in postgraduate medical education. *Medical Education, 53*(5), 477–493.
89. De Meuse, K., Dai, G., & Lee, R. (2009). Evaluating the effectiveness of executive coaching: Beyond ROI? *Coaching: An International Journal of Theory, Research and Practice, 2*(2), 117–134.
90. Trathen, S. (2011). Executive coaching: Implications for developing leaders in the Middle East and Africa. *Career Planning and Adult Development Journal, 27*(1), 138–154.
91. Hicks, R., & McCracken, J. (2010). Three hats of a leader: Coaching, mentoring and teaching. *Physician Executive, 36*(6).
92. Hiatt, J. (2006). *ADKAR: A model for change in business, government and our community: How to implement successful change in our personal lives and professional careers*. Prosci Research.
93. Hall-Ellis, S. (2014). Accept, coach, and inspire: A formula for success. *The Bottom Line, 27*(3), 103–106.
94. Megginson, D., & Clutterbuck, D. (2009). *Further techniques for coaching and mentoring*. Routledge.
95. Kolb, D. (1984). *Experiential learning experience as a source of learning and development*. Prentice Hall.
96. Kolb, A., et al. (2014). On becoming an experiential educator: The educator role profile. *Simulation & Gaming, 45*(2), 204–234.
97. Knowles, M. (1980). *The modern practice of Adult education: From pedagogy to andragogy* (2nd ed.). Cambridge Books.
98. Knowles, M. (2004). *The Adult Learner: A neglected species* (3rd ed.). Gulf.

99. Knowles, M. (1975). *Self-directed learning: A guide for learners and teachers.* Follett Publishing.
100. Knowles, M., Holton, E., & Swanson, R. (2015). *The Adult Learner: The definitive classic in adult education and Human Resource Development.* Routledge.
101. Knowles, M., Holton, E. I., & Swanson, R. (2011). *The adult learner* (6th ed.). Elsevier.
102. Borton, T. (1970). *Reach, touch, and teach.* McGraw Hill.
103. Gonzalo, J., et al. (2019). A developmental approach to internal medicine residency education: Lessons learned from the design and implementation of a novel longitudinal coaching program. *Medical Education Online, 24*(1), 1–5.
104. Sargeant, J., Lockyer, J., & Mann, K. (2018). The R2C2 model in residency education: How does it foster coaching and promote feedback use? *Academic Medicine, 93*(7), 1055–1063.
105. Davies, F., et al. (2020). Training in health coaching skills for health professionals who work with people with progressive neurological conditions: A realist evaluation. *Health Expectations, 23*(4), 919–933.
106. Dyrbye, L., et al. (2019). Effect of a professional coaching intervention on the well-being and distress of physicians: A pilot randomized clinical trial. *JAMA Internal Medicine*, 1–13.
107. Turner, C., & McCarthy, G. (2015). Coachable moments: Identifying factors that influence managers to take advantage of coachable moments in day-to-day management. *International Journal of Evidence Based Coaching and Mentoring, 13*(1), 1–13.
108. Westcott, L. (2016). How coaching can play a key role in the development of nurse managers. *Journal of Clinical Nursing, 25*(17–18), 2669–2677.
109. Maini, A., et al. (2020). Coaching skills for medical education in a VUCA world. *Medical Teacher, 42*(11), 1308–1309.
110. Grant, A. M., et al. (2017). The impact of leadership coaching in an Australian healthcare setting. *Journal of HealthOrganization Management, 31*(2), 237–252.
111. Singh, H. K., Kennedy, G. A., & Stupans, I. (2020). Pharmacist health coaching in Australian community pharmacies: What do pharmacy professionals think? *Health & Social Care in the Community, 28*(4), 1190–1198.
112. Morey, J. C., et al. (2002). Error reduction and performance improvement in the emergency department through formal teamwork training: Evaluation results of the MedTeams project. *Health Services Research, 37*(6), 1553–1581.
113. McQueen, A., et al. (2018). Perceptions of health coaching for behavior change among Medicaid and commercially insured adults. *Health Promotion Practice, 10*, 1524839918790936.
114. Thompson, L., et al. (2021). Clinical coaches and patient safety—Just in time: A descriptive exploratory study. *Nurse Education in Practice, 54*, 103134.
115. Wolever, R. Q., et al. (2011). Integrative health coaching: An organizational case study. *The Journal of Science and Healing, 7*(1), 30–36.
116. Sudore, R. L., & Schillinger, D. (2009). Interventions to improve care for patients with limited health literacy. *Journal of Clinical Outcomes Management, 16*(1), 20.
117. McMillan, S. S., et al. (2014). Is the pharmacy profession innovative enough?: Meeting the needs of Australian residents with chronic conditions and their carers using the nominal group technique. *BMC Health Services Research, 14*(1), 476.
118. Singh, H. K., Kennedy, G. A., & Stupans, I. (2019). A systematic review of pharmacy health coaching and an evaluation of patient outcomes. *Research in Social and Administrative Pharmacy, 15*(3), 244–251.
119. Scott, I. (2014). Ten clinician-driven strategies for maximising value of Australian health care. *Australian Health Review, 38*(2), 125–133.
120. Maynard, L. (2012). Using clinical peer coaching for patient safety. *Association of Operating Room Nurses (AORN) Journal, 96*(2), 203–205.
121. Parker, P., Kram, K., & Hall, D. (2014). Peer coaching: An untapped resource for development. *Organizational Dynamics, 43*(2), 122–129.
122. Beattie, R., et al. (2014). Managerial coaching: A review of the empirical literature and development of a model to guide future practice. *Advances in Developing Human Resources, 16*(2), 184–201.

Chapter 5
Coaching to Increase Leader Capability

This chapter explores the first purpose of coaching in a healthcare setting—to increase leadership capability so leaders can prevent the occurrence of adverse events and keep patients safe from harm (Fig. 5.1). Staff in healthcare organizations are critically aware of the importance of keeping patients safe. They have the clinical (technical) skills to do so but not always the personal (nontechnical) skills to render compassionate, person-centered care, especially in difficult situations or when working in interdisciplinary teams. Coaching can increase leaders' nontechnical capability to communicate and relate better with patients and other staff members. Leaders who are emotionally intelligent and adopt a coaching leadership style [1–3] are better able to motivate and inspire staff to emulate excellent clinical practice and learn from adverse events. Communication is enhanced when leaders actively engage in dialog with staff and patients and encourage others to do the same. Leaders who adopt a coaching leadership style listen to what staff members are saying and utilize the strengths of interdisciplinary teams. They encourage staff to analyze situations, think critically about possible outcomes, and take preventative action in relation to potentially adverse situations that may cause patients harm.

5.1 Leadership

In healthcare settings, leadership is a vital capability for managing complex interactions among clinical and multiprofessional teams in the provision of quality and safe patient care. Leaders act as guides, motivating and inspiring team members and modeling coach-like behaviors to create a social environment in which common tasks are solved without putting undue stress on team members. The result of effective leadership is better clinical outcomes for patients and enhanced staff well-being. Exceptional clinical progress is the ultimate goal, and patient communication and safety, harmonious teamwork, and inefficiency reduction are all key health

© The Author(s), under exclusive license to Springer Nature Switzerland AG 2024
S. Knowles, *Patient Safety Coaching*,
https://doi.org/10.1007/978-3-031-68722-8_5

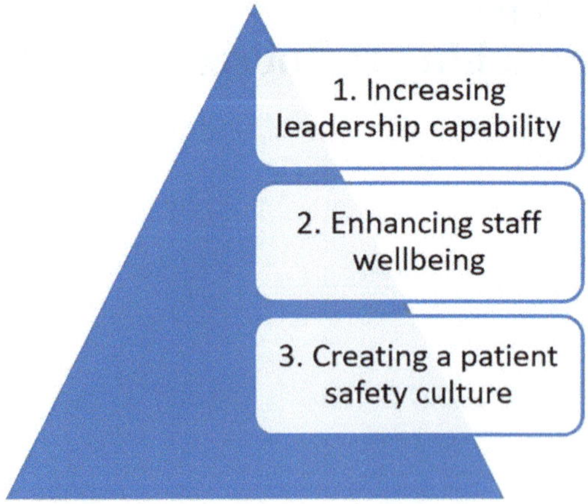

Fig. 5.1 Purposes of patient safety coaching

management outcomes required to achieve that goal [4]. In addition, one of the important tasks of leaders is to prepare team members for future roles as team leaders, irrespective of the career path they follow. A clinician or operating surgeon must be just as effective as a leader and influencer as they are an effective practitioner, ensuring the quality and flow of optimal patient care. This ability to lead and influence better is essential to ensure quality performance in patient care.

Workplace demands and resources have been found to influence the number of safety issues such as near misses, accidents, injuries, and adverse events. Caldwell [5] noted that leadership and management practices can have a positive but also negative impact on the uptake of safety procedures within an organization. She presented a model that emphasized the importance of authentic leadership behaviors in creating engaged fellowship and organizational trust, which leads to resilience in high-reliability organizations. Further, she called for research into how to "marry the functionalist and interpretive approaches to culture in a way that considers the multidimensional aspects of leadership" [5]. Nahrgang et al. [6] found that the engagement of motivated workers was positively related to workplace safety and that burnout was negatively related to workplace safety.

5.1.1 *Leadership Styles*

Effective healthcare delivery is highly dependent on multidisciplinary teamwork, drawing on the expertise of each discipline or team member and pooling this expertise to collectively diagnose and treat patients. Unfortunately, traditional hierarchical leadership models have done little to achieve synergy across disciplines. Hence, two alternative styles of leadership have been proposed in the literature to develop a patient safety culture—*transformational* leadership and *collective* leadership.

Seljemo et al. [7] proposed that a transformational leader's role is critical in the creation of a culture of patient safety. They describe transformational leadership as based on four defining characteristics: idealized influence, inspirational motivation, intellectual stimulation, and individualized consideration [8]. These leadership characteristics enable staff to act beyond their own needs and interests for the greater good of the team [9–11]. The transformational leader also works to change the team culture, which benefits the entire organization [7, 12, 13].

Drawing on emerging theories of leadership, McAuliffe et al. [14] developed a model of collective leadership which they proposed would enhance team performance in healthcare settings. The intervention they conducted in their study positioned the team as a dynamic leadership entity, with each team member accountable for the performance of the team as a whole. The results revealed that role clarity and understanding, trust, communication, and shared goals were key components for collective leadership to achieve integrated, quality patient care. Their conclusion was that it makes sense to engage team members in taking responsibility and being accountable for collective team performance as they drive the delivery of integrated, safe, patient care.

5.1.2 Leadership Competency Framework

Clinical leaders are skilled in the technical skills pertaining to their discipline area of expertise. However, to fulfill their role in relation to patient safety, they need to develop and embrace nontechnical skills as well—the behaviors, attitudes, and philosophies that are less visible yet instrumental in building trustworthy relationships with others and fostering effective communication. In other words, leaders need to possess or develop knowledge and competencies in the nontechnical skills of active and reflective listening, asking powerful questions, and summarizing—the *coaching* skills.

At the First Global Experts' Consultation in March 2014 to develop the World Health Organization (WHO)'s *Leaders Guide on Patient Safety and Quality of Care in Service Delivery*, a draft *Leadership Competencies Framework on Patient Safety and Quality of Care* [15] was developed by the WHO Patient Safety Education team through an extensive literature search and analysis of findings. The group recognized that, to ensure that the framework could be implemented successfully, several factors had to be addressed in unison, namely, patient safety strategies, policies, leadership capacity, data to drive safety improvements, skilled healthcare professionals, and the effective involvement of patients in their own care. The resulting framework focused on three key competency areas:

- The personal attributes of healthcare leaders.
- The core functions of healthcare leaders.
- Mise-en-place of healthcare leaders.

These are the three areas of focus in which leaders receive patient safety coaching. Coaches develop the leader's personal attributes, strengthen their core functionality as a leader, and ensure that they effectively meet the requirements of their role in a healthcare environment. Later iterations of this framework resulted in the publication of the *Global Competency Framework for Universal Health Coverage* (2022) [16], which reinforced the original three competencies and added specific others:

Domain 1: People-centeredness.
Domain 11: Decision-making.
Domain 111: Communication.
Domain IV: Collaboration.
Domain V: Evidence-informed practice.
Domain V1: Personal conduct.

An effective leader in patient safety is self-aware and adaptable, acts professionally and ethically, and avoids inappropriate blame when things do not go well. They listen to staff and patients and raise any concerns for discussion and resolution. They are a learner as well as a leader. They lead toward a set direction, deliver competently, and communicate effectively to transform the culture from one of blame to a culture of justice. They improve on policies and systems as performance dictates, as they transition their team toward high-quality, integrated, person-centered care.[1]

5.1.3 Leader Role in Patient Safety

Research has shown that the absence of quality clinical leadership in healthcare settings has a clear negative impact on patient and staff well-being, as well as on the development of a patient safety culture [17]. Over the last decade, the implementation of standardized clinical interventions, such as hand hygiene guidelines and surgical checklists, has reduced the incidence of preventable medication and diagnostic and surgical errors. In addition, a growing body of evidence suggests that contextual factors such as teamwork and culture can increase the likelihood of successfully implementing safety improvement interventions that positively influence patient safety [18]. Leadership support for safety has been found to have a positive impact on patient outcomes such as decreased falls, lower rates of medication errors, and a lower likelihood of hospital-acquired infections [19].

At a practical level, the role of the leader in relation to patient safety is multipurposed (Fig. 5.2):

1. Prevent adverse events from occurring.
2. Increase incident reporting.

[1]Appendix 5.1. Readers may like to complete the Healthcare Leadership Competencies Survey to identify areas for their own improvement

Fig. 5.2 The role of the leader in developing a patient safety culture

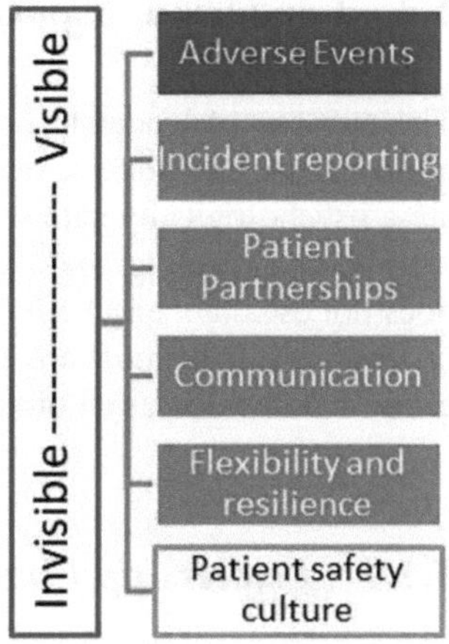

3. Facilitate patient partnerships where feasible to do so.
4. Develop effective communication within the team.
5. Support team members to become more flexible in managing change and resilient in navigating adversity and uncertainty.
6. Create a patient safety culture within their team.

The leader's attention is most frequently drawn to the adverse events or incidents—the behaviors that are most visible. A psychologically safe environment that, in itself, is not visible will be evidenced by increased reporting. As cultures transition from an incident and error focus (Safety-1) to a high-performing patient safety focus (Safety-11) [20], leaders need to become more observant, identify and understand the positive behaviors and interactions that prevent incidents from occurring, and then promote and reinforce these examples of excellent clinical practice. Patient partnerships based on trusting relationships in which patients are actively involved in their own care reduce the incidence of adverse events. Effective communication among team members and across multidisciplinary teams is imperative as care treatment progresses. Ineffective communication is sometimes evidenced as conflict, but, at times, ructions between individuals may also occur at deeper levels that are hidden from view. The attributes of flexibility and resilience may only become obvious as staff "soldier-on" without expressing the need to rest, especially in emergency situations. Underpinning all of these activities is the culture of the ward or department that either supports staff in their hours of greatest need or hinders them because of excessive workload, poor interpersonal relationships, power struggles, hierarchical gamesmanship, bullying, or harassment. Each of these elements in a leader's role in relation to patient safety is explored in this chapter. However, first, let us look at the role of leadership coaching in supporting leaders in the performance of their role.

5.2 Leadership Coaching

The purpose of leadership coaching in healthcare settings is to improve leaders' ability to prevent adverse events from occurring, support staff well-being, and create a psychologically safe workplace. Leaders play a crucial role in enabling team members to speak up and report errors, address errors quickly so that the situation does not escalate, and help the team learn from mistakes. The leadership coaching process and its benefits are explained below, and opportunities for leaders to learn, grow, and develop as an outcome of the coaching explored.

5.2.1 Leadership Coaching Process

Leadership coaching is the formal, one-on-one collaborative relationship between a coach and coachee that promotes and supports the leader's growth and development [21, 22]. It is focused on work-related issues with the purpose of improving the coachee's leadership effectiveness [23, 24]. "Leadership coaching is all about helping leaders to identify and define their specific goals, then organize themselves to find a way to attain them" [25] so that they become more effective leaders [26–28]. The coach and coachee collaborate to assess and understand the coachee's needs in relation to their leadership development tasks. The coach challenges current constraints and explores new possibilities with the coachee.

As a meta-process, coaching can be applied to any situation in which a coachee feels the need for improvement or to achieve a desired goal that they have been unable to achieve by themself. The coaching process is guided by (i) the needs, characteristics, and experiences of the coachee, (ii) the needs of the organization, and (iii) the knowledge, skills, abilities, and perspectives of the coach. Together, the coach and coachee determine the appropriate balance of time and effort spent on the various aspects of the coachee and organizational needs. Coaching is dynamic and interactive and seeks to maximize the positive transfer of learning to other contexts within the coachee's workplace by embedding the learning so that the coachee and others see positive results immediately [29].

During coaching, the coachee gains insight into their current and desired situations as they increase in self-awareness and discover their development needs via reflection, assessment, and feedback [30]. A number of changes may be desired or required in relation to their behavior, attitude, beliefs, or perspectives, which impact the coachee's ability to develop trusting and collaborative relationships at work and deliver on performance expectations. In addition to these personal reasons for individuals being coached, healthcare organizations generally expect improved outcomes in terms of the coachee's leadership skills and ability to achieve better performance outcomes from their team in relation to patient safety and care [31].

Techniques based on developmental, humanistic, and positive psychology approaches inform the coaching process when coachees bring issues to the surface to be resolved, thereby enabling mental and emotional well-being [22, 32]. These techniques are founded on the psychological construct of "unconditional positive regard" [33, 34], which involves reality-checking to ensure that the coachee's needs, drives, and expectations are realistic and attainable [35, 36], and the exploration of limiting beliefs that are holding them back from becoming authentically happy and achieving "flow" [37, 38]. Social psychology techniques recognize the importance of the social environment in reinforcing individual learning [39] and assisting coachees to develop self-regulation, goal attainment, and emotional competence [40–45].

Two styles of leadership coaching—guidance and facilitation—have been reported in the literature [46]. The guidance style combines clear expectations of performance requirements with observational learning, behavioral realignment, and role modeling to achieve performance mastery. The facilitation style enables adaptive learning from the environment, one-on-one feedback, and the adoption of a transformational leadership style. A focus on coaching new leaders to integrate multiple identities as they settle into their role adds further dimensions to the discussion [47].

5.2.2 Benefits of Leadership Coaching

Research has examined the impact of coaching on a number of variables including leadership development [10, 48–53], personality traits [54–56], self-identity [57, 58], compassion [59], and workplace behavior [9, 60–63]. How coaching impacts psychological variables such as metacognition, mental health, and the desire for goal attainment, has also been investigated by researchers [64–70].

Apart from these personal benefits of coaching, one of the major benefits of leadership coaching is that leaders learn how to grow and develop each member of their team. Leaders who learn how to distribute power to team members benefit from their increasing ability to work independently to mastery level in this supportive environment. In today's social workplace, leadership is associated with the recognition that individuals can complement each other by using social networks for collective action [71]. For example, the leader's ability to engage and support frontline teams was highlighted as a key facilitation skill in the SCQIRE project [17]. As leaders are coached, they come to understand that structure and hierarchy may impede a team or team member's ability to perform to their best and that they would instead benefit from an atmosphere that was more collaborative [72]. This changed model of care influences the culture in which the team operates and impacts the degree of clinical care provided in the healthcare unit [73].

Coaching for leadership development encourages healthcare leaders to draw on their clinical expertise, skills, and strengths to help them become even more effective [10, 48–53]. Leaders discover better ways to communicate, build trusting relationships, solve problems, and make decisions. They develop critical reflexivity and cognitive agility as well as emotional intelligence, which motivates and drives them to change their behavior and improve their performance [3, 74]. Limiting beliefs and assumptions are replaced by a positive mindset developed from personal insights, resulting in a more optimistic view of the future. Leaders role model their changed outlook to others and become more constructive in their interactions with staff. They more readily resolve conflict and engineer jointly negotiated outcomes based on collaborative relationships. Research suggests that a critical component for future-proofing the healthcare workforce is empathetic leadership, which allows leaders to understand the needs of staff outside of the workplace such as caretaking responsibilities for children or elderly parents [75]. A focus on collective and compassionate leadership, where everyone is a leader of something, has been found to be a key aspect of good clinical leadership [76, 77].

5.2.3 Learning, Growth, and Development

Leadership coaching from a positive psychology perspective takes a broader, strategic approach than performance coaching, dealing with issues relating to how the coachee can develop both personally and professionally in their role and in preparation for future roles within their profession or the healthcare organization. As coachees respond to coaching, they start to question their assumptions and behavioral patterns, actively construct meaning based on new perspectives, and explore creative possibilities for innovation. Coachees grow independently in socially and emotionally fulfilling ways [78, 79]. Reflective practice stimulates individuals to engage in single-loop learning to discover what they intuitively know or have learned from experience [80]. When they are able to meta-reflect or step back and review, single-loop learning is converted to double-loop learning, which impacts their future work situations more deeply as they make corrections to their behavior and performance, which may change their governing values [81].

Leadership coaching also focuses on how leaders can work more effectively with their team [82]. The coach challenges current constraints and explores new possibilities with the coachee. As coaching stimulates cognitive and behavioral change in leaders, their learning triggers ways in which their team can also learn. They encourage the sharing of new beliefs and behaviors that support the implementation of innovations in multiple arenas, including clinical practice [83]. As the coaching process unlocks learning opportunities for growth and development, it can lead to transformational change which is "explicitly and intentionally created and reflective in approach" [84]. Transformational change relates to the entirety of leaders' personal, professional, emotional, and social life and work, and takes into account the possible consequences of the change for the team and organization.

When skills or performance enhancement is needed, education and training interventions followed by leadership coaching are most effective in producing change [85–88].

5.3 Leading Effectively

The best way that leaders can prevent adverse events from occurring and ensure the well-being of patients and staff is by delivering effective leadership. Leadership is effective when leaders observe objectively, provide constructive feedback, and consider adverse events to be opportunities for individuals and teams to learn. Team members are encouraged to become more responsible parties to ensure that patients are free from harm [89]. Specifically, leaders become more effective when they:

- Become more emotionally intelligent.
- Adopt a coaching leadership style with their team members and others in the organization.
- Critically reflect on their leadership and clinical practice, seeking opportunities for improvement (Fig. 5.3).

5.3.1 Emotional Intelligence

An early study on emotional intelligence (EQ) highlighted the impact of self-awareness, self-management, social awareness, and social skills on an individual's ability to communicate and maintain significant relationships [3]. Each of these fundamental capabilities of leaders comprises specific sets of competencies and their corresponding traits. An emotionally intelligent person is able to manage themselves and their relationships effectively.

When the EQ construct was first proposed in the leadership literature [90], it brought into focus the development opportunity for leaders to examine their behavior and interaction with others so that they could become more self- and socially aware and better able to self-manage. Leaders who are emotionally intelligent start to think about how staff both know and feel that they are respected, and how they communicate that their work is valued. They aim to engage, motivate, and support team members to manage their level of stress so that it does not impact clinical outcomes.

Goleman proposed that there are six leadership styles, each of which is associated with different organizational outcomes—coercive, authoritative, affiliative,

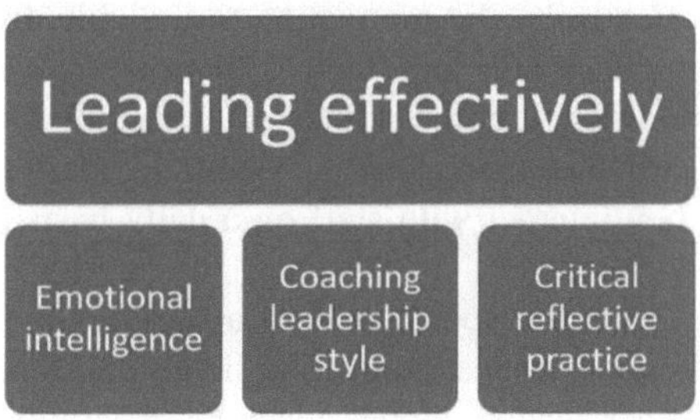

Fig. 5.3 Leading effectively

democratic, pacesetting, and coaching [3]. The leader who is emotionally intelligent has mastered the art of utilizing each of these styles as they are appropriate for the situation. Goleman's team found that all six leadership styles have a measurable effect on culture—the most positive being authoritative, affiliative, democratic, and coaching. He concluded that the most effective leaders switch flexibly between these four leadership styles. Later, Goleman, and Cherniss [91] compared the predominant leadership styles of that time with those found to be the most effective in promoting a healthy organizational culture and reconfirmed that *coaching* is one of the most effective leadership styles for creating a positive organizational culture.

In a recent study, undergraduate nursing students about to start a placement in a mental health facility were trained in emotional intelligence [92]. Researchers found that they experienced greater resilience during placement as a result of prior training. They used their improved nontechnical skills to respond positively to mental health patients and showed greater empathy and compassion for them. These findings suggest that the majority of healthcare staff would benefit from emotional intelligence training and coaching.

5.3.2 Coaching Leadership Style

According to Goleman's research, the second way that leaders can become more effective is by adopting a *coaching leadership style* [22] to create a patient safety culture within their healthcare team and organization. A coaching leadership style helps team members develop emotional intelligence in themselves and others, build long-term relationships, and improve their performance. Leaders who make a personal commitment to using coaching skills in their interactions with others serve as important role models for integrating coaching into the organization [93]. Team members also develop greater self-awareness and a more mindful presence when treating patients. They come to better address the everyday, practical challenges they face in delivering care services to patients.

Leaders who "let go" of their *command-and-control* management style and adopt a coaching leadership style share a common language, philosophy, and model of coaching with their team members. By doing so, they begin to learn new ways of interacting with each other. A leadership coaching style incorporates the essential aspects of the coaching process—the use of reflective dialog to communicate more effectively, the motivation to individually and collectively learn and succeed, and the desire for an effective "partner" relationship with others, including patients. In addition, it embeds feedback coaching loops within the organization's existing performance management system. Leaders who use a coaching leadership style when they interact with staff on a daily basis preempt and prevent adverse events from occurring.

A key responsibility of a leader is to model coach-like behaviors that reach the heart of issues, build team bonds and relationships, and support peak performance. When leaders model coaching behaviors, team members start to adopt these same behaviors which they can see are more effective in achieving the desired results. As all team members become more coach-like in their behavior, they start to peer-coach others [94], resulting in powerful outcomes for staff and patients. Coaching and corridor conversations become routine [22]. Feedback conversations improve individual and team performance almost immediately. The best way for leaders to guarantee that they are continuing to model coach-like behaviors is for them to regularly reflect on their communication and relationships with team members.

5.3.3 Critical Reflective Practice

The third way that leaders become more effective is by critically reflecting on their leadership style as they support team members in their daily practice. Reflective practice derives its origins from education when it was introduced as a critical, problem-solving mechanism, challenging individuals to think differently to effect change [95–97]. Coaching is an active and purposeful journey of exploration and discovery in which coachees engage in reflective practice that reinterprets their experiences and creates new knowledge from unanticipated insights. Coachees envision their best possible future and, together with their coach, identify a plan to change their behavior and communicate the changes [98]. Coachees' long-held assumptions are challenged as they become more receptive to alternative ways of thinking and doing [99]. Leaders who engage in self-reflexivity of their own leadership practice are also more likely to be comfortable in assisting team members to do the same.

Reflection may be learned in formal classroom contexts or facilitated through developmental processes such as coaching and mentoring [84, 99]. Reflective coaching practices have been used to improve professional leadership practices [100], ease frustrations associated with the pace of change, reduce pressure from conflicting demands, and overcome feelings of isolation [101]. To aid reflection, the use of storytelling, metaphors, reflective journals, and mind mapping tools may prove useful [102].

Research shows that leaders who are self-reflective facilitate team meta-processes that trigger critical discussion about team objectives and progress and foster information sharing and learning [103, 104]. Team reflection is positively related to team performance because, although habitual routines can be advantageous in terms of saving time and energy during task performance, reflection enables team members to be more aware of problems and constraints, which may impact their ability to meet schedules and operate within budgets. Team reflection has been found to enhance team effectiveness and goal attainment to the degree that work processes become free from errors, and the services provided by the team are increasingly aligned with targeted performance expectations [105].

Addressing the tensions between the team's immediate goals, and important wider-system issues and pressures, helps team members reflect on how they work together, why they do what they do, and how they can improve. This kind of reflection can prompt significant changes in individuals' and teams' understanding of their direction and purpose, and the nature of the activities in which they engage on a daily basis. It can also support long-term views or visions of improvement, encouraging persistence and resilience in major improvement projects.

Engaging in critical self-reflexivity as a routinized habit is to be applauded since team members can find it difficult to look beyond themselves to recognize what might be startlingly obvious to an external viewer. The Johari window provides a model that staff can use for self-reflection in relation to three of the four quadrants [106–108]. It is reflection on the Unknown quadrant (not known to self/not known to others) which can surface significant insights, although sometimes these insights can only be uncovered by interaction with a coach who helps unpack this "black box."

5.4 Patient Safety Coaching to Increase Leader Capability

The purpose of patient safety coaching for leaders is to (i) improve their ability to prevent adverse events from occurring, (ii) support staff wellbeing, and (iii) create a psychologically safe workplace. Leading more effectively is achieved when leaders are more emotionally intelligent, adopt a coaching leadership style, and encourage critical reflection on clinical practices. Leadership coaching can assist leaders in these three special ways. Staff well-being is enhanced when leaders attend to individuals who have experienced or witnessed adverse events and take the time to consider the best ways to support them as they return to everyday work.[2] Leaders develop a patient safety culture when they create conditions in which staff feel psychologically safe to report incidents and near misses so that everyone can learn from them.[3]

Patient safety coaching is delivered by healthcare leaders and clinical coaches who have been formally trained to deliver coaching to individuals in organizations by using, e.g., the ©AIPC COACH model.[4] Leaders become more effective when, during the coaching process, they reflect on their successes and failures to examine what led them to and influenced the decisions they made in relation to their own and their team's performance. The coaching process supports leaders in testing their assumptions and beliefs against reality. Reflection leads to constructive conversations that provide insights into how things could have been done differently. Reflection allows for new and novel options to emerge regarding processes and procedures that may work better in the future and reveals actions that can be taken immediately to improve team performance.

Ongoing coaching from a qualified coach keeps patient safety front-of-mind in importance for both leaders and team members. The monthly coaching of leaders

[2] Coaching for Staff Well-Being in discussed in Chap. 6.

[3] Coaching to develop a Patient Safety Culture is discussed in Chap. 7.

[4] The ©AIPC COACH model was explained in Chap. 4.

reveals how they are progressing in their quest to reduce incidents and errors within their team and provides insights for future action. Investing in ongoing patient safety coaching enables leaders to reinforce patient safety behaviors within their team, engage staff in taking responsibility and being accountable for their own actions, reduce errors and near misses, and improve the team's clinical performance.

Leaders who have been coached or witnessed the positive benefits of coaching are particularly amenable to receiving training in patient safety coaching.[5] Then, using their coaching skills, they can better assist team members and others in the organization to achieve personal goals such as work/life balance, as well as clinical performance goals that move them professionally forward while also supporting the healthcare agenda.

Key Takeaways

- Leaders increase their nontechnical capability when they learn how to coach.
- Leaders who coach their team members help them discover their own solutions to overcome problems at work, and more easily and quickly achieve their professional goals.
- When leaders adopt a coaching leadership style, staff are more engaged, motivated to do their best work, and enthusiastic to learn how to improve their clinical practice.
- Leaders who are emotionally intelligent use a coaching leadership style to help staff succeed and ensure that patients receive the best care.
- Leaders who engage in critical reflective practice enhance their leadership capability and encourage staff to critically reflect on their own clinical practice to keep patients safe.

5.5 Case Study 5: Clinical Leadership Leader Capability

Dr. Alex Johnson is a technically competent neurosurgeon known for his exceptional surgical skills and precision. However, he struggles with social and relational skills, often failing to recognize the impact of his behavior on team members or patients. He has a habit of reprimanding staff and colleagues publicly, unaware of the emotional toll it takes on them. In addition, the hospital has received complaints from families about the doctor's attitude and approach to patients, and complaints have even been made to the regulatory body.

Dr. Johnson's continued negative behavior has led to a significant decline in team morale and tension between team members. Several staff members have either

[5] Training in patient safety coaching is delivered by the Australian Institute of Professional Coaches. www.professionalcoachtraining.com.au

applied for transfer or refused to cross-cover his patients—one has even resigned. Dr. Johnson has been made aware that he is under observation for his behavior and that it needs to change. In response to this crisis, a performance management plan has been developed and shared with him. A leader trained in coaching will be brought in to help Dr. Johnson develop better interpersonal skills and improve the overall work environment in the unit.

After discussion with Dr. Johnson, it is agreed that coaching will focus on developing his leadership skills through several key strategies:

1. *Self-awareness:* Coaching will help Dr. Johnson become more aware of his behavior and its impact on others. Through feedback and reflective exercises, coaching will help him recognize how his actions affect team dynamics and morale. He will discover that his motivation at work lies in performance, and he will come to understand that the team will perform more effectively when he relates more interpersonally with them as individual team members.
2. *Emotional intelligence:* Coaching sessions involving mindfulness and reflection will help Dr. Johnson understand and manage his emotions, as well as empathize with his team members. As he develops this skill, he will increase his enjoyment and satisfaction with work. His increasing empathy for team members will foster a desire to deal with issues privately and professionally, rather than publicly reprimanding staff.
3. *Leadership development:* Through coaching, Dr. Johnson will learn how to develop a more collaborative and supportive leadership style. He will learn how to set clear expectations, provide positive reinforcement, and foster a team-oriented environment.

By addressing these areas, coaching helps Dr. Johnson to become a more effective leader and team member, improve team cohesion, and create a more positive, productive work environment. These changes, in turn, have a tangible effect on the quality of care given to patients, the effectiveness of handovers, and the overall patient experience. Over time, Dr. Johnson works hard to build up the team morale, leading to a stable team workforce.

For discussion

1. Clinical leaders are highly qualified and experienced in their technical field of excellence.
   - How can using coaching skills enhance their capability?
   - What happened in this case study, and what could have been done differently?
2. Leaders who are emotionally intelligent are self-aware and engage in critical self-reflection of their clinical practices.
   - Is critical reflective practice followed where you work?
3. Leaders who adopt a coaching leadership style with staff motivate and inspire them to improve their performance.

- Do you agree or disagree with this statement?
- Provide examples to support your views based on your observations of and reflections on the leadership styles of those you work with.

4. How could coaching improve your leadership capability and that of those you work with?

Appendix 5.1 Healthcare Leadership Competencies

Instructions:

1. Self-reflects on the healthcare leadership competencies that you display within your team and within interdisciplinary teams. Provide examples to support your self-reflection.
2. Then, imagine that you do possess these attributes. What would you need to do differently to possess all of these attributes? What are your ideas for improvement? [15]

		Leadership competency	Self-reflection	Ideas for improvement
Personal attributes	1	Exhibits a coaching leadership style, self-awareness, and adaptability		
	2	Is a leader in professional and ethical conduct		
	3	Is a learner as well as a leader		
Core functions	4	Sets the direction		
	5	Communicates effectively		
	6	Leads positive transformation		
Mise-en-place	7	Delivers competently and effectively		
	8	Has political and social astuteness		
	9	Establishes crisis systems		
	10	Uses evidence and information for policy decision		

Overall conclusions to be discussed with your coach:

1.
2.
3.

What actions will you take to improve your leadership capability?

1.
2.
3.

References

1. Karlsen, J. T., & Berg, M. E. (2020). Coaching leadership style: A learning process. *International Journal of Knowledge and Learning, 13*(4), 356–368.
2. Knowles, S. (2022). *Coaching culture*. Springer Nature.
3. Goleman, D. (2000). Leadership that gets results. *Harvard Business Review, 78*(2), 78–90.
4. Khan, R. N., Aziz, A., & Siddiqui, N. A. (2022). Clinicians as leaders: Impact and challenges. *Pakistan Journal of Medical Sciences, 38*(4), 1069–1072.
5. Caldwell, C. (2018). *Safety culture and high-risk environments: A leadership perspective* (Ebscohost, Ed.). CRC Press, Taylor; Francis Group.
6. Nahrgang, J., Morgeson, F., & Hofmann, D. (2011). Safety at work: A meta-analytic investigation of the link between job demands, job resources, burnout, engagement, and safety outcomes. *Journal of Applied Psychology, 96*(1), 71–94.
7. Seljemo, C., Viksveen, P., & Ree, E. (2020). The role of transformational leadership, job demands and job resources for patient safety culture in Norwegian nursing homes: A cross-sectional study. *BMC Health Services Research, 20*(1), 1–12.
8. Bass, B. (1985). *Leadership and performance beyond expectations*. Free Press.
9. Avolio, B., et al. (2004). Unlocking the mask: A look at the process by which authentic leaders impact follower attitudes and behaviors. *The Leadership Quarterly, 15*(6), 801–823.
10. Avolio, B., & Gardner, W. (2005). Authentic leadership development: Getting to the root of positive forms of leadership. *The Leadership Quarterly, 16*(3), 315–338.
11. Bass, B., et al. (2003). Predicting unit performance by assessing transformational and transactional leadership. *Journal of Applied Psychology, 88*(2), 207–218.
12. Veiseh, S., et al. (2014). The relation between transformational leadership and organizational culture (Case study: Medical school of Ilam). *Journal of Business Studies Quarterly, 5*(3), 113–124.
13. Jha, S. (2014). Transformational leadership and psychological empowerment. *South Asian Journal of Global Business Research, 3*(1), 18–35.
14. McAuliffe, E., DeBrun, A., & Cunningham, U. (2019). Collective leadership and safety cultures: Developing an alternative model of leadership for healthcare teams. *International Journal of Integrated Care (IJIC), 19*(S1), 1–2.
15. Leotsakos, A., et al. (2014). *Leadership Competencies framework on patient safety and quality of care (DRAFT)*. WHO.
16. WHO. (2022). *Global Competency framework for universal health coverage*. World Health Organization.
17. Manley, K., & Jackson, C. (2019). Microsystems culture change: A refined theory for developing person-centred, safe and effective workplaces based on strategies that embed a safety culture. *International Practice Development Journal, 9*(2), 1–21.
18. Zaheer, S., et al. (2018). Importance of safety climate, teamwork climate and demographics: Understanding nurses, allied health professionals and clerical staff perceptions of patient safety. *BMJ Open Quality, 7*(4), e000433.
19. Mardon, R. E., et al. (2010). Exploring relationships between hospital patient safety culture and adverse events. *Journal of Patient Safety, 6*(4), 226–232.
20. Hollnagel, E., Wears, R., & Braithwaite, J. (2015). *From safety-I to safety-II: A white paper*. University of Southern Denmark, University of Florida, USA, and Macquarie University.
21. Ely, K., et al. (2010). Evaluating leadership coaching: A review and integrated framework. *The Leadership Quarterly, 21*(4), 585–599.
22. Knowles, S. (2021). *Positive psychology coaching*. Springer Nature.
23. Stajkovic, A., & Luthans, F. (1998). Self-efficacy and work-related performance: A meta-analysis. *Psychological Bulletin, 124*(2), 240.
24. Feldman, D., & Lankau, M. (2005). Executive coaching: A review and agenda for future research. *Journal of Management, 31*(6), 829–848.

25. Kets de Vries, M. (2011). Leadership coaching and high performance teams. In *Reflections on groups and organizations: On the Couch with Manfred Kets de Vries*. John Wiley & Sons, Incorporated.
26. Kilburg, R. (1996). Toward a conceptual understanding and definition of executive coaching. *Consulting Psychology Journal: Practice and Research, 48*(2), 134–144.
27. Hicks, M., Peterson, D., & Mobley, W. (1999). Leaders coaching across borders. *Advances in Global Leadership, 1*, 297.
28. Witherspoon, R. (2014). Double-loop coaching for leadership development. *The Journal of Applied Behavioral Science, 50*(3), 261–283.
29. Foley, J., & Kaiser, L. (2013). Learning transfer and its intentionality in adult and continuing education. *New Directions for Adult and Continuing Education, 37*(5), 15.
30. Schlosser, B., et al. (2006). The coaching impact study: Measuring the value of executive leader coaching. *International Journal of Coaching in Organizations, 4*(3), 8–26.
31. Fletcher, K., & Meyer, M. (2016). Coaching model + Clinical playbook = Transformative learning. *Journal of Professional Nursing, 32*(2), 121–129.
32. Snowling, M., et al. (2010). *Mental capital and mental wellbeing* (p. 775). Wiley-Blackwell.
33. Rogers, C. (1951). *Client-centred therapy: Its current practice, implications and theory*. Houghton Mifflin.
34. Bartlett, J. (2007). Advances in coaching practices: A humanistic approach to coach and client roles. *Journal of Business Research, 60*(1), 91–93.
35. Adler, A., Ansbacher, H., & Ansbacher, R. (1956). *The Individual Psychology of Alfred Adler: A systematic presentation in selections from his writings*. Basic Books.
36. Jung, C. (1921). *Personality theory*. Rascher.
37. Seligman, M. (2011). *Authentic Happiness: Using the new positive psychology to realise your potential for lasting fulfilment*. Nicholas Brealey Publishing.
38. Csikszentmihalyi, M. (1990). *Flow: The psychology of optimal experience*. Harper & Row.
39. Bandura, A., Davidson, H., & Davidson, J. (2003). *Bandura's social cognitive theory: An introduction*. Davidson Films, Inc.
40. Allard-Poesi, F. (1998). Representations and influence processes in groups: Towards a socio-cognitive perspective on cognition in organisation. *Scandinavian Journal of Management, 14*(4), 395–420.
41. Johan, S. (1997). How institutions learn: A socio-cognitive perspective. *Journal of Economic Issues, 31*(3), 729–740.
42. Bandura, A. (2006). *Toward a psychology of human agency. perspectives on psychological science* (Vol. 1, pp. 164–180). Sage Publications, Inc.
43. Bandura, A., & Locke, E. (2003). Negative self-efficacy and goal effects revisited. *Journal of Applied Psychology, 88*(1), 87–99.
44. Dweck, C., & Leggett, E. (1988). A social-cognitive approach to motivation and personality. *Psychological Review, 95*(2), 256–273.
45. Mizokawa, A., & Koyasu, M. (2015). Digging deeper into the link between socio-cognitive ability and social relationships. *British Journal of Developmental Psychology, 33*(1), 21–23.
46. Hui, R., & Sue-Chan, C. (2018). Variations in coaching style and their impact on subordinates' work outcomes. *Journal of Organizational Behavior, 39*(5), 663–679.
47. Yip, J., et al. (2020). Coaching new leaders: A relational process of integrating multiple identities. *Academy of Management Learning & Education, 19*(4), 503–520.
48. Ann, C., & Carr, A. (2011). Inside outside leadership development: Coaching and storytelling potential. *Journal of Management Development, 30*(3), 297–310.
49. Carey, W., Philippon, D., & Cummings, G. (2011). Coaching models for leadership development: An integrative review. *Journal of Leadership Studies, 5*(1), 51–69.
50. Day, D., et al. (2014). Advances in leader and leadership development: A review of 25 years of research and theory. *The Leadership Quarterly, 25*(1), 63–82.
51. Ladegard, G., & Gjerde, S. (2014). Leadership coaching, leader role-efficacy, and trust in subordinates. A mixed methods study assessing leadership coaching as a leadership development tool. *The Leadership Quarterly, 25*(4), 631–646.

52. Roberts, C. (2013). Building social capital through leadership development. *Journal of Leadership Education, 12*(1), 54–73.
53. Mason, C., Griffin, M., & Parker, S. (2014). Transformational leadership development: Connecting psychological and behavioral change. *Leadership & Organization Development Journal, 35*(3), 174–194.
54. De Fruyt, F., Wille, B., & Furnham, A. (2013). Assessing aberrant personality in managerial coaching: Measurement issues and prevalence rates across employment sectors. *European Journal of Personality, 27*(6), 555–564.
55. Sliter, K., & Christiansen, N. (2012). Effects of targeted self-coaching on applicant distortion of personality measures. *Journal of Personnel Psychology, 11*(4), 169–175.
56. Baumeister, R., et al. (2006). Self-regulation and personality: How interventions increase regulatory success, and how depletion moderates the effects of traits on behavior. *Journal of Personality, 74*(6), 1773–1802.
57. Bachkirova, T. (2011). *Developmental coaching: Working with the self.* McGraw-Hill Education.
58. Bachkirova, T. (2012). The role of the self and identification with an organisation as factors influencing work-related stress: Implications for helping. *Counselling Psychology Quarterly, 25*(1), 49–62.
59. Boyatzis, R., Smith, M., & Blaize, N. (2006). Developing sustainable leaders through coaching and compassion. *Academy of Management Learning & Education, 5*(1), 8–24.
60. Kim, S., et al. (2013). The impact of managerial coaching behavior on employee work-related reactions. *Journal of Business and Psychology, 28*(3), 315–330.
61. Beattie, R., et al. (2014). Managerial coaching: A review of the empirical literature and development of a model to guide future practice. *Advances in Developing Human Resources, 16*(2), 184–201.
62. Burke, C., et al. (2006). What type of leadership behaviors are functional in teams? A meta-analysis. *The Leadership Quarterly, 17*(3), 288–307.
63. Hagen, M., & Peterson, S. (2015). Measuring coaching: Behavioral and skill-based managerial coaching scales. *Journal of Management Development, 34*(2), 114–133.
64. Grant, A. (2003). *Towards a psychology of coaching: The impact of coaching on metacognition, mental health and goal attainment*. Macquarie University.
65. Van der Horst, C., & Albertyn, R. (2018). The importance of metacognition and the experiential learning process within a cultural intelligence–based approach to cross-cultural coaching. *South African Journal of Human Resource Management, 16*(1).
66. Grant, A., Curtayne, L., & Burton, G. (2009). Executive coaching enhances goal attainment, resilience and workplace well-being: A randomised controlled study. *The Journal of Positive Psychology, 4*(5), 396.
67. Ives, Y., & Cox, E. (2012). *Goal-focused coaching: Theory and practice*. Routledge.
68. Megginson, D. (2014). Goal-focused coaching: Theory and practice. *Action Learning: Research and Practice, 11*(2), 243–245.
69. Locke, E., & Latham, G. (2013). *Goal-setting theory* (pp. 313–317). Sage Publications.
70. Martin, A., et al. (2014). The psychosocial work environment, employee mental health and organizational interventions: Improving research and practice by taking a multilevel approach. *Stress and Health, 32*(3), 201–215.
71. Stodd, J. (2016). *The social leadership handbook* (2nd ed.). The Printing House.
72. Kastor, J. (2011). Accountable care organizations at academic medical centers. *New England Journal of Medicine, 364*(7), e11.
73. Kim, C. S., et al. (2014). Unit-based interprofessional leadership models in six US hospitals. *Journal of Hospital Medicine, 9*(8), 545–550.
74. Leban, W., & Zulauf, C. (2004). Linking emotional intelligence abilities and transformational leadership styles. *Leadership & Organization Development Journal, 25*(7), 554–564.
75. Radick, L. E. (2022). Ready for what's next: Future-proofing the healthcare workforce. *Healthcare Executive, 37*(3), 16–24.

76. West, M., et al. (2014). *Developing collective leadership for healthcare*. King's Fund.
77. West, M., et al. (2017). *Caring to change: How compassionate leadership can stimulate innovation in health care*. King's Fund.
78. Durlak, J., et al. (2015). *Handbook of social and emotional learning: Research and pactice*. Guilford Publications.
79. Boyatzis, R., Stubbs, E., & Taylor, S. (2002). Learning cognitive and emotional intelligence competencies through graduate management education. *Academy of Management Learning & Education, 1*(2), 150–162.
80. Argyris, C., & Schön, D. (1997). *Organizational Learning: A theory of action perspective*. Addison-Wesley Pub. Co.
81. Argyris, C. (2002). Double-loop learning, teaching, and research. *Academy of Management Learning & Education, 1*(2), 206–218.
82. Grant, A., & Hartley, M. (2013). Developing the leader as coach: Insights, strategies and tips for embedding coaching skills in the workplace. *Coaching: An International Journal of Theory, Research and Practice, 6*(2), 1–14.
83. Gray, D. (2006). Executive coaching: Towards a dynamic alliance of psychotherapy and transformative learning processes. *Management Learning, 37*(4), 475–497.
84. Brockbank, A., & McGill, I. (2012). *Facilitating Reflective Learning: Coaching, mentoring and supervision* (2nd ed.). Kogan Page Ltd.
85. Dutton, J., et al. (2001). Moves that matter: Issue selling and organizational change. *Academy of Management Journal, 44*, 716–736.
86. Showers, B. (1987). Synthesis of research on staff development: A framework for future study and a state-of the art analysis. *Educational Leadership, 45*(3), 77–87.
87. Goldman, A. (2008). Consultant and critics on the couch. *Journal of Management Inquiry, 17*(3), 243–249.
88. Shuffler, M., et al. (2018). Developing, sustaining, and maximizing team effectiveness: An integrative, dynamic perspective of team development interventions. *Academy of Management Annals, 12*(2), 688–724.
89. Lee, S. (2007). *The effects of group coaching on emotional intelligence and self-efficacy of the nurses* (Dissertation). Yonsei University.
90. Goleman, D., Boyatzis, R., & McKee, A. (2001). Primal leadership: The hidden driver of great performance. *Harvard Business Review, 79*(11), 42–51.
91. Goleman, D., & Cherniss, C. (2001). *The Emotionally Intelligent Workplace: How to select for, measure, and improve emotional intelligence in individuals, groups, and organizations*. Jossey-Bass.
92. Hurley, J., et al. (2020). Emotional intelligence as a mechanism to build resilience and non-technical skills in undergraduate nurses undertaking clinical placement. *International Journal of Mental Health Nursing, 29*(1), 47–55.
93. Gormley, H., & Van Nieuwerburgh, C. (2014). Developing coaching cultures: A review of the literature. *Coaching: An International Journal of Theory, Research and Practice, 7*(2), 90–101.
94. Parker, P., Hall, D., & Kram, K. (2008). Peer coaching: A relational process for accelerating career learning. *Academy of Management Learning & Education, 7*(4), 487–503.
95. Dewey, J. (1993). *How We Think: A restatement of the relation of reflective thinking to the educative process*. Heath.
96. Dewey, J. (1938). *Experience and Education*. Macmillan.
97. Schön, D. (1987). *Educating the reflective practitioner: Toward a new design for teaching and learning in the professions*. Jossey-Bass.
98. Stober, D., Grant, A., Coaching, E. B., & Handbook: Putting best practices to work for your clients. (2006). *Hoboken*. John Wiley & Sons.
99. Gray, D. (2007). Facilitating management learning: Developing critical reflection through reflective tools. *Management Learning, 38*(5), 495–517.

100. Nicolaidou, M., Karagiorgi, Y., & Petridou, A. (2018). Professional learning through reflection promoted by feedback and coaching (PROFLEC) in Cyprus. *International Journal of Leadership in Education, 21*(4), 412–426.
101. Anthony, D., & van Nieuwerburgh, C. (2018). A thematic analysis of the experience of educational leaders introducing coaching into schools. *International Journal of Mentoring and Coaching in Education, 7*(4), 343–356.
102. Ramsey, C. (2005). Narrative: From learning in reflection to learning in performance. *Management Learning, 36*(2), 219–235.
103. Lyubovnikova, J., et al. (2017). How authentic leadership influences team performance: The mediating role of team reflexivity. *Journal of Business Ethics, 141*(1), 59–70.
104. Akella, D. (2010). Learning together: Kolb's experiential theory and its application. *Journal of Management and Organization, 16*(1), 100–112.
105. Van Woerkom, M., & Croon, M. (2009). The relationships between team learning activities and team performance. *Personnel Review, 38*(5), 560–577.
106. Luft, J. (1969). *Of human interaction*. Mayfield.
107. Luft, J., & Ingham, H. (1955). *The Johari window: A graphic model of interpersonal awareness in Proceedings of the Western Training Laboratory in Group Development*. University of California.
108. Koca, G. Ş., & Erigüç, G. (2020). The effects of communication skills levels of health professionals on the dimensions of the Johari Window model. *International Journal of Healthcare Management, 13*, 434–446.

Chapter 6
Coaching for Staff Well-Being

This chapter explores the second purpose of patient safety coaching in a healthcare setting—to improve staff well-being and job satisfaction so that staff are fully "present" with patients and alert to their care needs (Fig. 6.1). Keeping patients safe from harm relies on clinical staff being focused and on-purpose every minute of their shift. A concentration failure could result in dire consequences. Leaders have an obligation to ensure that all staff are fully "present" as they work, mindful of patient needs and concerns, and aware of any organizational barriers or constraints that may impede progress or cause patients harm. Staff who present to shift alert, self-aware, and confident in their ability to perform well are able to navigate through the trauma that may result following an adverse event. Coaching is a developmental process that helps staff overcome this trauma. It nurtures physical, mental, and emotional well-being so that staff can provide excellent patient care. Staff well-being is the sum of their resourcefulness, resilience, and emotional commitment to compassionate care. Staff who are motivated, enthusiastic, and empowered demonstrate the emotional strength that inspires confidence in all around them. Patients benefit when staff operate "in the flow" on a daily basis, supported by leaders who coach them when necessary to help them learn, grow, and develop to become excellent clinical practitioners.

6.1 Occupational Stress and Patient Safety

Occupational stress has been identified in the literature as a key factor contributing to the occurrence of adverse events in healthcare. Stress is a harmful physical and emotional response that occurs when healthcare workers are confronted with job demands and pressures that are outside of their current knowledge, skills, and abilities, making it difficult for them to cope. It is one of the leading reasons for physical and mental problems among healthcare staff and leads to lower productivity in

© The Author(s), under exclusive license to Springer Nature Switzerland AG 2024

S. Knowles, *Patient Safety Coaching*,
https://doi.org/10.1007/978-3-031-68722-8_6

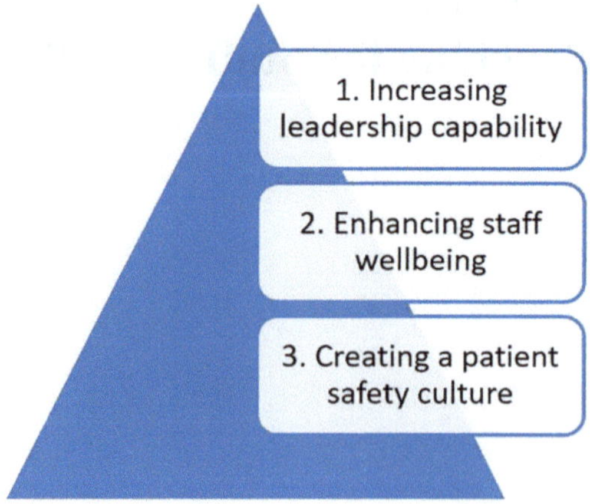

Fig. 6.1 Purposes of patient safety coaching

healthcare organizations. Staff shortages, work pressures, and underreporting of adverse events, all have an impact on the emergence of stress and the occurrence of adverse events, leading to an environment in which mistakes are more frequently made and patients suffer more harm [1]. Research has shown that job-related stress affects organizational performance, service delivery, and outcomes [2].

Reduced service delivery may impact the effectiveness and quality of the care provided by staff, particularly nurses who are generally at the forefront of patient treatment. Zabin et al. [3] reviewed the extant literature which examined the relationship between job stress and patient safety culture among nurses. The results showed a significant relationship between job-related stress and patient safety culture, since nurses who are stressed are more likely to make mistakes. Similarly, Suptitz Carneiro et al. [4] reported that nurses, who spend most of their time with patients, play a crucial role in maintaining patient safety within their workplace. They care for and about patients and may become mentally, emotionally, and physically exhausted when overwhelmed and stressed by job demands, which may negatively impact patient safety. These researchers concluded that effective stress management measures need to be implemented to enable nurses and other healthcare staff to cope with job stress. They recommended that nursing managers and administrators take action to minimize nursing job stress to improve the healthcare work environment and provide the best possible outcomes for patients. Furthermore, they suggested that nurses should receive training in how to remain resilient, particularly when working in trauma-related care areas.

Another study by Malinowska-Lipień et al. [5] used the Polish adaptation of the *Safety Attitudes Questionnaire* (SAQ) to evaluate 606 nurses' and 527 physicians' attitudes toward patient safety in surgical and medical wards in 21 Polish hospitals. They found that both nurses and physicians scored highest in stress recognition, with staff working in surgical wards experiencing more stress than those working in medical wards. The study revealed that 87% of nurses and almost 80% of physicians rated working conditions as a significant factor influencing patient safety—principally staffing resources, which may be a trigger to indicate the need to increase the number of nurses in medical and surgical wards to optimize patient safety. Aiken et al. [6] reported that even increasing the workload of nurses by one patient increased the risk of death within 30 days of admission to the hospital. These results indicate the importance of implementing strategies to assist staff in coping with occupational stressors and workload to improve patient safety. The World Health Organization (WHO)'s *Global Patient Safety Action Plan: 2021–2030* was produced to provide managers with strategies that can be adapted to the local context to do just this [7].

6.2 Categories of Stress in Healthcare

Everyone responds differently to stress depending on their personality, cultural background, social circumstances, past experiences, stage of life, support networks, and the situation in which they find themselves. Life stressors that may add to workplace stressors include relationship issues, personal/family illness, social isolation, and financial pressures. These situations cause particular stress when there is a mismatch between the situation and the person's ability to deal with it.

As a reflective practice, coaching transforms behavior by developing coachees' awareness of the need to change [8]. Coaching supports individuals and teams to discover solutions to issues where, in the past, they have been constrained by established ways of thinking and doing, to the detriment of patients. A meta-analysis investigating the effectiveness of individual coaching in an organizational setting revealed that coaching has significant, positive high correlations with individual-level outcome categories of coping and goal-directed self-regulation, and three intermediate correlations with performance/skills, well-being, and work attitudes [9].

In an increasingly globalized, complex environment, healthcare professionals are experiencing unprecedented levels of occupational stress—from work trauma, overload, fatigue, and exhaustion—which may lead to burnout [10]. Leaders who learn how to deliver patient safety coaching[1] are able to provide team members with exceptional support during times when they need it the most. The causes of stress in the healthcare environment are usually due to work-related issues or to the trauma staff have experienced as a result of being involved in or witnessing an adverse event.

[1] To find out more about coaching and how to deliver patient safety coaching, go to www.professionalcoachtraining.com.au and download the course brochure.

6.2.1 Work Induced

Work-induced stress factors in the healthcare environment often relate to factors beyond an individual's control such as work hours, workload, work rosters, staffing ratios, shift changes, availability of resources, and equipment conditions. Challenges may also be triggered by stress related to excessive changes in routine and varied procedures, as well as possibly bullying and harassment [11–14]. Team members at all levels need to be flexible so that they can respond faster and more effectively to organizationally generated patient safety challenges, because higher stress and burnout in healthcare professionals has been linked with the delivery of poorer quality, less safe, patient care across healthcare settings [3, 4, 15, 16].

Stress is a natural reaction as the body tries to deal with demands or pressures imposed on it by external forces, internal intentions, or goals, e.g., meeting a work deadline or preparing for an exam. Positive stress can lead to productive outcomes. However, too much stress or prolonged stress can negatively affect both physical and mental well-being. Long-term exposure to stress and exposure of the body to high levels of stress hormones such as cortisol and adrenaline can lead to increased vulnerability to illnesses such as depression, obesity, and heart disease. Taking steps to cope with stressful situations is important so that individuals can function and live productive lives.

When stress becomes too much for individuals to cope with, it can lead to burnout [4, 17, 18]. Burnout develops when individuals are unable to replenish personal energy resources to effectively address workplace challenges. This state can lead to emotional exhaustion, cynicism, and inefficacy [19, 20]. Emotional exhaustion is experienced as a result of both physical and mental exhaustion. Feeling burnt-out often leads to depersonalization which can result in a significant reduction in personal fulfillment, and insensitive and distant attitudes toward patients [21]. The healthcare professional feels incompetent and incapable of performing even their regular, daily work functions. Hence, burnout poses risks not only to clinicians themselves but also to their patients.

Dunbar et al. [17] recruited 41 cardiologists across five ambulatory cardiology clinics into a randomized controlled trial. They used the *Maslach Burnout Inventory* [19, 20] to assess levels of burnout and found that the clinicians most prone to burnout are those performing high-risk procedures, working in emergency departments, having serious discussions with patients about their condition, and treating diseases that are likely to result in significant risks of mortality or even morbidity. Compared with their male colleagues, female cardiologists reported lower emotional exhaustion scores. Those with 15 years or more in practice experienced high levels of emotional exhaustion, indicating moderate burnout. They concluded that mid-level cardiologists might be at the highest risk of emotional exhaustion.

Healthcare organizations that focus on creating a positive and supportive work environment for staff ensure that they receive proper training and support, feel able to speak up about any problems or concerns, and are empowered to take on additional responsibilities only if desired. Additionally, they ensure that staff are provided with adequate breaks and time off to help them maintain their physical and mental health.

6.2.2 *Trauma Induction*

Trauma-induced stress factors in the healthcare sector can refer to both the physical and psychological trauma experienced by healthcare workers due to their work. Physical trauma may include occupational injuries and illnesses acquired while performing their duties. This can range from needle stick injuries and burns to musculoskeletal disorders resulting from sustained physical activity. Psychological trauma may include the psychological stress associated with long and unpredictable hours, the emotional toll of caring for critically ill patients, and the challenges of providing care in an environment with ever-changing regulations and standards. Healthcare workers may experience additional trauma due to being involved in, witnessing, or hearing about traumatic events experienced by patients [22].

The body deals with trauma by activating the primal "fight-flight-freeze" mechanism [23] which releases chemicals that tell the body that it is in danger and needs to prepare for a response. A surge in these chemicals causes increased heart rate, rapid breathing, dry mouth, and sweating. These short-term responses do not harm physical health and are generally useful in assisting people manage the demands placed on them by making them more alert, energized, and attuned to external cues. However, in cases of severe psychological distress, medications and counseling might be prescribed by the individual's doctor.

Traditionally, to support staff experiencing trauma, healthcare organizations have implemented workplace strategies to reduce occupational injuries and illnesses, provided access to counseling and support services, and delivered education and training about how staff can recognize and manage stress. These are all Safety-1 strategies. Organizations adopting a Safety-11 perspective [24] also use coaching to encourage open dialog and respect for staff and their needs.

6.3 Coaching for Staff Well-Being

The healthcare sector is one of the most demanding and challenging professions, and as such, it is imperative that staff feel supported and valued by their employers. Coaching is a Safety-11 [24] strategy that addresses staff well-being issues caused by working conditions or trauma from adverse events. Through coaching, healthcare organizations can help to create an environment that is conducive to positive staff well-being.

Coaching has been found to be particularly beneficial in reducing trauma reactions to adverse events. It helps coachees process their feelings and thoughts about the event and allows them time and "head space" to better manage their emotions

[25]. Coachees learn how to recognize signs of stress, trauma, and burnout, and how to create healthy boundaries between work and personal life [26]. Coaching helps them regain a positive mindset and outlook on life following a traumatic event. This process is enhanced when leaders create a supportive work environment that encourages healthy communication [27].

Patient safety coaching can alleviate the effects of work-related and traumatic stress when coaches listen empathetically to coachees and help them understand what happened, come to terms with the situation, and take action to make change. Coaching helps staff overcome adversity, become more compassionate in relation to themselves and others, and become more resilient in the face of seemingly constant change [27, 28]. Through coaching, staff become more self-aware, mentally strong, emotionally resilient, happy, and confident. They are supported in identifying the things that are going *right* in their life and doing more of these things, while not neglecting the necessities of what sustains them in life and work.

In a research study, nurses who experienced being coached described it as helping them recognize and modify behaviors that hampered their performance; in doing so, they were able to improve their effectiveness and that of their team [29]. In another study, the coaching behaviors of nurse leaders were measured using the *Coaching Behavior Scale*, a survey tool designed to assess leadership coaching behavior (LCB) among nurses, first developed by Stowell [30] and revised by Ko and Yu [31]. The LCB is composed of 13 questions scored on a 5-point Likert scale measuring four behavioral factors: direction (3 items), development (3 items), performance evaluation (3 items), and relationships (4 items). The total scores range from 13 to 65 points. Higher scores indicate that the coaching behavior of a leader is perceived as positive. The overall perception of LCB for each respondent was calculated by taking the average scores of the 13 items in the LCB questionnaire. Individuals with a high score were placed in the high-performance coaching group, and the rest were placed in the low-performance coaching group. High-performing nurses were more likely to report errors than were their low-performing counterparts. Researchers concluded that a flexible culture can promote patient safety and error reporting within a healthcare organization by developing trust and improving the leadership capabilities of nurses.

6.4 Purposes of Coaching for Staff Well-Being

When staff are stressed and close to burnout, they often need patient safety coaching to assist them in taking back control of their life so that they can stay focused and centered on their job and live a happy life. The issues that confront them can be categorized into a number of areas that relate to how they feel and what they think they are able to do to bring their lives back to "normal". These issues are areas for possible coaching. Patient safety coaching begins by identifying the coachee's most important issue at that time, which may be one of the seven main purposes of coaching for staff well-being (Fig. 6.2).

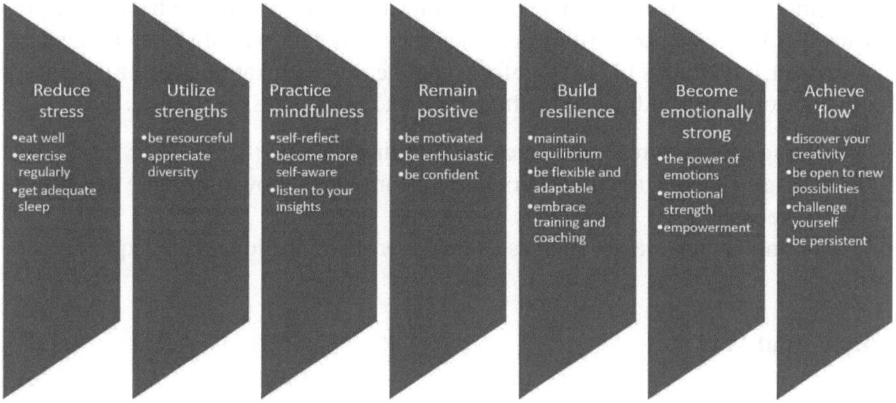

Fig. 6.2 Purposes of coaching for staff well-being

6.4.1 Reduce Stress

The first area that patient safety coaching explores with coachees is the level of stress they are experiencing and ways to reduce it. Stress can manifest as sleeplessness, headaches, excessive eating and drinking, lack of motivation and concentration, lethargy and listlessness, moodiness, feeling overwhelmed or anxious, and inability to cope with daily demands or responsibilities. Broadly speaking, there are two approaches to reducing occupational stress: (i) reduce work demands or (ii) increase workplace support [32]. Interventions that focus on reducing work demands aim to change the job factors and workplace conditions that create stress. Recommendations for strategies to do this, conducted separately or in concert, include the following:

- Having an open-door policy where staff can approach leaders with any concern or issue.
- Establishing clear expectations for staff performance and providing regular feedback to ensure that they are meeting expectations.
- Creating a supportive workplace environment by encouraging open communication and collaboration among colleagues.
- Encouraging staff to maintain a healthy work-life balance by limiting overtime, allowing flexible scheduling, and encouraging vacation time.
- Investing in technology that can help reduce stress levels by streamlining processes and simplifying tedious tasks.
- Implementing team building exercises to help foster positive relationships and communication among colleagues.

These are everyday recommendations to reduce stress in the workplace. In addition, organizational support is generally available via training programs, employee assistance programs, and access to counseling services. However, these interventions, while well-documented as ways to reduce burnout in healthcare professionals [33], have been criticized, since they may fail to address the real causes of stress for individuals [34]. Therefore, healthcare organizations with a Safety-II [24] perspective use additional methods to reduce staff stress including:

- Providing access to resources such as coaching.
- Encouraging healthcare professionals to prioritize their own self-care and mental health needs.
- Promoting healthy habits such as exercise, proper nutrition, and adequate sleep.

6.4.1.1 Eat Well

Stress is one of the main psychological factors that leads to overeating. People who are stressed often experience a change in appetite—often an increased drive to eat unhealthily—e.g., by choosing sweet or processed foods such as desserts or burgers which could lead to obesity. Research has shown that increased stress is associated with a number of biomarkers for obesity including binge eating, disinhibited eating, and ineffective efforts to regulate eating.

Patient safety coaching explores the coachee's attitude toward and approach to food and drink. Poor nutrition can lead to reduced immunity, increased susceptibility to disease, impaired physical and mental development, and reduced productivity. The coach encourages coachees to eat a healthy balanced diet as dictated by their cultural norms, noting that they may also have spiritual reasons and beliefs for choosing a certain nutritional regimen. Regardless of their food preferences, coachees are encouraged to choose whole foods rather than processed or fatty foods and to limit their intake of convenient, prepackaged foods. Discretionary foods that are high in saturated fats, added salt, added sugars, or alcohol should be avoided because they tend to be low in fiber and lack important nutrients such as vitamins and minerals. These foods are best consumed in small amounts on special occasions such as when celebrating a particular event, e.g., birthday, wedding, or public event.

6.4.1.2 Exercise Regularly

Exercise is the second self-care method by which stress can be managed. A regular exercise routine helps coachees structure their environment and reestablish familiar ways of coping. Exercise prompts the body to release hormones such as endorphins which helps individuals feel less stressed. The exercise does not have to be extreme. A simple walk around the block for 20 minutes will be enough to reduce stress levels as the stress hormones are released. Muscles that may contract subconsciously can relax with exercise.

National guidelines for exercise recommend that any form of exercise is better than none, that exercise should be conducted daily if possible, and that exertion should gradually increase as fitness levels improve. They recommend strength and muscle training 2–3 times per week plus moderate or vigorous physical activity. For adults aged 18–64, 150–300 min of moderate-intensity physical activity per week or 75–150 min of vigorous-intensity physical activity improves health. Pedometers should record approximately 10,000 steps per day.

It is recommended that coachees keep an exercise journal so that they become more aware of the way they are exercising and moving their body. Progress can be recorded and compared with baseline data; patterns of exercise and movement will emerge to inform the coaching sessions.

6.4.1.3 Get Adequate Sleep

The third aspect of self-care that patient safety coaching addresses is sleep—specifically, the number of hours that coachees sleep and their sleep pattern. Shift workers in healthcare settings often face challenges in maintaining a healthy circadian rhythm due to irregular work schedules and exposure to artificial light at night. This disruption can lead to a lack of sleep or disturbed sleep patterns which may be a major contributor to stress levels, with potential long-term health consequences. A good indicator of whether the coachee is getting enough sleep is how they feel in the morning (bright/alive or groggy/unsettled). If the latter, or if they find themselves falling asleep at work, needing a coffee fix to get through the day, or feeling drowsy driving to or from work, they are definitely not getting enough sleep—or good quality sleep. Light therapy, which is specifically tailored for shift workers, has been shown to be beneficial for managing circadian rhythm disruption. At times, however, coachees may need a professional assessment of their sleep patterns to rule out conditions such as sleep apnea.

Overall, patient safety coaching to reduce stress encourages coachees to:

- Energize their body through what they eat and drink.
- Exercise their body to experience improved mood and energy—physical movement oxygenates the blood, clears the mind, and stimulates "feel good" endorphins.
- Get enough sleep at night to recharge for the next day—research has shown that sleep deprivation impairs immune regulation, metabolic control, and neurocognitive processes such as learning and memory.
- Establish consistent, daily health routines such as rising at the same time each morning—this will develop stable and predictable circadian rhythms that will put their body in the best biochemical state to deal with any emotional incidents during the day.

6.4.2 Utilize Strengths

The second area that patient safety coaching explores is how coachees' strengths are utilized at work. This is because when coachees are stressed, they can become uncertain, lack confidence, and forget their strengths and internal capacity. Patient safety coaching can bring coachees back to who they were (and still are really!) by taking them back to first base—the time when they were fully functional—and felt that they were making a meaningful contribution to life and work. The coach does this by reigniting their passion for doing more of the things they love and are good at—that utilize their strengths—just as they used to do.

Coachees' strengths in the healthcare setting typically relate to their technical capabilities as clinical professionals—although they may have lost some confidence in their ability to perform to peak performance due to an adverse event. Nontechnical strengths may include their ability to relate well to others, be supportive of team members, and express compassion. Coaches help coachees reconnect with their innate strengths and abilities and acknowledge ownership of these strengths without the prospect of obvious reward. For example, nonphysical strength is any trait or psychological characteristic that the coachee displays across different situations and over time such as courage, conviction, and persistence. Moral strengths that the coachee has learned and developed over time may include kindness, supportiveness, and concern for others. People choose to acquire a strength and then to retain it, often as a result of reinforcement of the display of this strength. Coaches ask coachees to identify those strengths they consider strong as well as those they may consider lesser strengths and remind them that, as people are not always self-aware, others may see strengths in them that they do not recognize in themselves.

The Johari window (Fig. 6.3) is a useful tool for explaining this concept [35, 36]. Coachees self-reflect on their strengths according to two dimensions—"Known to Self" and "Known to Others." Strengths that are "Open" are known to both the self and others. "Blind" strengths are known to others but not to the self. "Hidden"

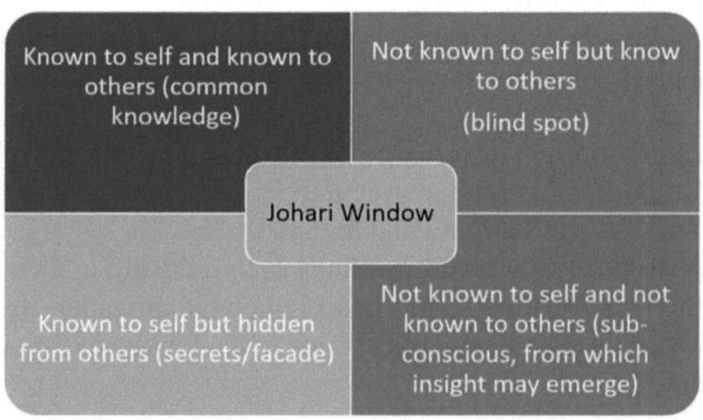

Fig. 6.3 Johari Window (Luft and Ingham [36])

strengths are those that one keeps to oneself. Strengths that are "Unknown to Self and Others" only come to be known under exceptional circumstances, e.g., a person being able to lift a car off a road accident victim. Coachees may ask others such as friends and family members to give them feedback on what they see as their greatest strengths. Patient safety coaching helps coachees rebuild the strengths they may have forgotten or relegated in priority.

6.4.2.1 Be Resourceful

When coachees utilize their strengths, they are being resourceful—possibly in new or novel ways. Being resourceful requires persistence, not taking "No" for an answer, and trusting that the desired outcome is in their best interests. The solutions they develop from "out-of-the-box" thinking are both creative and unique. Resourceful people are confident, explorative, proactive, and persistent. They "back themselves" and have the backing and support of significant others.

It is important that coachees are flexible in terms of the outcomes or goals they desire from life/work, as these may need to be adjusted if internal or external circumstances change. For example, setting goals and actions cannot be a linear process unless timelines are short and nothing in the external environment changes—which is unlikely in work environments. Individuals can only control their actions, not the actions or timelines of others.

Resourcefulness can be built in coachees when they:

- Use problem-solving skills to look at a situation, challenge, or goal in a different, unexpected way.
- Are open-minded to new and different possibilities, opportunities, people, views, suggestions, and experiences.
- Focus on what they "can do" rather than what they "cannot do."
- Expand their comfort zone by undertaking new experiences, meeting new people, and learning about new things.

The coach can ask questions such as the following to help coachees develop their resourcefulness:

- Is there another way to get what you want?
- Is the desired result truly the best result?
- Who else has information that might help you?
- What is something very similar to what you need that might also work?
- Who is an expert in this area?
- What is one more thing you can try?
- What would someone you admire do in this situation?

6.4.2.2 Appreciate Diversity

The healthcare workforce is multicultural. A diversity of clinical strengths, skills, and expertise is held by workers from a number of cultures with a variety of beliefs and perspectives. This cultural diversity adds richness to the healthcare system as staff learn and grow from observations of different clinical practices. It is important that coachees understand and value the diversity of cultures, beliefs, and perspectives within their team to successfully engage meaningfully with individuals. It is also essential that they recognize that cultural diversity is not limited to only race, ethnicity, and nationality but also encompasses gender, religion, sexual orientation, age, physical and mental abilities, and socioeconomic status.

Just as leaders need to appreciate the diversity within their healthcare team to ensure that all team members feel that they belong, they also need to respect and appreciate the diversity of the patients in their care. This is especially important so that patients receive equitable, high-quality care that is appropriate for their individual care needs. For example, staff may need to have training in the provision of culturally sensitive care. By understanding and respecting the cultural diversity of their patients, healthcare workers can provide better patient care and create a more inclusive environment.

Similarly, the healthcare sector is becoming increasingly aware of the need to recognize and honor spiritual diversity among its patients. Spiritual diversity can be observed in a variety of ways, from the recognition of faith-based healing rituals to the celebration of cultural holidays and traditions. Spiritual diversity in healthcare can provide comfort and support to patients who may struggle with difficult medical or emotional issues. It can also help to create an atmosphere of trust and understanding between healthcare organizations and patients. For example, if a patient is a member of a faith-based community, the organization may be able to provide appropriate resources and support in recognition of the importance of that faith to the patient's healing process. Similarly, if the patient celebrates a particular holiday or tradition, the healthcare organization may be able to provide a safe and supportive space in which the patient can express their beliefs. In this way, recognizing and honoring spiritual diversity in healthcare can help to create an atmosphere of mutual respect and understanding between healthcare organizations and their patients.

In addition, healthcare organizations may include a number of staff and patients with neurodiversity. These individuals may have been diagnosed with conditions such as autism, ADHD, dyslexia, dyspraxia, or psychological/psychiatric conditions. These people provide unique perspectives on patient care and treatment. The challenge for healthcare leaders is to recognize, understand, and accept the neurological differences that exist among staff and patients. Examples of how the healthcare sector can better accommodate neurodiversity include the following:

- Developing an understanding of the different types of neurodiversity as well as the unique needs of neurodiverse individuals.
- Offering patient-centered care tailored to the needs of neurodiverse individuals.
- Encouraging staff and patient education and self-advocacy.

- Providing specialized patient care and services such as sensory integration therapy to address the needs of neurodiverse individuals.
- Incorporating neurodiversity into medical education and training to ensure that healthcare professionals are prepared to recognize and respond to the needs of neurodiverse individuals.
- Developing policies and procedures to ensure that neurodiverse individuals, their families, and caregivers are provided with equitable access to quality patient care.

In summary, an inclusive healthcare organization maximizes the diversity of its workforce so that staff members feel that they "belong" to the team, department, and organization, i.e., they have a sense of being accepted, and respected. Their strengths are recognized and valued. Their differences are used to explore other ways of working. They are included in discussions on patient care and treatment options and are involved in the decision-making process. At all times, they know they are supported by senior management, believe they are important members of the team, and feel valued by colleagues. Belonging helps staff feel motivated and engaged in their work which tends to lead to improved patient care and satisfaction.

6.4.3 Practice Mindfulness

The third area that patient safety coaching explores with coachees is the degree to which they are mindful. Mindfulness has been defined as attention to, and awareness of, the present moment which does not seek to react to or classify experience [37]. Individuals who are mindful accept their everyday momentary thoughts, feelings, and perceptions without censure [38]. Mindfulness enhances their ability to express respectful attitudes and behaviors in everyday life. By fostering emotional detachment to thoughts and feelings that constantly flow through one's mind without self-evaluation [39], mindfulness increases self-reflection and self-regulation, reduces stress, and promotes empathy for others including patients [40]. Mindfulness training encourages individuals to focus their attention and observe their thoughts, emotions, and behaviors at a particular point in time [41].

Individuals who practice mindfulness become more alert to, and observant of, stimuli in their external environment as they work [42]. Mindfulness practices have been shown to have a positive effect on well-being [37] and long-term quality of life [43]. The beneficial effects of mindfulness practices on mental health [44], task persistence and performance-related stress [45], and proactivity [46] have also been demonstrated. When healthcare staff are not mindful, unconscious biases, perceptions, and judgments may form in relation to colleagues and patients [47]; consequently, they may dehumanize others or treat them with less respect [48]. Hence, mindfulness practice is important in healthcare settings so that staff are fully "present" with patients as they deliver care. The *Mindful Attention Awareness Scale* [37] may be used to measure the relationships between mindfulness and psychological health and functioning.

Contemporary mindfulness training techniques (such as mindful breathing and body scan techniques) have been shown to have therapeutic effects on clinical conditions such as depression, anxiety, and chronic pain [49, 50]. Mindfulness training programs have also been found to exercise, strengthen, and remediate dysfunctional brain networks that regulate frontostriatal circuits, restoring an adaptive balance between top-down and bottom-up processes [51]. They facilitate cognitive control over drug-related automaticity, attentional bias, and drug cue reactivity while enhancing responsiveness to natural rewards [51]. Cognition manipulation enables the mind to create new neural behavior pathways because of its malleability and neuroplasticity [52, 53].

6.4.3.1 Self-Reflect

Mindfulness practice is based on the meditative practice of self-refection which is "the extent to which an individual pays attention to and evaluates [their] internal states and behaviors" [46]. It is a deliberate process aimed at reducing personal biases [54] and now widely accepted as a valuable developmental tool [55]. Self-reflection allows individuals time and space to examine and review past feelings, actions, and their consequences and reevaluate prior beliefs and thoughts to develop insight for future responses [56, 57]. Self-evaluation during self-reflection creates a cycle of growth and development [58] which promotes well-being and life satisfaction [59, 60] and leads to self-awareness and insight.

6.4.3.2 Become More Self-Aware

Self-awareness was originally viewed as a therapeutic tool to alleviate psychological distress in clinical patients. However, more recently, researchers have focused on self-awareness as an important component of self-development in nonclinical populations [46]. Self-awareness has been variously defined as the awareness of one's own feelings and ability to recognize, manage, and control these feelings [61], an overarching awareness of one's mental states and environments [59], and "a conscious awareness of one's internal states and interactions with others" [46]. The practice of self-awareness includes the observation and management of feelings and thoughts to protect and improve the *self* [55].

When individuals are self-aware, they have the ability to see themselves as others do [62]. Those with a higher level of self-awareness have increased self-knowledge [63] and a stronger sense of identity [64], are less influenced by external factors [65], are more likely to acknowledge responsibility for their actions [66], and have a greater sense of well-being [59]. They can take an external perspective since focusing on the *self* necessitates understanding the perspective of others [67].

Healthcare staff who have a heightened sense of self-awareness generally have increased awareness and understanding of others, including their patients.

6.4.3.3 Listen to Your Insights

Insight is the clarity generated when individuals self-reflect on their internal states and external visible behaviors. It has been defined as "the reorientation of one's thinking, including breaking of the unwarranted 'fixation' and forming of novel, task-related associations among the old nodes of concepts or cognitive skills" [68]. Those with cognitive flexibility are able to increase their psychological well-being [59] by cognitively restructuring their approach to a problem or how they interpret it to generate insight [69].

The insight generated from using conventional problem-solving methods is usually a gradual, incremental process [70, 71]. However, when unconventional methods are used, insight experience may appear "like dynamite … [exploding] on the solver's cognitive landscape with breathtaking suddenness" [72]. The "Aha!" experience, which generates insight and one-time learning, comes from "out-of-the-box" thinking, which changes how the problem is viewed or constructed [73, 74]. Insight experiences have been associated with feelings of ease, pleasure, and confidence when a problem is solved [75].

In summary, patient safety coaching shows coachees how to use mindfulness techniques in their daily lives to promote self-reflection, generate self-awareness and insight, enrich their life/work experiences, and support a positive mental state.

6.4.4 Remain Positive

The fourth area that patient safety coaching explores with coachees is the degree to which they have a positive approach to life and work. Addressing the coachee's mindset is important because strengthening the body will not sustain change unless the mind is also strengthened. Hence, the role of the coach is to assist coachees in adopting a positive mindset and attitude toward life and work.

The patient safety coaching process is underpinned by the following coaching practices that support the development of a positive mental mindset:

1. *Challenge mental model.* Positive psychology coaching challenges the coachee's mental model of the world from one that is *against* them to one that is *for* them—a negative to a positive—to assist coachees in understanding how they can take action to create a more positive future. The coach also challenges the coachee's underlying assumptions and limiting beliefs to create an understanding of how they can do things *right*. Self-determination theory [76] proposes that we are in charge of our own thoughts and feelings and, as such, we determine our future.

2. *Reframe mental mindset.* Patient safety coaching encourages coachees to consider what they *can* do rather than what they *cannot* do to reorient their thinking into a positive mental mindset. A fundamental tool of positive psychology is the focus on strengths to promote learning, growth, well-being, and happiness.
3. *Practice mindfulness.* Coachees are encouraged to practice mindfulness to increase their *self-awareness* of who they are and what they stand for, and to generate *insight* into how they can move forward to achieve their dreams.
4. *Promote self-efficacy.* Ultimately, it is the coachees' belief in themselves that will get them through. Self-efficacy [77] acknowledges what cannot be changed (e.g., due to illness, past experiences, or external factors such as a pandemic) and recognizes that we must try and possibly fail, to succeed.
5. *Encourage openness, honesty, and flexibility.* The coach's role is to support the coachee in becoming more creative and to explore and discover new perspectives. These attributes are the prerequisites for the development of new knowledge, learning, and growth. There is no denial, justification, or externalization of blame during the patient safety coaching process—simply the coachee's acceptance of responsibility for their actions and the outcomes.

Coachees can develop a stronger and more positive mental attitude toward life when they adopt the following principles.

1. Seek to find what's *right* in their life rather than what's *wrong*.
2. Look on the "bright side"—be open to discovery, creativity, and possibilities—learn to "live in the grays."
3. Learn from mistakes that are never "failures"—just learning opportunities. If we never made a mistake, we would be "perfect"—which nobody is.
4. Make goals SMART (specific, measurable, attainable, realistic, time-bound)—which gives purpose and meaning to life. Even small goals, when achieved, make us feel good.
5. Surround themselves with a supportive network of family and friends—those who listen, acknowledge how they feel, and are there for them no matter what.
6. Meditate—to channel a higher-order spirit as their guide to improved mental strength.
7. Utilize and build on their strengths.
8. Develop resourcefulness and resilience.[2]
9. Live true to their values, to find their authentic self.
10. Believe in themselves so they can become the person they truly want to be.

[2] Discussed later in this chapter.

6.4.4.1 Be Motivated

Being and remaining positive is sometimes difficult to do. Life and work demands can get in the way. Experiencing happiness and looking after your health and well-being every day requires a degree of determination and motivation. Happy people generally do not need to be motivated to maintain their self-worth. However, at times, they do need to "reboot" their system, e.g., if they feel overwhelmed and their self-esteem drops, or they become demotivated. On these occasions, the role of patient safety coaching is to help coachees reconnect with their motivation and purpose, identify their next step, and take action toward achieving it. The very act of taking action is, in itself, motivating since that first step typically leads to the next and the next… until they return to their former self. Take action, and the motivation will follow.

According to Daniel Pink [78], motivation comprises three key elements: autonomy, mastery, and purpose. Autonomy is our "default" setting. We strive to be autonomous and self-directed. People need autonomy over what they do and how they do it. Unfortunately, circumstances do not always allow such freedom as we are frequently constrained by forces outside of our control, e.g., policies and procedures, regulations, and laws. Learning how to identify which rules and regulations are "necessary" for the coachee's health and well-being and which ones are "optional" (perhaps self-imposed) is an outcome of the coaching. Mastery is the drive to become better at something that matters—a mindset that requires individuals to view their capacity and abilities as subject to improvement; as such, mastery is never attained because we can always keep improving. Purpose is the driving force that propels us to do and be our best; it gives us the motivation to keep going even against all odds to achieve a certain goal or reach an end-point. Purpose gives meaning to our daily activities and a reason to live.

Most people are familiar with Maslow's basic drive for "self-actualization" which we all strive for [79] and with the three motivations that drive people principally at work: achievement, affiliation, and power [80]. Csikszentmihalyi [81] suggested several other ways in which individuals are motivated at work including: being challenged by feasible tasks that require the skills they possess, being encouraged and trusted to carry out tasks, and receiving regular feedback to clarify how to progress these tasks. In addition, people value being listened to and supported, having a sense of control over their life and work, being kept informed and appreciated, and having assistance in developing their skills and abilities.

6.4.4.2 Be Enthusiastic

Enthusiasm is the energy we bring to a task. When we are motivated, we invest energy to reach the desired outcome. When we are disinterested, we conserve our energy for something more interesting. People enjoy being around enthusiastic people. Their zeal and inspiration are contagious. Enthusiasm is created by our thinking so, if the coachee is disinterested, there are a few techniques that coaches can use to increase their level of enthusiasm for a particular task, including the following:

1. *Revisit why the task matters*. Why is it important (to the coachee or to others) that the task gets done? What do they want to accomplish, achieve, or obtain by completing the task?
2. *Pretend.* Act "as if" they are enthusiastic. The mind tells the body what to do so if the coachee adopts a mindset of enthusiasm, a stronger posture and presence will follow. Furthermore, posture can influence hormone production so when individuals stand tall and confidently approach a task, enthusiasm generally follows.
3. *Briefly do something they love* before they tackle the necessary task. This will get them into a better frame of mind, and the feelings of happiness and enthusiasm will flow over into the task that they have to do next.
4. *Avoid energy drainers*. Surround themselves with enthusiastic, supportive, and energetic people. Talk to someone who loves performing that task and find out what they love about it.
5. *Practice gratitude*. What opportunity (for learning, growth, development, or something else) does this task present? Who would be grateful to have the opportunity to complete this task? Who will be grateful for having the task completed? How will the coachee feel when it is done?
6. *Undertake random acts of kindness*. Ask the coachee to do something nice for someone else without any thought of reward or favor coming their way.

6.4.4.3 Be Confident

Confidence is not something that can be learned like a set of rules. Confidence is a state of mind—the outcome of feeling secure in oneself and your abilities and being able to trust yourself. One way for coachees to become more confident is for them to breakdown tasks into smaller achievable goals. Confident people know that they can experience any emotion (including "failure") without losing their overall opinion of themselves. Confidence comes from feelings of well-being, acceptance of one's body and mind (one's self-esteem), and belief in one's own ability, skills, and experience.

What you think of yourself is what generates or depletes self-confidence. Hence, the way we think about ourselves determines whether we feel confident or not. Fear does not prevent self-confidence; rather, the unwillingness to feel fear does. People are not born with self-confidence; you have to learn it by keeping your word and doing what you say you are going to do. The ability to trust yourself comes from consistent follow-through on your word to yourself and others. Unfortunately, too many people spend too much time in self-doubt because they do not know whether they can handle everything that comes their way. The outcome of not being able to handle a situation may be an emotional upset—but at least you've tried! When coachees are willing to experience any emotion and know that it is the worst that can happen, this is a great starting point for developing self-confidence.

Coachees become more confident when they receive criticism and reply in a non-defensive way so as not to lower their self-esteem. They consider the criticism, make sure that they understand what is being said, and then use this information as feedback and a way to learn and improve. However, remember that criticism is just the opinion of somebody else so, rather than simply accepting it, encourage coachees to think about whether the criticism is about them and their behavior or whether it is a projection based on the other's personal experience. Alternatively, when they receive a compliment, have them thank the person and ask what exactly they liked. This will help coachees recognize their own achievements and celebrate them with family and friends.

Above all, coachees should be encouraged to believe in themselves—that they can achieve a particular task or perform to a certain level—and utilize their strengths to do so. This will stop their critical self-talk, which they can replace with positive messages of self-encouragement.

6.4.5 Build Resilience

The fifth area that patient safety coaching explores is how to build resilience in the face of adversity. Life and work often throw us "curve balls"—things and events we didn't expect and have to respond (or react) to—sometimes very quickly. Patient safety coaching supports coachees who continually work in stressful environments such as healthcare, which requires precision care in what could be life-threatening situations, to become more resilient.

Resilience interventions are one type of workplace support intervention that are generally acceptable and effective at increasing coping ability across populations and occupational groups [93, 94]. They proactively develop the psychological skills that contribute to the maintenance of staff well-being. Several studies have shown that resilience interventions may confer a range of benefits to healthcare professionals, including lower levels of depression and burnout, and increased well-being [98–100]. However, resilience interventions cannot fix problems endemic in healthcare systems; other types of organizational change interventions are required to make these corrections.

6.4.5.1 Maintain Equilibrium

Resilience is the term used to describe an individual's capacity to maintain equilibrium in response to difficult experiences [82]. Resilient individuals are more likely to be open to new experiences and more flexible and emotionally stable in the face of adversity [83]. They are typically more amenable to change, experience fewer negative emotional and physical consequences when faced with change, and are more likely to adapt to and implement the required changes. Resilience is fundamental to managing stress and anxiety in an emotionally challenging environment [95]. At extreme levels, low resilience has been associated with mental health issues and even death [96, 97].

Leadership is perceived as a key component in the promotion of resilience and the control of burnout within organizations. Hence, the way that leaders manage their own stress and potential burnout is an important role model for staff. In essence, leader burnout has negative trickle-down effects as it impacts employees' communication, relationships, cognitive performance, decision-making skills, and productivity [106]. Therefore, healthcare leaders need to understand their own ability to lead actively and productively when excess pressure is applied, which may cause them and others to stretch beyond their endurable limits. Instead, their role is to model resilient behavior and support team members in doing the same. One way to increase resilience is by receiving patient safety coaching.

In an attempt to establish and measure biomarkers for resilience, researchers conducted a control study to explore the possibility of estimating personal resilience using physiological and speech signals measured during human–robot conversations [101]. The physiology-based predictors included the galvanic skin response (GSR), electrocardiogram (ECG), and heart rate variability (HRV). This study confirmed the possibility of estimating personal resilience from HRV data which can be conveniently collected from wearable devices. This would allow medical practitioners to be informed of the data prior to patient consultations to avoid putting too much pressure during hospital interactions on those who have registered low in resilience and may quickly become stressed.

6.4.5.2 Be Flexible and Adaptable

Within healthcare settings, resilience has been described as the capacity to adapt to challenges and changes at different system levels to maintain high-quality patient care. Research has explored how stakeholders and systems adapt and cope with a large range of variations to enable high-quality care [86]. Researchers coined the term "adaptive capacity" which is the ability to adapt to external and internal demands by reframing, aligning, coping, and innovating [87]. From their research, Fagerdal et al. [88] concluded that leaders are key actors in everyday healthcare systems and facilitate organizational resilience by supporting adaptive capacity in hospital teams. Leaders enhance their teams' adaptive capacity by a number of means including building sufficient competence in their teams; balancing workload, risk, and staff needs; providing relational leadership; and emphasizing situational understanding and awareness through the provision of timely and relevant information.

Resilience has been variously defined as an individual trait-like capacity, an adaptive process for overcoming adversity, and an outcome of successful event adaptation [89]. As a trait, resilience is the ability to resist or positively manage individual stress [90]. As a process, resilience is derived from experiencing and surviving an unexpected, generally adverse, event [91]. As an outcome, resilience is achieved as a result of increased competence and confidence after a traumatic event, which can have positive impacts such as being better able to deal with future competing demands and enhancing work relationships [92].

As a phenomenon, resilience is related to organizational responses to disruptions, turbulence, and discontinuities, and involves the ability of individuals to endure and adapt to new risk environments [84]. Given that organizational change may represent an "adverse" situation for many staff, the ability to adapt to and even thrive during change could offer significant benefits for both healthcare workers and organizations [85].

6.4.5.3 Embrace Training and Coaching

The value of resilience training for healthcare workers to help them balance academic and clinical application pressures is widely acknowledged [102, 103], although researchers are divided as to when such training should be conducted. Some researchers recommend that resilience training be conducted as part of the early career curriculum in preparation for later professional life, since newly qualified healthcare professionals are particularly vulnerable to the psychological impact of stressful healthcare events and may need to be prepared for an adverse event before it arises [15, 104, 105]. However, it is possible that these early clinicians may be less likely to comprehend the impact of adverse events when they have never witnessed one; hence, they may not be able to fully appreciate the value of this training at the beginning stage of their career.

Within the healthcare literature, a number of studies have reported that healthcare organizations have attempted to provide better support for healthcare professionals from a resilience perspective. For example, several studies have utilized the *Promoting Resilience in Stress Management* (PRISM) intervention which is a resilience-coaching program that has been shown to mitigate distress and improve quality of life among adolescents and young adults with serious illness [107–110]. PRISM is a skill-based training program in which recipients learn to develop and apply key resilience skills during challenging circumstances.

An approach initiated by North Memorial Health in the USA during the COVID-19 pandemic was to employ a new category of worker called a Resilience Coach whose role was to alleviate high levels of staff stress and burnout and promote well-being through flexible, evidence-based, peer-focused support options. It was reported that more than one-third of North Memorial Health's 6,400 staff members sought assistance from the Resilience Coach during the first six months of this role [111].

Additionally, during the pandemic, resilience coaching was introduced to an academic hospital in Toronto, Canada, to support the psychological well-being of staff [112]. The coaching was delivered by 13 Resilience Coaches from an interdisciplinary team including psychiatrists, mental health nurses, allied health staff, and a senior bioethicist. The Resilience Coaches provided positive psychosocial support to colleagues but also noted the challenges to delivering coaching such as finding time within busy work schedules, balancing role tensions, and working while experiencing burnout. They concluded that hospital-based mental health professionals are well positioned to support colleagues' wellness during acute crises and that this work is meaningful. Researchers have suggested that paired coaching and peer support among the coaching group may mitigate some of the challenges they experienced.

Another study in 2020 focused on a prevention-based approach to adverse events, aimed at emotionally preparing healthcare professionals before they occurred, to reduce negative impacts [34]. The intervention was designed to provide generalizability to a range of healthcare professional disciplines. A tailored resilience coaching intervention comprising a workshop followed by one-on-one coaching sessions was implemented to address the specific challenges in participants' workplaces. Following the intervention, participants reported greater confidence in coping with adverse events as well as greater relevant knowledge and greater levels of general resilience. This gain was maintained at each post-baseline time point. The feedback data following the workshop were overwhelmingly positive; all participants agreed or strongly agreed that the training was engaging and relevant to their discipline and said they had learned useful skills. The researchers concluded that these results support the feasibility of delivering a psychological resilience intervention to multidisciplinary healthcare professionals, and provide preliminary evidence that this may be an effective method to improve practitioners' confidence in their ability to cope with adverse events, and enhance their general resilience.

Another example of a resilience training program incorporating coaching is that developed through collaboration between Imperial College London and Harvard Medical School. Researchers trained cohorts of medical students and faculty members in coaching skills to help them mitigate burnout, maintain more rewarding, person-centered conversations in clinical practice, and personally enable them to respond flexibly and adapt constructively to change [15]. They encouraged participants to use coaching skills in virtual consultations with patients to support health behavior changes during the COVID-19 pandemic when in-person consultations were considerably reduced. A key aspect of the training involved participants working in pairs to coach each other on an issue that they would like to address (e.g., an approach to studying, well-being, improving interactions with patients). Subsequently, Imperial College London launched a freely accessible short massive online open course (MOOC) in *Coaching Skills for Learner-Centered Conversations* to provide further support to their students and faculty as well as to support educators and students worldwide who wanted to learn how to incorporate coaching approaches into teaching and learning programs.

Coaching was also used as an intervention by researchers who conducted a brief, structured coaching program of three 90-minute coaching sessions over a six-week period to investigate whether a coaching intervention could increase a coachee's level of resilience and confidence to address organizational change [85]. The coaching was skill based to develop resilience rather than developmental, which is usually delivered by more experienced coaches. The researchers concluded that brief, skills (behavior)-focused coaching is a potentially effective method to enhance an individual's resilience and change their personal orientation. It was also an accessible and affordable means of providing support to workers in adverse conditions. Subsequently, one of the researchers replicated the study but added a workbook and learning goals to the methodology [113]. She concluded that new realizations, insights, and opportunities for self-reflection were critical in assisting coachees to look beyond their current solutions and mindset to achieve greater openness, flexibility, and different perspectives.

6.4.6 Become Emotionally Strong

The sixth area that patient safety coaching explores with coachees is how to support them in becoming emotionally strong. The coach will have already addressed with them how to eat well, exercise, and get enough sleep. They will have identified how to utilize their strengths and become more resourceful, be more mindful every day, and maintain a positive mindset in the face of adversity. Now, it is time to address how they can develop their emotional strength which will allow them to stay resilient even in the most horrific situations as can occur in healthcare settings. Feeling emotionally secure in themselves and being able to manage their emotions while maintaining their sense of care and humanity are essential characteristics of healthcare workers.

6.4.6.1 The Power of Emotions

Emotions are derived from conscious or subconscious thoughts and experiences that trigger a positive or negative reaction to an event. They all have meaning and value as triggers to our awareness of what is currently happening in our world and what we need to do differently.

As human beings, we may be cognitively aware of a situation that triggers an immediate reaction or, alternatively, an awareness may "creep up on us" as the event unfolds, triggering a delayed reaction. We may express our emotions immediately, or we may try to hide them so that they are not obvious to others. If the latter, we may need to express those emotions at a later time to family or friends so that the emotions do not take over our thought processes and subsequent actions. As part of their journey to become emotionally well, coachees may need to share with the coach the details of an event that caused them to express or repress deep emotions, such as being involved in or witnessing an adverse event.

The most useful approach that the coach can take is to allow coachees' emotions to surface, assist them in embracing the discomfort they feel, and discourage avoidance of the issue. As emotions surface, these previously "Unknown" emotions become known to "Self" and "Others" [35] in the quiet, confidential coaching space. The goal of the coach is to bring coachees back to a state of emotional and psychological well-being, so that they can regain their equilibrium and ability to perform their normal daily functioning. If the emotion is more deep-seated, a referral to their doctor or counseling support services may be needed.

During coaching about an emotional issue, the first step is getting coachees to recognize, label and accept the emotion, and understand the positive intention of the emotion in bringing an important issue to their consciousness so that it can be dealt with. Often, unhealthy habits are created through the desire to resist, deny, or avoid uncomfortable emotions. Developing emotional intelligence [114] is one of the most significant tasks that coaches can guide coachees toward—the ability to identify and label emotion, allow the experience of that emotion to surface, and constructively address ways to manage it now and in the future. Coachees can develop the ability to monitor their emotions, create useful emotions on purpose, and adjust their mindset and behavior accordingly.

The next step is to work with coachees to ensure that they are not defined by their emotions, i.e., that they do not consider themselves to be weak, insignificant, or unworthy. The coach's role is to separate the emotion from the individual and work with the coachee as an individual who is able to manage their emotions in appropriate ways. This is an active process that involves thinking about the emotion and its trigger as separate from *Self*, looking at it in the plain light of day, and identifying the source of the trigger and dealing with it—be that a stressor, a person or an event. The coach aims to reframe how the coachee thinks about the stressor, person, or event in a way that defines it as an "object" that they can manage next time it is encountered. Shaping how they think about the "object" into a learning experience will surface actions to address future events. Mind you, some events cannot be changed and must be "lived with," e.g., significant illness or death. Some ways that coachees may learn to deal with emotions include drawing on their inner strength, utilizing external resources, being flexible, remaining resilient, and seeking support from family and friends.

6.4.6.2 Emotional Strength

People who are mentally strong generally feel emotionally strong. Emotionally strong means that their basic needs for love and belonging are met. They like themselves and others like them too. They feel safe and secure "in their own skin" and are confident about who they are and what they stand for. Those coachees who do not feel emotionally strong have somehow lost their way, and it is the role of the coach to guide them back to who they truly are or toward who they want to become.

People who feel emotionally strong have learned to look to the future, learn from the past, and live in the present. They are confident in themselves and their decision-making ability and open to new ways of living and being. They have dreams, hopes, and aspirations about what might lie ahead for them and are realistic about what is in their control to act upon or do. Their inner power is grounded in creating a renewed future based on a philosophy of "If it's not yet attained, it just needs more time, or a different perspective, or a different approach." There is no blame, justification, or recrimination for goals not yet achieved. If they are meant to be, they will form part of their future.

Investing highly in trying to create this future in the short term may lead to burnout and possibly despair. Hence, coachees are encouraged to take a slower, moderated approach to the attainment of their innermost dreams so they can sustain for the long term. In the meantime, coaches support them in gaining meaning, purpose, and happiness from the everyday activities they engage in now, as they live in the present. Negative thinking, e.g., "the world is skewed against people like me," or "I just haven't been trying hard enough," will bring them down. Positive thinking will align their thoughts, feelings, intentions, and desires with that future state and maintain mental and emotional wellbeing. Remember that dreams, hope, and aspirations do not have to be SMART (specific, measurable, attainable, realistic, time bound) [115]. They can seem unattainable and yet still be motivational (e.g., to win $1M on the lotto) as long as the coachee does not act as if the dream has already become a reality (e.g., resign from their job). The dreams may include the coachee's fondest wishes and desires—the things they would like to be, do or have—but are not yet ready or able to create in their life.

If coachees are ready to work on creating their dreams, hopes, and aspirations, it can be helpful for them to consider them as projects rather than as specific goals to be achieved. Projects have a shorter lifespan and are focused on the day-to-day activities that need to be performed. They are things to work on, not toward. Projects have actions that can be carried out every day, culminating in the achievement of longer-term goals, e.g., studying for 2 h a day (project) to obtain a qualification within 12 months (goal). Every day is a success when the 2 h have been completed. Of course, there will be challenges along the way, so coachees should be realistic in not aiming to study every day but pledging to study for, say, 5 days out of 7. In this way, they have a short-term, weekly target to aim for and do not need to find excuses when they miss a day. In addition, they have choice and control over the activity in terms of which days they study.

6.4.6.3 Empowerment

Once coachees have identified their major stressors and ways to overcome them, they can apply these strategies to their current lifestyle. Personal empowerment comes from setting realistic goals to fulfill one's potential and then taking action. People who feel empowered are in control of their life. They capitalize on their strengths and refuse to focus on their weaknesses unless that is necessary. They are self-aware and make positive choices based on the available evidence coupled with personal intuition. Building personal empowerment involves coachees reflecting on their personal and core values and beliefs and being prepared to adjust their behavior to achieve their desired goals.

Some strategies to help coachees achieve their hopes, dreams, and aspirations much sooner than they ever thought possible include the following:

1. *Take full responsibility for where they are now*. Their current state is the result of the choices they made with the information that was available to them at that time. However, as time has passed, they now know more and can do more and are able to do things differently. They cannot change the past; there is no going back. The role of the coach is to help them live in the present and envisage a more positive future. Change can only occur after people stop looking outside for someone to blame and start to take full responsibility for their past actions. This is when they reclaim ownership of their life and let in abundance as they accept everything that they have done—the good and the bad—as the entirety of their life's work and journey thus far.
2. *Visualize the future they desire as vividly as they possibly can*. Visualization is a powerful technique for creating abundance. Making a physical reminder of their goal can help (e.g., by constructing a vision board or collage, painting a picture of what the future looks like for them, or assembling a model or slide presentation). The coach asks them to express the energy and happiness behind each action they take as they move further toward their end goal, and to note what actions work for them and what actions do not—then reflect, adjust, and continue.
3. *Specify a "reward" they will give themselves once the goal has been achieved*. The "reward" needs to be specific (e.g., frame the graduation certificate, celebrate with friends). Each week, they might meditate for, say, 15 min to visualize claiming this reward—being "in the moment" when it is attained. They might also include "progress claims" toward achieving this reward to maintain the study momentum—small goals to keep them motivated and indicate success.
4. *Hold a positive mindset and use positive, active language* to express their needs and desires. Research into language suggests that a person's self-image is reflected in the words they use. For example, when people say they "should" behave in a certain way, this implies passivity and can detract from their seeming to be in control and taking responsibility for their actions. Alternatively, talking about oneself in a positive way and acknowledging strengths and weaknesses can be empowering. The coach encourages coachees to use words that imply positive action rather than vague statements, particularly when talking about the future, e.g., use "I am..." and "I can..." to start positive proclamation rather than negative statements.

6.4.7 Achieve "Flow"

The seventh area that patient safety coaching explores with coachees is how they can live their best life in "flow." What does this mean? It means searching for what gives your life joy and meaning, being open to new possibilities, challenging yourself, and being persistent.

6.4.7.1 Discover your Creativity

Mihaly Csikszentmihalyi was a contemporary psychologist who studied happiness and creativity, optimal experience, and the evolving self. He coined the term "flow" [116] which he described as a state of being when a person gives their fullest attention to a task that is performed for intrinsic reasons (i.e., for the pure pleasure that it gives the person rather than as a means to an end). The activity takes the person's complete attention, and as a result, their mind is totally absorbed in what they are doing to the exclusion of events and people around them. They are in a state of "flow."

Think back to a situation when you were totally absorbed in an activity and completely lost track of time; you missed your next appointment. When you are in a state of "flow," your entire being is immersed in the activity and everything seems to be working together in complete harmony. Your performance is at its peak, and you achieve an optimum level of clarity and focus without even thinking about it. You are not judging every move or planning your next move—you are just letting it unfold.

In "flow," your ego withdraws, making way for the process to happen, unimpeded. You are not conscious of hunger, thirst, fatigue, or anything outside of the activity. All worries, thoughts, and memories have melted away. Time flies by and you are completely unaware of it, as if you have stepped outside of it for the moment. You become one with what you are doing when you are in that state of "flow."

> *Flow is important both because it makes the present instant more enjoyable and because it builds the self-confidence that allows us to develop skills and make significant contributions to humankind* [116].

Csikszentmihalyi noted that artists fell into a particular state of mind while they were working, characterized by an intense focus and great concentration on the task at hand, to the point of losing track of time for hours on end. He observed six factors that characterize a "flow" experience.

- You are completely involved in what you are doing—completely focused and concentrated.
- There is a sense of ecstasy—of being outside of everyday reality.
- There is great inner clarity. You know what needs to be done, and you receive immediate feedback on how well you are doing it.
- You know that the activity is doable—that you have the necessary skills to complete the task successfully.

- You lose your sense of self, and all your worries and concerns drift away.
- You lose track of time—you are completely focused on the present moment.
- There is an intrinsic motivation—whatever produces "flow" becomes its own reward.

6.4.7.2 Be Open to New Possibilities

Earlier we discussed the concept of burnout when a person is over-challenged and under-resourced to achieve a particular task. They may lack the time or resources to complete the task, or the skill required may be beyond their current level of expertise. For these reasons, they "fail" the task, and their self-esteem and confidence plummet. Csikszentmihalyi "unpacked" this concept of burnout when he proposed eight possible categories of "state" that people may experience in relation to a task to be achieved, based on the level of challenge that the task presents, and the person's ability to achieve it.

His framework suggests that if the degree of challenge and the person's ability to perform the task are both low, they will experience *apathy*. If their ability to perform is more advanced, they may be *bored* as they perform the task or see the task as a recreational challenge. As the level of challenge increases, individuals may start to *worry* that they may not be able to complete the task, which could result in *anxiety* as their level of *arousal* increases. However, if they find that the task is within their ability to perform, they take *control* of themselves and the task which, with full concentration and focus and the absence of external distractions, leads to *flow*—a state in which they feel *relaxed* and confident. Think about scientists "holed up" in their laboratories for days on end as they conduct experiments that may change the world. They do not think about eating, sleeping, or personal hygiene. All they think about is what they are doing *in that moment*. Their "flow" state drives them to continue the task regardless of what is happening around them.

6.4.7.3 Challenge Yourself

Because the "flow" state can be all-consuming and most people do not have the luxury of staying focused and concentrating for too long, it is wise for coachees to establish smaller "chunks" of goals that they can complete in one session and feel satisfied with the result (e.g., reading the next chapter of a book, researching a particular topic). Coachees may have to learn new skills before they tackle the task. The task should be challenging enough to require their full concentration but not too challenging that they cannot even begin to think about how to get started.

Setting clear goals gives coachees a sense of control over the outcome and a sense of "reward" when they are achieved. The coach encourages coachees to identify a time and place to complete the task so that they will not be disturbed. When and where is the best time and place to read the latest Journal? If they choose a busy thoroughfare in their home, they are setting themselves up for "failure." The role of the coach is to help coachees select the time and place that will most likely lead to successful completion of the task. Coachees are encouraged to turn off their computer and phone for the duration of the activity, since it takes about 25 minutes to regain full attention once people are distracted.

Before the coachee starts on a task, the coach recommends that they declutter their mind from all thoughts and distractions that may bother them while they complete the task (e.g., use the bathroom, return a phone call). The best way to keep their brain hydrated is by drinking water during the task so that their energy level remains high, and they do not become fatigued or "foggy-brained." Coachees are encouraged to make a list of things "to-do" later on to get these thoughts out of their mind. Then, they may like to perform a short visualization meditation, a focused body scan, or breathing exercises for a few minutes—whatever makes them feel good. Background meditative music may assist them to concentrate and eliminate low-level distractors.

6.4.7.4 Be Persistent

Coaches usually recommend that coachees choose the most appropriate time of day to complete a task. Mornings are best because the mind is fresh and energy levels are high. However, if this is not possible, an alternative is after a break of 15–30 min, which has given the brain time to regenerate 50% of its capacity. It may assist coachees to have their brain give them a mental reminder that it is time to go into a state of "flow" by having them devise and anchor a mantra each time they wish to go into this state. Their brain adjusts and recognizes this cue on subsequent occasions. Practicing "flow" will help them get better at it. They may start with a simple task and, after a while, build to tasks of more importance as time goes by and as they gain in competence and confidence. Achieving a state of "flow" is a skill that can be acquired with practice.

6.5 Patient Safety Coaching for Staff Well-Being

As we have seen from the above discussions, the second purpose of patient safety coaching is to enhance staff well-being by first addressing their stress level and then supporting them in developing strategies to utilize their strengths, practice mindfulness, remain positive, build resilience, become more emotionally strong, and achieve a state of "flow."

Patient safety coaching is delivered by healthcare leaders and clinical coaches who have been formally trained to deliver coaching to individuals in organizations by using, e.g., the ©AIPC COACH model.[3] When *Coaching for Staff Well-Being*, the coach focuses on and reinforces the following:

---

[3] The ©AIPC COACH model is explained in Chap. 4.

- Coachees' strengths, interests, and passions.
- What is going *right* in their life.
- What brings them most joy and happiness in life.
- What sustains them and what makes their heart sing.

To begin the coaching session, the coach seeks information about the coachee's physical body activities in relation to daily/weekly food and drink intake, exercise, and sleep. One or more of these areas may be the critical issue that the coachee is grappling with or, alternatively, the discussion may reveal how well the coachee is managing in relation to these areas given the stress they are experiencing. Thereafter, the coaching session continues by asking: "What's the most important thing we should be talking about today?" and proceeds from there to discover what's on the coachee's mind for which they seek resolution. The agenda is coachee-driven, with no preconceived expectations regarding outcomes, except as expressed by the coachee as their desired goal, e.g., becoming more enthusiastic about work, utilizing a particular strength, achieving a professional milestone, or becoming more confident in their ability to lead. Coaching continues for as many sessions as required to achieve this goal.

Key Takeaways

- Leaders who coach their staff can relieve them of stress which, at the extreme, may result in burnout and limit their retention in the healthcare sector.
- Occupational stress is a debilitating condition that not only impacts negatively on healthcare staff but also reduces the level of care that patients receive.
- Stress may be either work-related by factors such as work overload, staff shortage or equipment failure, or trauma-induced when staff are involved in or witness an adverse event.
- There are multiple purposes for healthcare staff to receive coaching including to: reduce work-related or trauma-induced stress; find ways to better utilize their strengths; show them how to practice mindfulness and remain positive; help them build resilience, become emotionally strong, and achieve a state of flow.
- When staff are coached for their own well-being, they feel valued and acknowledged for the work they do and their commitment to patient care.

6.6 Case Study 6: Staff Well-Being After a Significant Incident

Dr. Samantha Lee, an experienced anatomical pathologist, received a call one Friday afternoon from Dr. Singh, a senior oncologist at the hospital. He had important information regarding a recent case. "Samantha, I need to discuss a patient, Mr. John Roberts. He initially presented with gastric discomfort some months ago, and we have now diagnosed him with advanced gastric cancer. Upon reviewing his initial biopsy, it appears there was an adenocarcinoma section that was missed."

Dr. Lee felt a growing sense of anxiety as she listened. Her mind was racing. She vividly remembered the case, having carefully examined the slides. The realization that she had missed a critical diagnosis was deeply troubling. Dr. Singh continued: "Unfortunately, this event has delayed Mr. Roberts' diagnosis and subsequent treatment. As a result, his options for life-prolonging therapy are now limited." It became apparent that the hospital was going to commence an investigation into this outcome for Mr. Roberts and that Dr. Lee would need to be involved in a family meeting.

Dr. Singh took time to explain that an investigation was needed to identify everything along the course of Mr. Roberts' medical journey that did not go to plan. He shared his experience that poor outcomes were rarely the result of one thing going wrong; more often, they were the result of a series of failures, omissions, or errors that went unnoticed or unreported.

Dr. Lee acknowledged the situation's seriousness. She wondered if she would lose her job and felt responsible for Mr. Roberts' shorter life expectancy. The knowledge that her oversight had potentially impacted a patient's prognosis weighed heavily on her. That weekend she was distressed and had trouble sleeping.

On Monday, the hospital's medical governance coordinator, Dr. Namali, phoned Dr. Lee to advise her of the process for the investigation and family meeting. At the same time, it was Dr. Namali's standard practice to enquire about the well-being of staff involved in an investigation. Dr. Lee sounded tired and anxious. Dr. Namali listened attentively to hear her out completely, reflecting back how Dr. Lee was feeling and what her anxieties were. Over the course of the conversation, Dr. Lee understood that there were many unknowns about the situation and that the investigation was likely to find several issues. Dr. Namali was able to assist Dr. Lee reframe the events into an opportunity to connect with the patient and his family and apologize and, following the investigation, find ways to make the system even more robust. This gave Dr. Lee the strength to meet with the family face to face, with the intention of working together to prevent a future occurrence of diagnostic delay. This meant that the family could ask detailed questions about pathological processes and felt that they were being supported through this event.

For Discussion

1. Discuss the various purposes of coaching for staff well-being.
    - How would you coach healthcare leaders to put supportive processes in place for staff who have experienced or witnessed an adverse event?
2. How would you coach someone experiencing trauma associated with a work-related event?
    - What happened in this case study? What, specifically, did Dr. Namali do to support Dr. Lee's well-being?
    - What could have been done differently?

3. Let us assume that part of the reason for this error was later discovered to be high workload for the anatomical pathologists.
   - How would you coach someone experiencing work overload?

References

1. Wami, S. D., et al. (2016). Patient safety culture and associated factors: A quantitative and qualitative study of healthcare workers' view in Jimma zone hospitals, Southwest Ethiopia. *BMC Health Services Research, 16*(1), 495.
2. Chatzigianni, D., et al. (2018). Occupational stress experienced by nurses working in a Greek regional hospital: A cross-sectional study. *Iranian Journal of Nursing Midwifery Research, 23*(6), 450–457.
3. Zabin, L. M., et al. (2023). The relationship between job stress and patient safety culture among nurses: A systematic review. *BMC Nursing, 22*(1), 1–7.
4. Suptitz Carneiro, A., et al. (2021). Occupational stress, burnout and patient safety culture among workers from critical care and non critical care units in a hospital in Brazil. *Intensive Critical Care Nursing, 63*, 102978.
5. Malinowska-Lipień, I., et al. (2021). Nurses and physicians attitudes towards factors related to hospitalized patient safety. *PLoS One, 16*(12), 1–13.
6. Aiken, L. H., et al. (2014). Nurse staffing and education and hospital mortality in nine European countries. A retrospective observational study. *Lancet, 383*, 1824–1830.
7. WHO. (2021). *Global Patient Safety Action Plan 2021–2030:Towards eliminating avoidable harm in health care*. World Health Organization, License: CC BY-NC-SA 3.0 IGO.
8. Hiatt, J. (2006). *ADKAR: A model for change in business, government and our community: How to implement successful change in our personal lives and professional careers*. Prosci Research.
9. Theeboom, T., Beersma, B., & van Vianen, A. (2014). Does coaching work? A meta-analysis on the effects of coaching on individual level outcomes in an organizational context. *The Journal of Positive Psychology, 9*(1), 1–18.
10. Long, J. C., et al. (2021). The pace of hospital life: A mixed methods study. *PLoS One, 16*(8), 1–12.
11. Arnetz, J. E., et al. (2019). Organizational determinants of bullying and work disengagement among hospital nurses. *Journal of Advanced Nursing, 75*(6), 1229–1238.
12. Schlitzkus, L. L., et al. (2014). Workplace bullying of general surgery residents by nurses. *Journal of Surgical Education, 71*(6), e149–e154.
13. Quine, L. (1999). Workplace bullying in NHS Community Trust: Staff questionnaire survey. *British Medical Journal, 318*, 228–232.
14. PSC. (2010). *Trends in bullying in the Victorian Public Sector: People matter survey 2004–2010*. Victorian Public Sector Commission.
15. Maini, A., et al. (2020). Coaching skills for medical education in a VUCA world. *Medical Teacher, 42*(11), 1308–1309.
16. de Lima Garcia, C., et al. (2019). Association between culture of patient safety and burnout in pediatric hospitals. *PLoS One, 14*(6), 1–14.
17. Dunbar, T. K., et al. (2022). Characteristics associated with burnout among cardiologists in an academic medical setting: Baseline survey results from a Communication Coaching RCT. *Behavioral Sciences, 12*(10), 362.
18. LeNoble, C. A., et al. (2020). To address burnout in oncology, we must look to teams: Reflections on an organizational science approach. *JCO Oncology Practice, 16*(4), e377–e383.
19. Maslach, C., & Jackson, S. (1981). The measurement of experienced burnout. *Journal of Occupational Behavior, 2*, 99–113.

20. Maslach, C., Schaufeli, W., & Leiter, M. P. (2001). Job burnout. *Annual Review of Psychology, 52*, 397–422.
21. Franca, F. M., et al. (2012). Burnout and labour aspects in the nursing teams at two medium-sized hospitals. *Revista Latino-Americana de Enfermagem, 20*(5), 961–970.
22. Hyland, P., et al. (2014). Rational beliefs as cognitive protective factors against post-traumatic stress symptoms. *Journal of Rational-Emotive & Cognitive-Behavior Therapy, 32*(4), 297–312.
23. Corr, P. (2016). Reinforcement sensitivity Theory of personality questionnaires: Structural survey with recommendations. *Personality and Individual Differences, 89*, 60–64.
24. Hollnagel, E., Wears, R., & Braithwaite, J. (2015). *From safety-I to safety-II: A white paper*. University of Southern Denmark/University of Florida/Macquarie University.
25. Williams, H., Palmer, S., et al. (2013). *The Coaching Psychologist, 9*, 45–47.
26. Nixon-Witt, C. (2008). A coaching approach for Work/life balance. *Business & Economic Review, 54*(2), 8–11.
27. Grant, A., Curtayne, L., & Burton, G. (2009). Executive coaching enhances goal attainment, resilience and workplace well-being: A randomised controlled study. *The Journal of Positive Psychology, 4*(5), 396.
28. Boyatzis, R., Smith, M., & Blaize, N. (2006). Developing sustainable leaders through coaching and compassion. *Academy of Management Learning & Education, 5*(1), 8–24.
29. Ponte, P. R., et al. (2006). Using an executive coach to increase leadership effectiveness. *Journal of Nursing Administration, 36*(6), 319–324.
30. Stowell, S. (1986). *Leadership and coaching*. University of Utah.
31. Ko, Y., & Yu, S. (2017). The relationships among perceived patients' safety culture, intention to report errors, and leader coaching behavior of nurses in Korea: A pilot study. *Journal of Patient Safety, 13*(3), 175–183.
32. Demerouti, E., et al. (2001). The job demands resources model of burnout. *Journal of Applied Psychology, 86*(3), 499.
33. Panagioti, M., et al. (2017). Controlled interventions to reduce burnout in physicians: A systematic review and meta-analysis. *JAMA International Medicine, 177*(2), 195–205.
34. Johnson, J., et al. (2020). Can we prepare healthcare professionals and students for involvement in stressful healthcare events? A mixed-methods evaluation of a resilience training intervention. *BMC Health Services Research, 20*(1), 1–14.
35. Koca, G. Ş., & Erigüç, G. (2020). The effects of communication skills levels of health professionals on the dimensions of the Johari window model. *International Journal of Healthcare Management, 13*, 434–446.
36. Luft, J., & Ingham, H. (1955). The Johari window: A graphic model of interpersonal awareness. In *Proceedings of the Western Training Laboratory in group development*. University of California.
37. Brown, K., & Ryan, R. (2003). The benefits of being present: Mindfulness and its role in psychological well-being. *Journal of Personality and Social Psychology, 84*(4), 822–848.
38. Baer, R., et al. (2006). Using self-report assessment methods to explore facets of mindfulness. *Assessment, 13*(1), 27–45.
39. Shapiro, S., et al. (2006). Mechanisms of mindfulness. *Journal of Clinical Psychology, 62*(3), 373–386.
40. Thomas, J. (2017). Brief mindfulness training in the social work practice classroom. *Social Work Education, 36*(1), 102–118.
41. Lynn, R. (2010). Mindfulness in social work education. *Social Work Education, 29*, 289–304.
42. Brown, K., Ryan, R., & Creswell, J. (2007). Mindfulness: Theoretical foundations and evidence for its salutary effects. *Psychological Inquiry, 18*(4), 211–237.
43. Morgan, L., et al. (2014). Relationships between amount of post-intervention mindfulness practice and follow-up outcome variables in an acceptance-based behavior therapy for Generalized Anxiety Disorder: The importance of informal practice. *Journal of Contextual Behavioral Science, 3*(3), 173–178.

44. Gu, J., et al. (2015). How do mindfulness-based cognitive therapy and mindfulness-based stress reduction improve mental health and wellbeing? A systematic review and meta-analysis of mediation studies. *Clinical Psychology Review, 37*, 1–12.
45. Feldman, G., et al. (2014). Mindfulness and rumination as predictors of persistence with a distress tolerance task. *Personality & Individual Differences, 56*, 154–158.
46. Sutton, A. (2016). Measuring the effects of self-awareness: Construction of the self-awareness outcomes questionnaire. *Europe's Journal of Psychology, 12*(4), 645–658.
47. Heotis, E. (2018). Cultivating self-awareness: Dual processes in social cognition. *Journal for Spiritual & Consciousness Studies, 41*(1), 22–28.
48. Prati, F., et al. (2016). Humanizing outgroups through multiple categorization: The roles of individuation and threat. *Personality and Social Psychology Bulletin, 42*(4), 526–539.
49. Goyal, M., Singh, S., & Sibinga, E. (2014). Meditation programs for psychological stress and Well-being: A systematic review and meta-analysis. *Journal of AMA Internal Medicine, 174*(3), 357–368.
50. Chiesa, A., & Serretti, A. (2011). Mindfulness-based interventions for chronic pain: A systematic review of the evidence. *Journal of Alternate Complementary Medicine, 17*(1), 83–93.
51. Garland, E., et al. (2016). Mindfulness training applied to addiction therapy: Insights into the neural mechanisms of positive behavioral change. *Neuroscience and Neuroeconomics, 5*, 55–63.
52. Fox, K., Nijeboer, S., & Dixon, M. (2014). Is meditation associated with altered brain structure? A systematic review and meta-analysis of morphometric neuroimaging in meditation practitioners. *Neuroscience Biobehavior Review, 43*, 48–73.
53. Holzel, B., Carmody, J., & Vangel, M. (2011). Mindfulness practice leads to increases in regional brain gray matter density. *Psychiatry Research, 191*, 36–43.
54. Schön, D. (1994). *The reflective practitioner: How professionals think in action*. Routledge.
55. Feize, L., & Faver, C. (2019). Teaching self-awareness: Social work educators' endeavors and struggles. *Social Work Education, 38*(2), 159–176.
56. Bennett-Levy, J., et al. (2001). The value of self-practice of cognitive therapy techniques and self-reflection in the training of cognitive therapists. *Behavioural and Cognitive Psychotherapy, 29*, 203–220.
57. Pompeo, A., & Levitt, D. (2014). A path of counselor self-awareness. *Counseling and Values, 59*(1), 80–94.
58. Furman, R., Coyne, A., & Negi, N. (2008). An international experience for social work students: Self-reflection through poetry and journal writing exercises. *Journal of Teaching in Social Work, 28*(1/2), 71–85.
59. Harrington, R., & Loffredo, D. (2011). Insight, rumination, and self-reflection as predictors of well-being. *The Journal of Psychology, 145*(1), 39–57.
60. Richards, K., Campenni, C., & Muse-Burke, J. (2010). Self-care and well-being in mental health professionals: The mediating effects of self-awareness and mindfulness. *Journal of Mental Health Counseling, 32*, 247–264.
61. Dulewicz, V., & Higgs, M. (1999). Can emotional intelligence be measured and developed? *Leadership & Organization Development Journal, 20*, 242–252.
62. Zhao, S. (2018). What is reflective self-awareness for? Role expectation for situational collaboration in alliance animal society. *Philosophical Psychology, 31*(2), 187–209.
63. Morin, A. (2011). Self-awareness part 1: Definition, measures, effects, functions, and antecedents. *Social & Personality Psychology Compass, 5*(10), 807–823.
64. Ickes, W., Layden, M., & Barnes, R. (1978). Objective self-awareness and individuation: An empirical link. *Journal of Personality, 46*, 146–161.
65. Lefcourt, H., Hogg, E., & Sordoni, C. (1975). Locus of control, field dependence and the conditions arousing objective vs subjective self-awareness. *Journal of Research in Personality, 9*(1), 21–36.
66. Duval, S., & Wicklund, R. (1972). *A theory of objective self-consciousness*. Academic.
67. Stephenson, B., & Wicklund, R. (1983). Self-directed attention and taking the other's perspective. *Journal of Experimental Social Psychology, 19*, 58–77.

68. Luo, J., & Niki, K. (2003). Function of hippocampus in "insight" of problem solving. *Hippocampus, 13*, 316–323.
69. DeYoung, C., Flanders, J., & Peterson, J. (2010). Cognitive abilities involved in insight problem solving: An individual differences model. *Creativity Research Journal, 20*, 278–290.
70. Gruber, H. (1995). Insight and affect in the history of science. In R. Sternberg & J. Davidson (Eds.), *The nature of insight* (pp. 397–431). MIT Press.
71. Perkins, D. (1981). *The mind's best work.* Harvard University Press.
72. Durso, F., Rea, C., & Dayton, T. (1994). Graph-theoretic confirmation of restructuring during insight. *Psychological Science, 5*, 94–98.
73. Ollinger, M., Jones, G., & Knoblich, G. (2008). Investigating the effect of mental set on insight problem solving. *Experimental Psychology, 55*(4), 269–282.
74. Köhler, W. (1959). Gestalt psychology today. *American Psychologist, 14*, 727–734.
75. Topolinski, S., & Reber, R. (2010). Gaining insight into the "Aha" experience. *Current Directions in Psychological Science, 19*(6), 402–405.
76. Ryan, R., & Deci, E. (Eds.). (2017). *Self-determination theory: Basic psychological needs in motivation, development, and wellness*. ProQuest/Guilford Press.
77. Bandura, A. (1977). Self-efficacy: Toward a unifying theory of behavioral change. *Psychological Review, 84*, 191–215.
78. Pink, D. (2011). *Drive: The surprising truth about what motivates us*. Riverhead Books.
79. Maslow, A. (1943). A theory of human motivation. *Psychological Review, 50*(4), 370–396.
80. McClelland, D. (1955). *Studies in motivation*. New York Appleton-Century-Crofts.
81. Csikszentmihalyi, M., & Csikszentmihalyi, I. (1988). *Optimal experience: Psychological studies of flow in consciousness*. Cambridge Press.
82. Johnson, J., et al. (2017). Resilience to emotional distress in response to failure, error or mistakes: A systematic review. *Clinical Psychology Review, 52*, 19–42.
83. Avey, J. B., Luthans, F., & Jensen, S. J. (2009). Psychological capital: A positive resource for combating employee stress and turnover. *Human Resource Management, 48*, 677–693.
84. Bhamra, R. (2016). *Organisational resilience concepts, integration and practice*. Taylor & Francis.
85. Sherlock-Storey, M., Moss, M., & Timson, S. (2013). Brief coaching for resilience during organisational change – An exploratory study. *Coaching Psychologist, 9*(1), 19–26.
86. Anderson, J., et al. (2020). Multi-level influences on resilient healthcare in six countries – An international comprarative study protocol. *BMJ Open, 10*, e039158.
87. Lyng, H. B., et al. (2022). Exploring the nature of adaptive capacity for resilience in healthcare across different healthcare contexts; a metasynthesis of narratives. *Applied Ergonomics, 104*, 103810.
88. Fagerdal, B., et al. (2022). Exploring the role of leaders in enabling adaptive capacity in hospital teams: A multiple case study. *BMC Health Services Research, 22*(1), 1–17.
89. Fletcher, D., & Sarkar, M. (2013). Psychological resilience. *European Psychologist, 18*, 12–23.
90. Wehner, A., Fick, J., & Dishman, L. *A systematic literature review of the relationship between resilience and burnout among healthcare executives*. A.T. Still University.
91. Bryce, C., et al. (2020). Resilience in the face of uncertainty: Early lessons form the COVID-19 pandemic. *Journal of Risk Research, 23*(7–8), 880–887.
92. Clohessy, N., McKellar, L., & Fleet, J. (2019). Bounce back—Bounce forward: Midwifery students experience of resilience. *Nurse Education in Practice, 37*, 22–28.
93. Robertson, I. T., et al. (2015). *Resilience training in the workplace from 2003 to 2014: A systematic review., 88*(3), 533–562.
94. Joyce, S., et al. (2018). Road to resilience: A systematic review and meta-analysis of resilience training programmes and interventions. *BMJ Open, 8*(6), e017858.
95. Grant, L., & Kinman, G. (2015). Emotional resilience in the helping professions and how it can be enhanced. *Health and Social Care Education, 3*(1), 23–34.

96. Hiroeh, U., et al. (2001). Death by homicide, suicide, and other unnatural causes in people with mental illness: A population-based study. *Lancet, 358*, 2110–2112.
97. Dembling, B. P., Chen, D. T., & Vachon, L. (1999). Life expectancy and causes of death in a population treated for serious mental illness. *Psychiatric Services, 50*, 1036–1042.
98. Henshall, C., Davey, Z., & Jackson, D. (2020). The implementation and evaluation of a resilience enhancement programme for nurses working in the forensic setting. *International Journal of Mental Health Nursing, 29*(3), 508–520.
99. Slatyer, S., et al. (2018). Evaluating the effectiveness of a brief mindful self-care and resiliency (MSCR) intervention for nurses: A controlled trial. *Mindfulness, 9*(2), 534–546.
100. Foster, K., et al. (2018). On PAR: A feasibility study of the Promoting Adult Resilience programme with mental health nurses. *International Journal of Mental Health Nursing, 27*(5), 1470–1480.
101. Hsu, M., Chen, H., & Huang, R. (2021). Personal resilience can be well estimated from heart rate variability and paralinguistic features during human–robot conversations. *Sensors, 21*(17), 5844.
102. Pietrzak, R. H., & Cook, J. M. (2013). Psychological resilience in older US veterans: Results from the National Health and Resilience in Veterans study. *Depression and Anxiety Journal, 30*(5), 432–443.
103. Epstein, R. M., & Krasner, M. S. (2013). Physician resilience: What it means, why it matters, and how to promote it. *Academic Medicine, 88*(3), 301–303.
104. West, C. P., et al. (2006). Association of perceived medical errors with resident distress and empathy: A prospective longitudinal study. *JAMA, 296*(9), 1071–1078.
105. Martinez, W., & Lo, B. (2008). Medical students' experiences with medical errors: An analysis of medical student essays. *Medical Education, 42*(7), 733–741.
106. Thomas, C. (2022). Coaching and mentoring skills: A complement to the professional midwifery advocate role. *British Journal of Midwifery, 30*(5), 290–296.
107. Rosenberg, A. R., et al. (2015). Promoting resilience in stress management: A pilot study of a novel resilience-promoting intervention for adolescents and young adults with serious illness. *Journal of Pediatric Psychology, 40*(9), 992–999.
108. Lau, N., et al. (2019). Exploratory analysis of treatment response trajectories in the PRISM trial: Models of psychosocial care. *Psycho-Oncology, 28*(7), 1470–1476.
109. Rosenberg, A. R., et al. (2018). Promoting resilience in adolescents and young adults with cancer: Results from the PRISM randomized controlled trial. *Cancer, 124*(19), 3909–3917.
110. Steineck, A., et al. (2019). A psychosocial Intervention's impact on quality of life in AYAs with cancer: A post hoc analysis from the promoting resilience in stress management (PRISM) randomized controlled trial. *Children, 6*(11), 124.
111. Radick, L. E. (2022). Ready for what's next: Future-proofing the healthcare workforce. *Healthcare Executive, 37*(3), 16–24.
112. Rosen, B., et al. (2022). Providers' perspectives on implementing resilience coaching for healthcare workers during the COVID-19 pandemic. *BMC Health Services Research, 22*(1), 1–10.
113. Timson, S. (2015). Exploring what clients find helpful in a brief resilience coaching programme: A qualitative study. *Coaching Psychologist, 11*(2), 81–88.
114. Goleman, D. (2000). Leadership that gets results. *Harvard Business Review, 78*(2), 78–90.
115. Raia, A. (1965). Goal setting and self-control: An empirical study. *Journal of Management Studies, 2*(1), 34–53.
116. Csikszentmihalyi, M. (1990). *Flow: The psychology of optimal experience*. Harper & Row.

Chapter 7
Coaching to Develop a Patient Safety Culture

This chapter explores the third purpose of patient safety coaching in a healthcare setting—to develop a patient safety culture within frontline teams and across the entire healthcare organization (Fig. 7.1). In a psychologically safe workplace in which there is no blame or recrimination, near misses are reported, and staff learn from their mistakes. Routinely, they pay attention to observe and learn from excellent clinical practices to prevent the occurrence of adverse events. A patient safety culture is formed when all staff members share the values of patient safety, understand and share the meaning behind the words, are focused on a common purpose, and behave in ways that demonstrate commitment to patient safety. As a subculture of organizational culture, a patient safety culture is developed when healthcare leaders display patient safety behaviors in every situation, utilize a coaching leadership style, and support a bottom-up approach to cultural change within their team.

Patient safety is "the absence of preventable harm to a patient and reduction of risk of unnecessary harm associated with health care to an acceptable minimum." [1, 2]. *Patient safety culture* focuses on aspects of organizational culture that either support or hinder patient safety. Patient safety culture has been variously defined as "a pattern of individual and organizational behavior, based upon shared beliefs and values that continuously seeks to minimize patient harm, which may result from the process of care delivery" [3], "the values shared among organization members about what is important, their beliefs about how things operate in the organization, and the interaction of these with work unit and organizational structures and systems, which together produce behavioral norms in the organization that promote safety" [4], and "a set of values attitudes, perceptions, beliefs, and behaviors that support the safe conduct of individuals' activities in health organizations" [5].

When operationalizing these definitions to a healthcare environment, a patient safety culture describes "management and staff values, beliefs and norms about what is important in a health care organization, how organization members are expected to behave, what attitudes and actions are appropriate and inappropriate, and what processes and procedures are rewarded and punished concerning patient

© The Author(s), under exclusive license to Springer Nature Switzerland AG 2024

S. Knowles, *Patient Safety Coaching*,
https://doi.org/10.1007/978-3-031-68722-8_7

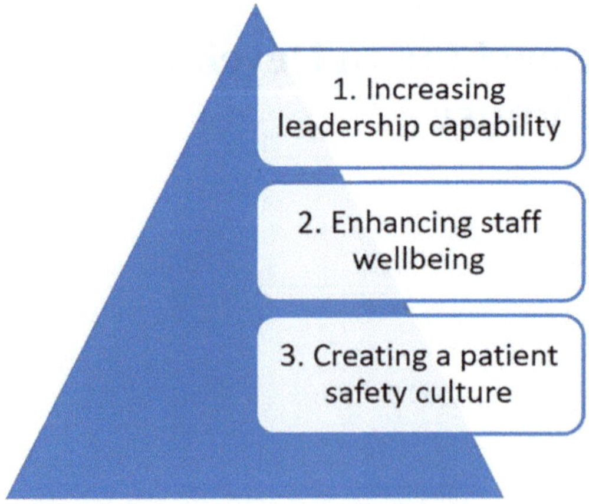

Fig. 7.1 Purposes of patient safety coaching

safety" [6]. In a patient safety culture, everyone is committed to the avoidance and prevention of patient injuries or adverse events resulting from the processes of healthcare delivery. Focusing on patient safety culture is crucial for minimizing adverse events and improving patient safety [7].

In an organizational context, the term "culture" refers to the "values, attitudes, norms, beliefs, practices, policies and behaviors of personnel" [8]. Research into organizational culture has identified the importance of four key components when developing a patient safety culture: shared meaning, common purpose, shared values and behaviors, and shared learning [9]. As a subculture of organizational culture, a patient safety culture can develop within frontline teams and across the entire healthcare organization when targeted strategies are implemented with the intent of facilitating error reporting without fear of blame or reprisal. These strategies also eliminate behaviors based on disciplinary hierarchies and create a psychologically safe workplace that prevents patient harm.

7.1 Organizational Culture

The foremost researcher of organizational culture was Edgar Schein, who described it as "a pattern of basic assumptions – invented, discovered or developed by a given group as it learns to cope with the problems of external adaptation and internal integration – that has worked well enough to be considered valid and therefore to be taught to new members as the correct way to perceive, think and feel in relation to these problems" [10]. An informal yet well-accepted definition of culture in the literature is "the way we do things around here" [10]. At times, the following addition is made: "… when no one is looking" [11].

Culture refers to the deep structure, normative beliefs, and shared behavioral expectations that work informally to coordinate and control behavior, actions, and decision-making within organizations. It reflects not only the written or explicit rules of the organization but also the implicit, unwritten, subconscious, intangible assumptions and beliefs that shape organizational behavior, as observed in all facets of day-to-day activities. Schein suggested that enculturation is simultaneously a behavioral, cognitive, and emotional process. The term *culture* has been used to indicate how values guide and constrain people in organizations [10], how individuals weave stories to obtain resources [12], or how individuals discriminately use tools to meet personal needs and interests [13, 14].

Schein identified three fundamental levels at which culture manifests: observable artifacts, values, and basic underlying assumptions. *Artifacts* are the external representations of what an organization holds dear. *Values* are represented by the behavioral norms that develop within an organization. Underlying *assumptions* are uncovered by a process of enquiry that brings them to the surface to create mutual understanding. The processes of reflective listening and powerful questioning unearth the cultural norms within an organization in relation to values and appropriate behaviors. Creating a common language and shared understandings enables the space for trust, inclusion, and belonging to evolve and grow. Reflective listening, powerful questioning, and developing a common language with shared understanding, are some of the basic processes that coaches use in their coaching practice.

7.1.1 Culture Characteristics

Research highlights that cultures thrive when there is shared meaning, a common purpose, shared values and behaviors, creating opportunities for shared learning by organizational members.

7.1.1.1 Shared Meaning

Attempts to uncover the underlying processes of the complex system of shared meanings contributing to culture emphasize the social and cultural aspects of organizational life evidenced by myths, values, and history as a means of understanding the exact nature of organizations. Alvesson [15] proposed that culture is not primarily "inside" people's heads but rather somewhere "between" the heads of a team of people where symbols and meanings are publicly expressed—in the language that is used in work teams and the stories that are told. Furthermore, researchers believe that organizational culture has a learning component since people learn in social situations within "macrosystem factors [e.g., technological shifts, globalization] that enable, constrain, or shape … developmental relationships" [16].

Research findings have revealed that opportunities to develop shared understandings exist based on shared meanings about what works in relation to reducing risks and harm in patient populations, and recognizing and acting on these signals [17].

Without the use of nontechnical coaching skills, it is more difficult to facilitate and enable shared direction and meaning to guide everyday actions. The importance of shared meaning was revealed when teams needed guidance about how to make sense of data from the *Texas Safety Culture Team Tool*—a tool used in the study to assess safety culture in frontline teams and how to work with the findings [18].

7.1.1.2 Common Purpose

Just as organizations are founded with a particular vision in mind, the work to be accomplished is organized around teams that each have their own purpose as contributing members to fulfill the organization's mission. The work of teams must address meaningful organizational needs and strive toward a compelling purpose for team members to believe that the work they do is important. The purpose of the team must be clearly established from inception and expressed as shared team goals to be achieved. Actioning team goals creates a shared experience that, if based on trust, cements cooperative and collaborative relationships within the team that stand the test of time.

7.1.1.3 Shared Values and Behaviors

All behaviors, thoughts, feelings, and actions are shaped and given direction, purpose, and meaning by the values and goals that individuals hold implicitly or explicitly [19]. Patient safety coaching techniques focus on identifying the behaviors and cognitions that support coachees' positive and enabling values and beliefs in relation to the patients in their care. An individual's values and beliefs are shaped by early childhood experiences; they are tested in the work environment. How staff respond in work situations to demonstrate these values is shaped by the role modeling they see around them. Leaders have an immense influence on the behaviors that staff members emulate as they care for patients and keep them safe.

From a coaching perspective, coachees gain insight into the behaviors that support their core values, both personal and professional, when they identify discrepancies between espoused and enacted behaviors in relation to patient safety. These discrepancies provide opportunities to discover their growth needs [20]. A number of changes may be desired or required in the coachee's behavior, attitude, beliefs or perspectives that impact their ability to develop empathy and compassion for patients and work collaboratively with colleagues. Coaching realigns their behaviors with patient safety values, unravels patterns of behavior that are not serving them well, and identifies ways that coachees can reinforce what they are doing *right* and should continue.

7.1.1.4 Shared Learning

Organizations learn as a result of individuals' collective learning. In patient safety coaching, the coach invites individual coachees to critically reflect and identify a "disorienting dilemma" [21] and then addresses the resulting discontent with them to evoke learning [22]. Individual learning that has resulted in productive outcomes is repeated and replicated throughout the organization. In time, these learnings are considered part of the organization's folklore and become cultural norms—established ways of thinking and behaving—and significant characteristics of the organization's culture. So it is with a patient safety culture; processes and procedures that work well to keep patients safe are replicated, and staff learn from observing excellent clinical practice.

At the collective level, learning takes place through individuals whose actions are based on shared models of values and expected behaviors, displaying and integrating them into practices [23]. This collective learning is transmitted via socially constructed cultural elements such as rituals and stories—an enculturation process. Commonly held values and beliefs create negotiated roles and norms as byproducts of the enculturation and socialization process [24].

When patient safety coaching is delivered across all levels, individual learning transitions to organizational learning and transformative cultural change [25]. Organizational learning enables organizations to adapt and transform in response to, or in anticipation of, change [26–28]. Transformative learning integrates existing knowledge with new thoughts and behaviors based on individual learnings and distributes this new information, processes, or practices among organizational members [29, 30].

In a hospital setting, Manley and Jackson investigated how a patient safety culture can promote shared learning in a clinical team and systemic transformation [17]. Across four hospitals, they found that a patient safety culture promoted a focus on learning within frontline teams; supported by quality clinical leadership, it was linked with successful change. Moreover, all incident reporting and learning systems, whether large or small, were found to create a positive culture in which reports of incidents are encouraged and valued, and staff are praised for participating in learning debriefs [31]. Feedback meetings facilitated the ability of staff to understand the actions that triggered the adverse event, better manage their reactions to it, and devise ways to prevent further occurrences. The resultant actions included feedback debriefing with staff; closing the loop by communicating back to the person who reported the adverse event; and arranging appropriate resourcing in that area to prevent future occurrences. These actions are all essential components of a patient safety management strategy at the Safety-1 level. When coaching is added to support staff through trauma, a Safety-11 [32] approach to patient safety has been adopted by the organization.

7.1.2 *Subcultures*

Subcultures constitute relatively cohesive social systems of "shared, learned behaviors which are common to a specific group or category" [33]. A subculture has been defined as "a distinctive subgroup of society that self-selects on the basis of a shared commitment to a particular product class, brand, or … activity" [34]. In contrast to Schein's views on culture, Geertz [35] believes that culture develops not as a function of the commonalities that groups experience, but because of their differences. He posited that culture is idiosyncratic to a particular group, which could explain the differences in culture across organizations and even divisions within an organization. Indeed, it could explain how, with different norms in operation based on different shared knowledge and understandings, several subcultures may emerge within an organization, e.g., safety culture, service culture, sales culture, and coaching culture [36, 37]. The development of subcultures has been linked to the adoption of the specific principles and processes necessary for that particular aspect of organizational culture to thrive.

Antonsen [38] suggested that subcultures emerge when attention is given to the principles and processes associated with a particular aspect of organizational culture in a coordinated fashion. Therefore, just as a safety culture has developed its own core principles and processes, a patient safety subculture operates from a shared philosophy and belief about how to communicate with and relate to patients and how to keep them safe. Antonsen believes that it is the interplay between structural aspects of the organization and the interactions of people within the organization that leads to the development of a shared language and cultural norms.

7.1.2.1 Safety Culture

A safety culture has been defined as "the product of individual and group values, attitudes, perceptions, competencies, and patterns of behavior that determine the commitment to, and the style and proficiency of, an organization's health and safety management" [18]. Antonsen's proposition that a safety culture is a subset of an organizational culture is consistent with the views of Clarke [39] and Parker et al. [40]. In an atmosphere of mutual trust, staff members can talk freely about safety problems and how to solve them without fear of blame or recrimination. A safety culture has both structural and cultural dimensions as a result of "the interplay between the different aspects of organizations … [hence, it is] impossible to study the cultural effects in isolation from the structural and interactional effects" [38]. Also, healthcare organizations do not exist in a vacuum; they are influenced by external events, culture, and political and economic landscapes.

The concept of a safety culture originated from studies on safety in high-risk organizations that constantly struggle to minimize adverse events while engaging in intrinsically complex and hazardous work. Safety in these organizations is achieved when all workers, from frontline deliverers to managers and executives, maintain a commitment to safety above all else. In a Safety-1 environment, safety is a key *priority* around which policies and procedures are formulated. Strict adherence to these policies and procedures is expected; any transgressions have serious consequences for the individual who supposedly triggered the event and could lead to their dismissal. A "blame" culture is typical in a Safety-1 environment.

In contrast, in a Safety-11 environment [32], safety is not only a key priority but also a key *value* held by all workers. The *values* are articulated, embedded, integrated, and observed in action. Manley and Jackson [17] suggested that these actions are based on the following:

- Person-centeredness in all relationships with patients, each other, and across disciplines.
- A focus on holistic safety and its integration with being person-centered with staff and service users.
- Ways of working that actively and appreciatively embrace learning.

In other words, in a Safety-11 workplace, every staff member knows that their behavior contributes to ensuring not only their own safety but also the safety of others. They operate safely in a blame-free environment in which individuals are able to report errors or near misses without fear of reprimand or punishment. There is collaboration across occupations and levels, as everyone seeks solutions to safety problems. The organization commits sufficient resources to ensure the safe operation of wards and departments. Leaders in frontline positions, who have a genuine commitment to safety, are recognized by their staff as having uncompromising standards for the delivery of care. This sends a clear message to all staff, which encourages and inspires similar standards across every department.

7.2 Patient Safety Culture

Patient safety culture is a subset of safety culture (Fig. 7.2). It has been defined as "a pattern of individual and organizational behavior, based upon shared beliefs and values that continuously seeks to minimize patient harm, which may result from the process of care delivery" [3]. Patient safety culture is focused on the aspects of organizational culture that relate to patient safety in all treatment settings and to all types of prevention, diagnosis, treatment, follow-up, and rehabilitation activities.

Just as every organization has its own organizational culture, a patient safety culture is developed as a subculture when all healthcare staff members hold the same philosophical belief in ensuring that patients are not exposed to "unnecessary harm or potential harm associated with health-care" [41]. Staff internalize safety beliefs, values and attitudes, translate them into healthcare practices, and commit to maintaining an error-free health environment [42]. Patient safety culture is a vital component in the provision of quality patient care.

In a patient safety culture—a Safety-11 environment [32]—staff are respected, processes are open and transparent, and relevant data/resources are available when

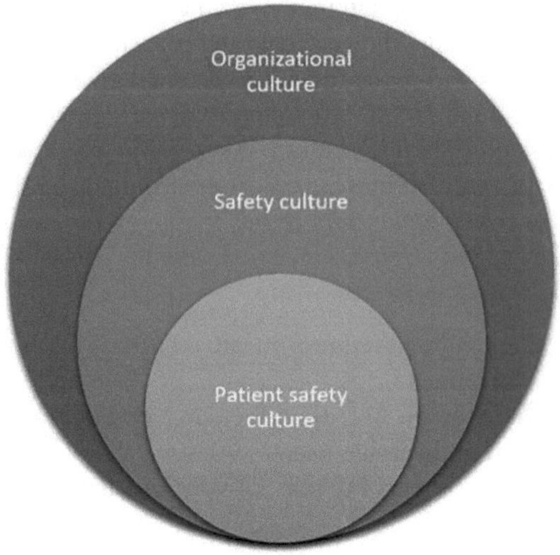

Fig. 7.2 Patient safety culture as a subset of organizational culture

needed. The organization cares less about hierarchy than it does about supporting staff and delivering quality patient care. A dedicated patient safety culture is sustained by staff who have a shared understanding of what patient safety means and by those who are committed to meeting the organization's vision of exemplary patient care.

Leaders in a patient safety culture share the value of patient safety and display the behaviors that underpin this value, such as open communication. They foster strong teamwork within care units and provide opportunities for organizational learning. They are ready and willing to change how they do things in their team and organization to keep both patients and staff safe. A common theme arising from a research study by Manley and Jackson [17] was the importance of senior managers and leaders having an approach that was bottom-up, nonhierarchical, non-power driven, and supportive of development, with *readiness to learn* being a characteristic of the organization as a learning organization.

Sammer et al. [43] reported the following elements to be important in a culture of patient safety: leadership; teamwork based on collaboration; evidence-based practice; an environment where individual staff members have the right and responsibility to speak up on behalf of the patient; a learning culture; a culture that recognizes errors as system failures; and an organization based on patient-centered care in which the patient is regarded as an active partner to the healthcare team. The key actors in this culture are senior leaders who design, foster, and nurture patient safety. Senior leaders must be committed to driving and prioritizing safety, as their actions and attitudes influence the perceptions, attitudes, and behaviors of the wider workforce.

Unfortunately, wide variations in the perception of what a patient safety culture is can exist within a single healthcare organization. The perception of safety culture might be high in one unit within a hospital and low in another unit, or high among management and low among frontline workers. Individual worker burnout negatively impacts perceptions of safety culture. These variations are likely to contribute to the mixed success of interventions intended to improve safety culture and reduce errors. Therefore, leaders must be deeply involved with, and attentive to, the issues frontline workers face, and they must understand the established norms and "hidden culture" that often guide behavior. Many determinants of a patient safety culture are dependent on interdisciplinary relationships and other local circumstances; thus, changing culture often starts at the microsystem level with incremental changes to frontline staff's everyday behaviors.

According to Vikan et al. [44], patient safety culture is a proxy for the quality of care experienced in a healthcare organization. They reviewed 1743 articles in the extant literature and found that in 76% of the studies, increased patient safety culture scores were associated with reduced adverse event rates, which is consistent with those of previous reviews reporting mostly significant associations between patient safety culture scores and patient safety outcomes [45–47]. They reported that increased patient safety culture scores were associated with a reduction in "intercepted near misses" [48], which previous research indicated may be related to an actual reduction in near misses [49].

7.2.1 *Enabling and Enacting Factors*

Lee et al. [50] tested a theoretical model of the relationships between what they proposed were three *enabling* factors of patient safety culture (supervisor/clinical leader support for patient safety, hospital management support for patient safety, and psychological safety) and four *enacting* factors of patient safety culture (handovers and information exchange, teamwork, error reporting intention, and withholding voice) by surveying 526 nurses in medical and surgical units in three Korean hospitals. Their findings revealed overall support for their proposition that enabling factors influence enacting factors which, in turn, lead to improved patient safety outcomes (Fig. 7.3).

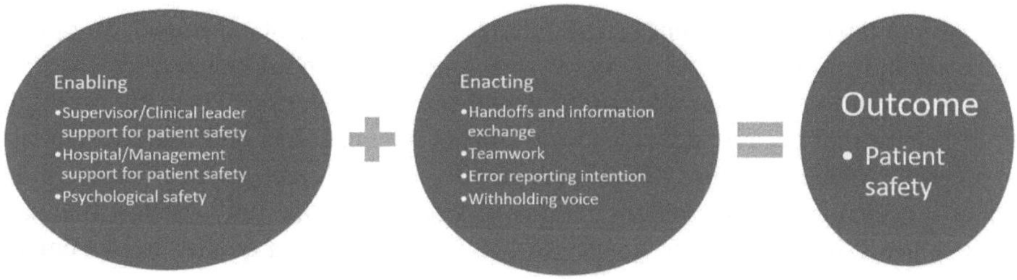

Fig. 7.3 Factors contributing to the development of a patient safety culture. (Adapted from Lee et al. [50])

Their results revealed that psychological safety is associated with all four enacting factors which, in turn, are all associated with overall patient safety, emphasizing the overarching effect and critical nature of psychological safety in ensuring patient safety. Drilling down, the researchers identified that hospital management support was associated with all enacting factors except teamwork, which was influenced only by psychological safety. Supervisor/clinical leader support was associated with only handovers and information exchange and withholding voice. The researchers concluded that these results provide further insight into the importance of support provided by hospital management and unit supervisors/clinical leaders for patient safety to motivate and enable hospital nurses to enact behaviors necessary for patient safety. Above all, such support must enhance psychological safety for hospital staff.

The findings from Manley and Jackson's SQUIRE project [17] emphasized the important role of skilled facilitators as organizational enablers of leadership, learning, development, and quality care. They also reinforced previous research that recommended the use of facilitators in transforming the workforce more broadly [51]. To be effective, these facilitators need to have a passion for the job and be embedded within frontline teams so they can develop a good understanding of the issues, relationships, and skillsets within the team and determine how to get the best out of team members. They need the skillsets and competences of clinical facilitation and transformational leadership, coupled with personal attributes of self-awareness and emotional resilience [52, 53].

At the team and individual levels, Manley and Jackson [17] described individual enablers of patient safety culture as follows: (i) quality clinical leadership based on an inclusive, participative, collaborative approach involving all stakeholders and (ii) facilitation that embraces all the skills required for learning, developing, and fostering person-centered values. They stated that it is particularly important for an organization to engage facilitators to support frontline teams and for senior organizational leaders to enable a bottom-up approach to supporting quality and innovation.[1]

7.3 Coaching as a Quality Organizational Strategy

The development of a patient safety culture is at the heart of *excellence* in patient care within frontline teams. Patient safety culture is also an important component of a *quality improvement strategy* within healthcare organizations [54]. Abousi et al. [55] believe that because adverse events impact patient safety and healthcare quality, a patient safety culture is a prerequisite for quality care. A safety problem is, therefore, also a quality problem. However, safety is not the only strategy that can be employed to improve the quality of healthcare; rather, a quality improvement

[1] Facilitators can be trained in patient safety coaching by the Australian Institute of Professional Coaches www.professionalcoachtraining.com.au

strategy encompasses a number of different initiatives that can support improvement. These initiatives can be viewed as components of a larger intervention that may be used to enable safer care within the entire organization. A quality management strategy that improves patient safety will focus on the following:

- Addressing adverse events to reduce their incidence.
- Learning from near misses.
- Ensuring psychological safety within the workplace so that staff speak up when incidents or near misses occur.
- Addressing unprofessional behavior that impacts staff well-being and their ability to deliver excellent patient care.

7.3.1 Addressing Adverse Events

Addressing adverse events is obviously the first step in starting the development of a patient safety culture. Adverse events provide rich data for learning and system improvement [56].[2] Patient safety is significantly strengthened through the coaching of leaders after adverse events have been reported [57]. In a Safety-11 environment [32], leaders collect data so they can focus on improving systems that lead to the prevention of adverse events and quality improvements [58, 59]. Coaching has emerged as a major developmental tool for promoting alternative perspectives, behavioral change, and positive, supportive team-based care [60, 61]. With the guidance and support of coaches, staff embrace improved clinical practices and develop an enhanced sense of patient safety and care.

Intensive care units (ICUs) are particularly high-risk areas for medical errors and adverse events due to patients' fragile medical conditions and the complexity of care needed. Taking a broad view of patient safety, Tlili et al. [62] assessed patient safety culture in 15 Tunisian ICUs using a mixed methods approach. They concluded that patient safety culture in these facilities is in need of improvement through the use of quality management and error reporting systems, and that quality improvement will not be achieved if it is not included in organizational policy and embedded in a comprehensive cultural change strategy. In high-risk areas such as ICUs, they believe that a well-developed patient safety culture is the key to improving patient safety and optimizing healthcare quality. The quality of care requires a combination of the commitment of healthcare professionals on the one hand, and management on the other hand [63].

[2] Adverse events are addressed in Chap. 3.

7.3.2 Learning from Near Misses

Many minor errors and near misses are unreported [64] and are often discounted since there was no harm done to the patient [65]. However, even if they do not lead to adverse events, near misses need to be reported so that they can be examined and quality improvements made. They are a valuable source of data into what processes and systems need to change. The cost of errors can be determined not only from the possible impact on patients' lives but also from the trauma caused to them and staff in making the recovery [66]. Moreover, the cost of additional medical treatment that may be required after a near miss can negatively affect the organization's bottom line. Reputational damage can also cost the organization. With a minimum of 210,000 deaths per annum in US hospitals associated with medical errors [67], 18,000 preventable deaths attributable to medical errors and at least 50,000 patients disabled in Australia each year [68], and 25,000 deaths resulting from 100,000 medical errors each year in Germany [65], reporting near misses needs to become a proactive patient safety and quality improvement strategy that is implemented each and every time an incident occurs, to prevent future patient harm [69].

It is the leader's role to work with team members to discover better ways to prevent harmful events from occurring. They can do this preemptively by focusing on excellence and what works *well* in healthcare and encouraging team members to collaboratively engage in learning new patient safety skills and behaviors. As a result of receiving constructive feedback and support from their leader, team members are better able to effectively implement safe care practices and help each other take personal responsibility for their performance in relation to safe practices in their clinical area of expertise.[3]

7.3.3 Ensuring Psychological Safety

Psychological safety plays a significant role in keeping people safe in high-risk work environments such as healthcare [70]. Psychological safety was found to be a direct predictor of the intention to report adverse events by physicians, highlighting its importance in creating safer care for patients [71]. Psychological safety is a construct first referred to by Amy Edmondson in the late 1990s [72]. She described it as a state in which individuals feel empowered to ask questions, admit mistakes, or voice concerns without fear of negative repercussions from their team. This concept applies to workers in all occupations but is particularly applicable to those in high-risk industries such as healthcare, where patient safety and quality of care are imperative.

Psychological safety creates an environment of trust and openness in which concerns can be discussed and errors raised without fear of retribution [73]. This enables

[3] Ways that leaders and teams can learn from near misses is addressed in Chap. 3.

healthcare staff to focus on providing high-quality care as opposed to worrying about voicing dissent and disagreement. It has also been shown that psychological safety increases physician engagement [74] and reduces burnout [75]. When there is an atmosphere of blame and retribution, reporting and learning will not flourish. Patients are likely to be at greater risk in such healthcare settings because mistakes will not be admitted [31].

In a systematic review of the literature, O'Donovan and McAuliffe [76] summarized the content, theoretical underpinnings, and outcomes of interventions that have targeted psychological safety, speaking-up, and voice behavior within healthcare settings. They identified several factors that researchers considered to be enablers of staff members' ability to speak up. Within a workplace that is open and trusting, welcomes participation, and shares power, they found that staff are willing to communicate and question established practices and make suggestions for improvements. Involving end-users in the design phase, targeting both group and organizational levels, ensuring visible leader support, and working across and within interdisciplinary teams are essential strategies to achieve a psychologically safe environment. When healthcare teams are psychologically safe, they are more likely to engage in quality improvement and team learning.

Remtulla et al. [77] explored the barriers to, and facilitators of, psychological safety in primary healthcare teams. They identified four barriers to psychological safety: hierarchy, perceived lack of knowledge, personality, and authoritarian leadership. Conversely, eight facilitators of psychological safety were revealed: leader inclusiveness, an open culture, a vocal personality, support in silos, a boundary spanner, chairing meetings, strong interpersonal relationships, and small groups. Shared beliefs support team functioning, providing an important background and context for the development of a psychologically safe team environment. Their findings support previous research which highlighted other factors facilitating psychological safety: inclusive behaviors displayed by a leader regardless of hierarchical differences, actively inviting participation, and showing appreciation of opinions [78].

Psychological safety is a phenomenon that also exists at the group level. It is built in a team environment through supportive workplace interactions [76] and has been found to be a key determinant of high-quality communication, trust, and decision-making within teams [79]. While the literature is clear that leaders are crucial in facilitating psychological safety in healthcare teams, there is less clarity around how team members contribute to the psychological safety of the environment in which they work [77]. Speaking up is a risky behavior in unsafe teams. Hence, more often, individuals choose silence over speaking up in healthcare environments [80]. It is one of the essential tasks of leaders to foster a team culture in which everyone feels safe to report.

It is well-known that the cultural hierarchy in healthcare organizations can lead to workers being afraid to speak up and not being able to do their best work [81, 82]. These findings may partly explain health professionals' perceptions of communication issues in Australian hospitals which are highly hierarchically organized [83]. In the USA, Appelbaum et al. [71] investigated the influences of power distance and leader inclusiveness on psychological safety among 106 medical residents. A greater perceived power distance predicted lower levels of psychological safety, while leader inclusiveness was positively correlated with psychological safety. Higher levels of psychological safety were positively correlated with the intention to report adverse medical events, further highlighting the importance of mitigating barriers to psychological safety to maintain and improve patient safety.

Sociological studies of nurse–doctor power relationships are particularly germane to policymakers and researchers as healthcare centers advance interdisciplinary care as the way to deliver quality patient care and ensure patient safety [84]. An inverse relationship between disengagement from work and psychological safety has been found following personally being bullied as well as from witnessing others being bullied [85].[4]

Leaders promote patient safety by performing three critical functions: (i) leading and guiding their team in the daily processes of delivering patient care, (ii) ensuring that patients and staff are safe at all times, and (iii) developing a psychologically safe culture in which team members feel that they are able to report near misses that could have been harmful to patients. Feeling psychologically safe encourages healthcare staff to speak up about errors and near misses.

Patient safety coaching supports healthcare staff in regaining trust in themselves and confidence in their abilities, and reignites their desire to deliver excellent patient care. It also supports teams in building trusting, internal relationships based on improved communication, cooperation, and collaboration. When leaders engage with staff through patient safety coaching, the result is beneficial not only to the staff member and team but also to patients, as evidenced by increased patient satisfaction with their care, fewer complaints, and a significant reduction in adverse events.

7.3.4 Addressing Unprofessional Behavior

Pavithra et al. [86] investigated the unprofessional behaviors of staff in seven hospitals in Australia. They found that unprofessional behaviors were perceived and experienced in different ways by staff across all professional groups and functions. Direct negative effects of unprofessional behaviors impacted patient safety, staff well-being, and organizational outcomes, while indirect negative effects impacted team cohesion, communication, and the quality of patient care. Moreover, conflicting priorities and diffuse responsibilities impact team dynamics, resulting in an increased likelihood of unprofessional behavior. A perceived lack of organizational action following staff reporting, and a lack of feedback to the reporter, eroded staff confidence in hospital leaders and staff members' ability to effectively address and eliminate unprofessional behaviors.

[4] Bullying and harassment are addressed in Chap. 9.

7.4 Coaching Individuals at a Practice level

At the practice level, poor patient safety culture has been linked to increased error rates in healthcare settings [7]. The characteristics of a poor patient safety culture include a lack of teamwork across units, fear of reporting adverse events, the existence of a blame culture, inconsistent response to errors, extreme shortage of staff, substandard handovers, lack of management support, and constrained resources [87]. Focusing on what went *wrong* when investigating an adverse event is a Safety-1 approach to patient safety. Rather, a Safety-11 approach [32] is to focus on the above combination of factors at the social/technical/systems levels related to the event to identify not only what went *wrong* so that improvements can be made, but also what went *right* so that learning from excellence can occur.[5]

The importance of improving patient safety culture at the organizational level as a foundation for success in patient safety within frontline teams has been noted by the World Health Organization [7]. Clinical leadership was found to be the pivotal enabler of effective team performance when team members embrace shared values and meaning as the norm for the way things are done in the team [88]. This shared learning and approach to clinical practice has a marked, positive effect on the safety behaviors of staff and their ability to work effectively in the workplace.

Changing an organization's culture is a key challenge for those interested in achieving transformation in healthcare provision at all levels of the organization. Believing that culture has the greatest potential to directly impact staff and patients in healthcare, Manley and Jackson [17] initiated the *Safety Culture Quality Improvement Realist Evaluation* (SCQIRE) project in England in 2019. This project aimed to refine the theoretical understanding of how to recognize and develop effective workplace cultures at the microsystem level, based on the premise that "attending to culture is central to developing workplaces that are safe and effective – those that prioritize learning to support continuing quality, person-centered relationships, and the well-being of providers and recipients of care" [17]. They concluded that the close relationship between person-centered values, ways of working, and continuing effectiveness makes it impossible to develop a patient safety culture without also being person-centered in relationships.

The findings of the SCQIRE project indicate a strong link between building relationships with patients and staff and living person-centered safety values through these relationships. This association suggests the need for congruence between values demonstrated in frontline teams by the behaviors and safety actions of team members, and the organizational values espoused as part of their culture. Manley and Jackson [17] developed a theory of cultural change within the healthcare industry based on the ten core values they identified as essential for a patient safety culture (Table 7.1).

---

[5] Differences between Safety-1 and Safety-11 approaches to patient safety are discussed in Chap. 2.

Table 7.1 Ten core values essential for a patient safety culture to exist [17]

Person-centered	Ways of working	Effective care
1. Person-centered approach to relationships	2. Open communication 3. High support/high challenge 4. Collaboration, inclusion and participation with stakeholders 5. Teamwork 6. Leadership development	7. Evidence use and development 8. Lifelong learning 9. Positive attitude to change 10. Safety (holistic)

According to their theory, cultural change in frontline teams involves embedding core values of holistic safety, person-centeredness, and teamwork and their associated behaviors, into formal organizational systems and processes. Cultural change also requires a flattened and transparent management structure that is ready to reinforce organizational values through an effective human resource management system. At the individual level, transformational leadership and skilled facilitation support role clarity. Evaluating the impact at the local level following learning and development opportunities assesses the extent to which frontline teams have adopted cultural change. When they do, an effective workplace culture is characterized by:

- The consistent achievement of standards and goals.
- Evidence-based and continuous development, improvement, and innovation in practice linked to the needs of patients.
- Empowered and committed staff.
- Flourishing of all involved.

Manley and Jackson [17] recommend that, for the full potential of patient safety initiatives to be optimized and sustained within frontline teams, there is a need for the following:

- Strong organizational values modeled by senior managers and leaders at every level.
- Buy-in from executive teams reflected in genuine organizational commitment.
- Integrated systems for learning, development, and improvement, in addition to support and capacity building for facilitators.

Healthcare organizations that commit to developing a patient safety culture adopt a holistic approach to unlocking their workforce's potential.

7.5 Patient Safety Coaching to Develop a Patient Safety Culture

The third purpose of patient safety coaching is to assist leaders in creating a patient safety culture within their team and/or organization. Patient safety coaching is delivered by healthcare leaders and clinical coaches who have been formally trained in a robust coaching methodology such as the ©AIPC COACH model.[6] In a team environment, shared meaning, direction, and purpose can be generated within the team by conducting a workshop to develop a patient safety culture.[7]

In a patient safety culture, all team members are responsible for patient safety which involves reporting incidents, errors, and omissions that may lead to adverse events. Patient safety coaching is the process that assists organizations in moving from a Safety-1 to a Safety-11 [32] mindset for patient safety (akin to a "growth mindset"). Healthcare organizations planning to implement patient safety culture initiatives need to be aware of, and put strategies in place to overcome, possible barriers to their development, such as rigidity of core beliefs, ineffective communication, a tendency toward scapegoating, and staff being unwilling to learn from negative experiences [89].

Leaders are responsible for the culture in which their team operates and for removing any institutional barriers to their effective functioning. When they receive patient safety coaching, leaders support and enable safe practices by facilitating team members' self-reflection and learning, and creating a shared sense of meaning, direction, and purpose in the team in relation to patient safety. When leaders are formally trained to deliver patient safety coaching, they use their enhanced nontechnical coaching skills to generate increased collaboration and inclusion within their team, create systematic improvements customized to specific contexts, and engage all team members in developing a patient safety culture.

Key Takeaways

- A patient safety culture is one in which staff share the same vision and values for healthcare, know and understand what it means to keep patients safe, share a common purpose to do whatever it takes to prevent adverse events, and share learnings from debriefs and observations of excellent clinical practice.
- Leaders develop a patient safety culture when they create a psychologically safe workplace in which staff feel able to speak up to report incidents or near misses without fear of blame or recrimination, and address them promptly to assist staff learn and prevent future events.
- In a patient safety culture, leaders address unprofessional behavior when it occurs so that it does not impact staff's ability to report near misses, which may cause adverse events to occur.
- Leaders who coach are better able to support the development of a patient safety culture within their unit, department, or organization.
- Implementing a patient safety culture is a quality management strategy that focuses on what staff do *well* and how they learn from *excellence*, to improve the provision of patient care.

---

[6] The ©AIPC COACH model is explained in Chap. 4.

[7] Appendix 7.1. Readers might like to use the PSC Facilitated Workshop process to develop a patient safety culture within their team.

7.6 Case Study 7: Patient Safety Culture

A critical element of patient safety culture that coaching positively influences is the ability of leaders and team members to listen actively and continue to communicate until a safe and satisfactory outcome is reached.

During a night shift in a busy hospital ward, an argument broke out between a nurse and a junior medical officer (JMO) over the prescribing of sleeping tablets for a patient. The JMO was not a part of the patient's standard team, did not know the patient, and was there prescribing antibiotics for another patient whose medication chart had expired without being written by the day team. The nursing station had plenty of activity with nurses updating charts and attending to call bells. The JMO silenced several pager calls while she was updating her patient's medication chart. Then, she was interrupted by a nurse with a request.

Nurse (Emily): "Dr. Black, Mr. George in bed 4 needs something to sleep. He is post-op day 3 and needs his rest. Can you write some temazepam up whilst you are here?".

Dr Black replied: "I don't want to prescribe any temazepam without reviewing the patient and I don't have time to review Mr. George for this right now. I have about 15 other calls from other wards with more important issues."

Emily became frustrated and insistent, feeling that Dr. Black didn't understand what she or her patient was dealing with. She continued: "It's not a big deal to write this up. You're here now. He's complaining that he can't sleep, and it's affecting his recovery. The tablets will help him rest and heal."

Dr. Black felt anxious, pressured and uncomfortable—she wouldn't usually prescribe a benzodiazepine for the first time without knowing more about the patient. She tried a different approach with the nurse: "We're seeing some patients becoming too drowsy, which increases their risk of falls, or pneumonia. Also, some of these patients are on medications that can interact with the sleeping tablets, leading to adverse effects."

Emily pushed further, frustrated at the lack of assistance: "The lack of sleep is causing him significant distress. We can't just ignore his complaints." She finished with: "You don't even care!"

Dr. Black, with her full bladder and sense of overwhelm at her busy shift, couldn't help herself and raised her voice: "Will you stand next to me in the Coroner's court when this situation goes to hell?"

At this point, the nursing shift coordinator stepped in, providing some reflections on what she had heard and offering an alternative solution: "I can hear you both care deeply about patients. Dr. Black is reluctant to prescribe a new medication to a patient she hasn't met, and Emily is keen that her sleepless patient gets the rest he needs to heal." The nursing supervisor then asked a series of questions, and they realized that they both had the patient's best interests at heart—but were coming from different mental models.

After further discussion, Dr. Black and Emily agreed to wait for Dr. Black to return after re-prioritizing other ward call jobs They would then review the patient's medication profile together and consider non-pharmacological methods as the first line of treatment. They decided to work collaboratively to ensure patient safety while addressing the need for adequate rest. The argument, though initially fractious, ended on a note of mutual respect and a shared commitment to patient care through the application of the nursing supervisor's coaching skills which resolved the situation.

For Discussion

1. What does the concept of a patient safety culture mean to you?
    - Do others you work with share this view?
2. What are the factors enabling the development of a patient safety culture?
3. What are the barriers to developing a patient safety culture?
4. Describe how a coach would assist a leader to develop a patient safety culture within their team.
    - What happened in this case study, and what could have been done differently?

Appendix 7.1: PSC Facilitated Workshop Process

To develop patient safety culture within a team at any level of the organization, team members must be aligned in relation to the following characteristics of a culture:

- Shared meaning.
- Common purpose.
- Shared values and behaviors.
- Shared learning.

A leader can facilitate a workshop with their team to discuss each of these areas and gain agreement on what each element means and how each contributes to the creation of a patient safety culture within their team, using the following process:

Critical Issue

- *Shared meaning*
    1. What does it mean to have a patient safety culture operating within our team? What does that look like? sound like? feel like?
    2. What would it take for everyone to feel psychologically safe to raise issues of concern in relation to patient safety?
- *Common purpose*
    3. What is the common purpose of this team? What are we here for? What is our overarching brief?
    4. Are we aligned in terms of the outcomes we want to achieve for our patients? Do we show up every day with that purpose in mind?

Shared values and behaviors

5. What values do we share as a team? What are the values we must hold to keep our patients safe?

6. How do we, as individuals and as a team, enact these values rather than just espouse them? What behaviors demonstrate these values?

Shared learning

7. What do we do *well*, as individuals and as a team? What can we learn from each other? What can we learn from other teams that are working *well*?
8. How do we respect each other's strengths and value their expertise?

Having discussed these critical issues in relation to what a patient safety culture means and how it is created and sustained, team members then consider how they can capitalize on what is going *well* within their team, what they can learn from other teams in which things are going *well*, and how the team can embrace opportunities for improvement based on *excellent* clinical practices.

Opportunities

9. What opportunities are available to us to create a patient safety culture within this team?

   The leader helps team members envisage the best possible future when a patient safety culture is operating within their team every day. What will team members be doing? How will they be communicating with and relating to each other as team members? What behaviors will they display? Are these coach-like? What behaviors will be called out for rectification (in a positive way)? How will the team be functioning when these issues have been resolved and the best possible outcome has been achieved?

Actionable Goals

10. What actions can the team reasonably take to create a patient safety culture right now and into the future?

    What goals will need to be achieved, and what actions will be taken to achieve this best possible outcome? Make the goals SMART. Who will take action? What resources or support does the team or team members need? Are there any systemic changes that need to be made or resources obtained? Who will take carriage of the outcomes? What are the timelines?

Commitment

11. What is the level of commitment to creating a patient safety culture within our team?

    Do all team members commit to taking action and achieving the desired goals? To the same degree? If, not, why not? If the exception is reasonable and/or justified, should additional actions be considered or taken, or resources obtained? What are they? Who will enact them?

Hold Accountals

12. How will we hold each other accountable for creating and developing a patient safety culture within our team?

    Team members determine how they will know when actions are on-track to reach the desired goals and what actions they will take to bring things back on-track if necessary. In other words, team members decide what success looks like when they can confidently say that a patient safety culture is operating within their team.

The responses to each of these questions are recorded as an indication of the team's commitment to this process. The leader ensures that the final document is displayed in a readily accessible place so that the decisions made by the team at this workshop can be referred to if required and actions monitored for completion over the next few months, with adjustments made as necessary.

References

1. WHO. (2019). *Medication safety in high-risk situations; Technical report*. World Health Organization.
2. WHO. (2009). *Conceptual framework for the International Classification for Patient Safety, Version 1.1: Final technical report*. World Health Organization.
3. Kristensen, S., & Bartels, P. (2010). *Use of patient safety culture instruments and recommendations*. European Society for Quality in Healthcare – Office for Quality Indicators.
4. Singer, S., et al. (2009). Relationship of safety climate and safety performance in hospitals. *Health Services Research, 44*(2 Pt 1), 399–421.
5. Khoshakhlagh, A. H., et al. (2019). Analysis of affecting factors on patient safety culture in public and private hospitals in Iran. *BMC Health Services Research, 19*(1), 1–14.
6. Sorra, J. S., & Dyer, N. (2010). Multilevel psychometric properties of the AHRQ hospital survey on patient safety culture. *BMC Health Services Research, 10*(1), 199.
7. WHO. (2015). *Patient safety tool kit*. World Health Organization, Regional Office for the Eastern Mediterranean.
8. Pronovost, P. J., & Sexton, B. (2005). *Assessing safety culture: Guidelines and recommendations*. BMJ Publishing Group Ltd.
9. Schein, E. (1990). Organizational culture. *American Psychologist, 45*(2), 109–119.
10. Schein, E. (1985). *Organizational culture and leadership: A dynamic view*. CA Jossey-Bass.
11. WHO. (2021). *Global patient safety action plan 2021–2030: Towards eliminating avoidable harm in health care*. World Health Organization, License: CC BY-NC-SA 3.0 IGO.
12. Lounsbury, M., & Glynn, M. (2001). Cultural entrepreneurship: Stories, legitimacy, and the acquisition of resources. *Strategic Management Journal, 22*(6), 545.
13. McPherson, C., & Sauder, M. (2013). Logics in action: Managing institutional complexity in a drug court. *Administrative Science Quarterly, 58*(2), 165–196.
14. Weber, K. (2005). A toolkit for analyzing corporate cultural toolkits. *Poetics, 33*(3), 227–252.
15. Alvesson, M. (2002). *Understanding organizational culture*. SAGE.
16. Chandler, D., Kram, K., & Yip, J. (2011). An ecological systems perspective on mentoring at work: A review and future prospects. *The Academy of Management Annals, 5*(1), 519–570.
17. Manley, K., & Jackson, C. (2019). Microsystems culture change: A refined theory for developing person-centred, safe and effective workplaces based on strategies that embed a safety culture. *International Practice Development Journal, 9*(2), 1–21.
18. Sexton, J. B., et al. (2006). The safety attitudes questionnaire: Psychometric properties, benchmarking data, and emerging research. *BMC Health Services Research, 6*(1), 1–10.
19. Grant, A. (2012). An integrated model of goal-focused coaching: An evidence-based framework for teaching and practice. *International Coaching Psychology Review, 7*(2), 146–165.
20. Schlosser, B., et al. (2006). The coaching impact study: Measuring the value of executive leader coaching. *International Journal of Coaching in Organizations, 4*(3), 8–26.

21. Gray, D. (2006). Executive coaching: Towards a dynamic alliance of psychotherapy and transformative learning processes. *Management Learning, 37*(4), 475–497.
22. Gonzalo, J., et al. (2019). A developmental approach to internal medicine residency education: Lessons learned from the design and implementation of a novel longitudinal coaching program. *Medical Education Online, 24*(1), 1–5.
23. Argyris, C., & Schön, D. (1978). *Organizational learning: A theory of action perspective*. Addison-Wesley Pub..
24. Cook, S., & Yanow, D. (1993). Culture and organizational learning. *Journal of Management Inquiry, 2*(4), 373–390.
25. Mezirow, J. (1997). Transformative learning: Theory to practice. *New Directions for Adult and Continuing Education, 1997*(74), 5–12.
26. Sun, H.-C. (2003). Conceptual clarifications for 'organizational learning', 'learning organization' and 'a learning organization'. *Human Resource Development International, 6*(2), 153–166.
27. Marsick, V., & Watkins, K. (2003). Demonstrating the value of an organization's learning culture: The dimensions of the Learning Organization Questionnaire. *Advances in Developing Human Resources, 5*(2), 132–151.
28. Ortenblad, A. (2001). On differences between organizational learning and learning organization. *The Learning Organization, 8*(3/4), 125–133.
29. Dixon, N. (1992). Organizational learning: A review of the literature with implications for HRD professionals. *Human Resource Development Quarterly, 3*(1), 29–49.
30. Huber, G. (1991). Organizational learning: The contributing processes and the literatures. *Organization Science, 2*(1), 88–115.
31. WHO. (2020). *Patient safety incident reporting and learning systems: Technical report and guidance*. World Health Organization, License: CC BY-NC-SA 3.0 IGO.
32. Hollnagel, E., Wears, R., & Braithwaite, J. (2015). *From Safety-I to Safety-II: A White Paper*. University of Southern Denmark/University of Florida/Macquarie University.
33. Young, K., & Mack, R. (1959). *Sociology and social life* (p. 472). American Book Co.
34. Schouten, J., & McAlexander, J. (1995). Subcultures of consumption: An ethnography of the new bikers. *Journal of Consumer Research, 22*(1), 43–61.
35. Geertz, C. (1973). Thick description: Toward an interpretive theory of culture. In C. Geertz (Ed.), *The interpretation of cultures*. Basic Books.
36. Schneider, B., Gunnarson, S., & Niles-Jolly, K. (1994). Creating the climate and culture of success. *Organizational Dynamics, 23*(1), 17–29.
37. Knowles, S. (2022). *Coaching culture*. Switzerland.
38. Antonsen, S. (2009). *Safety culture theory, method and improvement*. Ashgate Publishing Ltd..
39. Clarke, S. (1999). Perceptions of organizational safety: Implications for the development of safety culture. *Journal of Organizational Behavior, 20*(2), 185–198.
40. Parker, P., Lawrie, M., & Hudson, P. (2006). A framework for understanding the development of organisational safety culture. *Safety Science, 44*(6), 551–562.
41. WHO. (2014). *Regional strategy on patient safety*. World Health Organization, SEA-HSD-371.
42. Zaitoun, R. A., Said, N. B., & de Tantillo, L. (2023). Clinical nurse competence and its effect on patient safety culture: A systematic review. *BMC Nursing, 22*(1), 1–10.
43. Sammer, C. E., et al. (2010). What is patient safety culture? A review of the literature. *Journal of Nursing Scholarship, 42*, 156–165.
44. Vikan, M., et al. (2023). The association between patient safety culture and adverse events—A scoping review. *BMC Health Services Research, 23*(1), 1–27.
45. Lee, S. E., & Quinn, B. L. (2020). Safety culture and patient safety outcomes in East Asia: A literature review. *Western Journal of Nursing Research, 42*(3), 220–230.
46. Alanazi, F. K., Sim, J., & Lapkin, S. (2021). Systematic review: Nurses' safety attitudes and their impact on patient outcomes in acute-care hospitals. *Nursing Open, 9*(1), 30–43.
47. Braithwaite, J., et al. (2017). Association between organisational and workplace cultures, and patient outcomes: Systematic review. *BMJ Open, 7*(11), e017708.

48. Camargo, C. A. J., et al. (2012). Safety climate and medical errors in 62 US emergency departments. *Annals of Emergency Medicine, 60*(5), 555–63.e20.
49. Haugen, A. S., et al. (2013). Impact of the World Health Organization's Surgical Safety Checklist on safety culture in the operating theatre: A controlled intervention study. *British Journal of Anaesthesia, 110*(5), 807–815.
50. Lee, S. E., Dahinten, V. S., & Lee, J. H. (2023). Testing the association between the enabling and enacting factors of patient safety culture and patient safety: Structural equation modelling. *BMC Nursing, 22*(1), 1–8.
51. Manley, K., et al. (2016). Using systems thinking to identify workforce enablers for a whole systems approach to urgent and emergency care delivery: A multiple case study. *BMC Health Services Research, 16*(Article 368).
52. Day, H. (2014). Engaging staff to deliver compassionate care and reduce harm. *British Journal of Nursing, 23*(18), 974–980.
53. Martin, A., & Manley, K. (2017). Developing standards for an integrated approach to workplace facilitation for interprofessional teams in health and social care contexts: A Delphi study. *Journal of Interprofessional Care, 32*(1), 41–51.
54. Menear, M., et al. (2019). A framework for value-creating learning health systems. *Health Research Policy Systems, 17*(1), 1–13.
55. Abuosi, A. A., et al. (2022). Safety culture and adverse event reporting in Ghanaian healthcare facilities: Implications for patient safety. *PLoS One, 17*(10), 1–18.
56. Parand, A., Dopson, S., & Vincent, C. (2013). The role of Chief Executive Officers in a quality improvement initiative: A qualitative study. *BMJ Open, 3*(1), e001731.
57. DuPree, E., et al. (2011). Professionalism: A necessary ingredient in a culture of safety. *Journal of Quality Patient Safety, 37*(10), 447–455.
58. Manzi, A., et al. (2017). Mentorship and coaching to support strengthening healthcare systems: Lessons learned across the five population health implementation and training partnership projects in sub-Saharan Africa. *BMC Health Services Research, 17*(Suppl 3), 831.
59. Chegini, Z., et al. (2020). Exploring the barriers to patient engagement in the delivery of safe care in Iranian hospitals: A qualitative study. *Nursing Open, 7*(1), 457–465.
60. Morey, J. C., et al. (2002). Error reduction and performance improvement in the emergency department through formal teamwork training: evaluation results of the MedTeams project. *Health Services Research, 37*(6), 1553–1581.
61. Grant, A., et al. (2017). The impact of leadership coaching in an Australian healthcare setting. *Journal of Health Organization and Management, 31*(2), 237–252.
62. Tlili, M. A., et al. (2022). Assessing patient safety culture in 15 intensive care units: A mixed-methods study. *BMC Health Services Research, 22*(1), 1–9.
63. Biggs, S. E., et al. (2013). Safety leaders' perceptions of safety culture in a large Australasian construction organisation. *Safety Science, 52*, 3–12.
64. Kim, M. Y., et al. (2014). Nurses' willingness to report near misses: A multilevel analysis of contributing factors. *Social Behavior Personal International Journal, 42*(7), 133–146.
65. Durmus, S. Ç., et al. (2013). Medical errors: An important indicator of quality of care and patient safety. *Holistic Nursing Practice, 27*(4), 225–232.
66. Chen, L.-C., et al. (2018). A study on the reporting intention of medical incidents: A nursing perspective. *Clinical Nursing Research, 27*(5), 560–578.
67. James, J. T. (2013). A new, evidence-based estimate of patient harms associated with hospital care. *Journal of Patient Safety, 9*(3), 122–128.
68. Kohn, L. T., Corrigan, J. M., & Donaldson, M. S. (2000). Errors in health care: A leading cause of death and injury. In *To err is human: Building a safer health system*. National Academies Press.
69. Sinclair, J. E., et al. (2018). Barriers to self-reporting patient safety incidents by paramedics: A mixed methods study. *Prehospital Emergency Care, 22*(6), 762–772.
70. Newman, A., Donohue, R., & Eva, N. (2017). Psychological safety: A systematic review of the literature. *Human Resource Management Review, 27*(3), 521–535.

71. Appelbaum, N. P., et al. (2016). The effects of power, leadership and psychological safety on resident event reporting. *Medical Education, 50*(3), 343–350.
72. Edmondson, A. (1999). Psychological safety and learning behavior in work teams. *Administrative Science Quarterly, 44*(2), 350–383.
73. Ortega, A., et al. (2014). The influence of change-oriented leadership and psychological safety on team learning in healthcare teams. *Journal of Business Psychology, 29*(2), 311–321.
74. Yanchus, N. J., et al. (2019). How to make a job more than just a paycheck: Understanding physician disengagement. *Health Care Management Review, 45*(3), 245–254.
75. LeNoble, C. A., et al. (2020). To address burnout in oncology, we must look to teams: Reflections on an organizational science approach. *JCO Oncology Practice, 16*(4), e377–e383.
76. O'Donovan, R., & McAuliffe, E. (2020). A systematic review exploring the content and outcomes of interventions to improve psychological safety, speaking up and voice behaviour. *BMC Health Services Research, 20*(1), 1–11.
77. Remtulla, R., et al. (2021). Exploring the barriers and facilitators of psychological safety in primary care teams: A qualitative study. *BMC Health Services Research, 21*(1), 1–12.
78. Hirak, R., et al. (2012). Linking leader inclusiveness to work unit performance: The importance of psychological safety and learning from failures. *Leadership Quarterly, 23*(1), 107–117.
79. Edmondson, A. C., & Lei, Z. (2014). Psychological safety: The history, renaissance, and future of an interpersonal construct. *Annual Review of Organizational Psychology and Organizational Behavior, 1*(1), 23–43.
80. Brinsfield, C. T. (2013). Employee silence motives: investigation of dimensionality and development of measures. *Journal of Organizaional Behavior, 34*(5), 671–697.
81. Leape, L., et al. (2012). A culture of respect, Part 1: The nature and causes of disrespectful behaviour by physicians. *Academic Medicine, 87*, 1–8.
82. Leape, L., et al. (2012). A culture of respect, Part 2: Creating a culture of respect. *Academic Medicine, 87*, 853–858.
83. Draganović, Š., & Offermanns, G. (2022). Patient safety culture in Austria and recommendations of evidence-based instruments for improving patient safety. *PLoS One, 17*(10), 1–17.
84. Fernando, O., et al. (2016). Interprofessional communication between surgery trainees and nurses in the inpatient wards: Why time and space matter. *Journal of Interprofessional Care, 30*(5), 567–573.
85. Arnetz, J. E., et al. (2019). Organizational determinants of bullying and work disengagement among hospital nurses. *Journal of Advanced Nursing, 75*(6), 1229–1238.
86. Pavithra, A., et al. (2022). Unprofessional behaviours experienced by hospital staff: Qualitative analysis of narrative comments in a longitudinal survey across seven hospitals in Australia. *BMC Health Services Research, 22*(1), 1–15.
87. Tenza, I. S., et al. (2022). Hospital managers' views on the state of patient safety culture across three regions in Ghana. *BMC Health Services Research, 22*(1), 1–14.
88. Akhtar, M., et al. (2016). Leading the health service into the future: Transforming the NHS through transforming ourselves. *International Practice Development Journal, 6*(2), Article 5.
89. Paper, N. (2000). *An organisation with a memory: Report of an expert group on learning from adverse event in the NHS*, U.C.C. Chaired by the Chief Medical Officer, Editor. DH Department of Health.

Chapter 8
Measuring Patient Safety Culture

Assessing the patient safety culture of a healthcare organization at the beginning of a cultural change program is essential to its success. Baseline data can be collected using several validated instruments, principally the *Hospital Survey of Patient Safety Culture* (HSOPSC) which gathers staff perceptions of a patient safety culture in eight areas including how staff communicate with and relate to each other, and how *well* teams work together. Gaps in survey results become the focus of targeted interventions to improve patient safety culture. Medical and nonmedical staff may be selected to complete the survey. The results may be analyzed by ward or staff unit, occupation or position within the organization, and/or seniority within the ward or hospital. Other assessment instruments are available that measure staff attitudes toward patient safety, job satisfaction, and staff assessment of working conditions. Strategies to develop a patient safety culture based on a Safety-11 approach [1] include *coaching* to develop leadership capability, support staff well-being, and create a psychologically safe working culture. When the organization is ready for cultural change, measurements can be taken and strategies implemented, as part of a quality management strategy, to improve its patient safety record.

8.1 Beginning of Cultural Change

To ameliorate the risks of patient harm and maintain a reputation for person-centered care, healthcare organizations may implement a cultural change program as a key management strategy aimed at establishing a patient safety culture within their facility. First, assessment of the existing culture is essential [2, 3]. Quantitative or qualitative measures may be used to obtain baseline data, or a combination of both. Typical indicators of safety and quality include the frequency of complications acquired while in the hospital stay, the number of serious in-hospital incidents, the mortality rate, patient-reported measures of care, and accreditation outcomes.

© The Author(s), under exclusive license to Springer Nature Switzerland AG 2024

S. Knowles, *Patient Safety Coaching*,
https://doi.org/10.1007/978-3-031-68722-8_8

Quantitative measures utilize surveys to reveal basic understandings of the safety-related issues confronting leaders and frontline staff. They act as a diagnostic tool to identify areas for improvement, as well as a platform for launching patient safety initiatives at both the team and organizational levels. Surveys can "drill down" to measure the "pulse" of the overall patient safety culture in specific areas or within discrete groups. The metrics may be plotted and compared year after year. Organizations repeat these measures at the end of the cultural change program to determine the extent of the improvement as a result of the intervening patient safety intervention(s).

Qualitative approaches provide more nuanced, "real-time" data. Focus groups and brainstorming techniques are extremely helpful in capturing staff perceptions, feelings, and suggestions for improvement in relation to issues that may have been highlighted in surveys. For example, the nominal group technique is a structured process used for making group decisions [4]. It is designed to ensure that all members of the group have a chance to contribute their ideas and opinions. The technique involves a series of steps including the presentation of a problem or question, brainstorming of ideas, and voting on the best solutions. This technique is often used in organizational settings to make decisions more effectively and efficiently [5, 6].

Because hospital staff are often the first to notice patterns of unsafe practices and the conditions that increase or decrease these patterns, seeking their opinion about the patient safety culture in their team or ward is an important first step in a comprehensive quality improvement strategy. This process identifies *excellence* where the organization is doing *well* and areas where change is needed. However, it should be remembered that assessing the patient safety culture of a healthcare organization forms just one, albeit very important, component of a comprehensive quality improvement strategy. Assessing the status of the existing safety culture in a healthcare facility is the first step in the development of a strong patient safety culture [3, 7].

8.2 Measuring Patient Safety Culture

The report, *To Err is Human: Building a Safer Health System* [8], stirred the healthcare community to record the number of adverse events and deaths that occur within healthcare organizations and question how they could have been prevented. In the USA at that time, an estimated 44,000–98,000 deaths were caused annually by medical errors [8]. After the publication of this report, similar studies were conducted in France, England, Sweden, the Netherlands, Spain, Portugal, and the Republic of Ireland using the same research methodology—the Harvard Medical Practice Study [9]. The rate of adverse events in these countries ranged from 5.7% to 12.3%. Between 20% and 70% of these events were considered to be preventable. Since then, comprehensive global efforts have been made to assess the quality of care delivered in healthcare organizations [8, 10], mainly using the US *Agency for Research and Health Care* (AHRQ) HSOPSC. Since 2018, findings from locally administered versions of the HSOPSC in Canada [11], Austria [9], Sweden [12], Poland [13], Romania [14], Morocco [15], Jordan [16], South Africa [17], Saudi [18], Ethiopia [19], Korea [20], Indonesia [21], Ghana [22, 23], Iran [24, 25], Tunisia [26, 27], Brazil [28, 29], Kuwait [30], and Australia [31] have been published, and a number of literature reviews released [32–35].

8.3 Hospital Survey on Patient Safety Culture

In the USA, experts in the field of patient safety culture have agreed on certain characteristics (or dimensions) for assessment that apply to all levels of management, supervisors, and frontline leaders in healthcare organizations [36–38]. Based on their research, the AHRQ recommended that the following ten patient safety culture composite measures be used when assessing a patient safety culture [39]:

1. Communication about errors
2. Communication openness
3. Handovers and information exchange
4. Hospital management support for patient safety
5. Organizational learning
6. Reporting patient safety events
7. Response to error
8. Staffing and work pace
9. Supervisor, manager, or clinical leader support for patient safety
10. Teamwork

The most commonly used survey in the USA to measure these dimensions is the HSOPSC which was developed by the AHRQ in 2004, with an updated version being released in 2019. The survey was designed to measure staff opinions about patient safety issues, medical errors, and safety event reporting. Separate validated versions of the HSOPSC measure either the safety culture within a particular unit or within the entire healthcare organization. They are supported by User Guides to aid implementation.

- Hospital Survey on Patient Safety Culture
- Nursing Home Survey on Patient Safety Culture
- Medical Office Survey on Patient Safety Culture
- Community Pharmacy Survey on Patient Safety Culture
- Patient Safety Culture Resources
- Ambulatory Surgery Center Survey on Patient Safety Culture

The HSOPSC gathers staff perceptions of a patient safety culture in eight main sections:

1. Section A: Classification in the ward, department, or area in which the respondent carries out their main activity
2. Section B: Interaction with the direct hierarchical superior
3. Section C: Communication
4. Section D: Frequency of adverse events reported at the hospital level
5. Section E: Assessment of the general degree of patient safety
6. Section F: About the hospital in which the staff member works
7. Section G: Number of adverse events reported
8. Section H: General information about the respondents for inclusion in the structure characteristics

The HSOPSC consists of 42 items grouped over 12 dimensions. All items are measured on two scales: (i) a 5-point agreement scale (from 1—strongly disagree to 5—strongly agree) and (ii) a frequency scale (from 1—never to 5—always). The positive response rate (PRR) can also be calculated for each item from the responses of "strongly agree/agree" or "always/most of the time." Medical staff (e.g., doctors, pharmacists, biologists, biochemists, psychologists, nurses) and nonmedical staff (including administrative staff) may be selected to complete the survey. The results may be analyzed by the following:

- Ward or staff unit
- Occupation or position within the organization
- Seniority in the ward
- Seniority within the hospital

Once an assessment has been made of the organization's patient safety culture, leaders can use the AHRQ database to compare their *Surveys on Patient Safety Culture™ (SOPSC®)* results with those of others. The AHRQ provides yearly updated benchmarking data for hospital surveys; reports summarizing benchmarking data across cohorts nationwide are also available. The AHRQ Web M&M perspective discusses how to establish a safety culture.

8.3.1 HSOPSC Survey Results

The findings from more than 26 peer-reviewed academic research articles that have used the HSOPSC to assess patient safety culture in various hospital settings around the world and in various groups from 2018 to 2024 are reported in the following sections.

8.3.1.1 Primary Care Centers

In Kuwait, Alfadhalah et al. [30] used the medical version of the HSOPSC (MOSPSC) to investigate patient safety culture in primary healthcare centers and benchmarked the findings against regional and international results. They sought to establish the association between predictors and outcomes of patient safety culture in these settings. The results from 6602 staff at 94 centers (response rate 78.7%) revealed "Teamwork" (87.8% positive ratings) and "Organizational learning" (78.8%) as perceived areas that strengthen a patient safety culture. Several areas cited for improvement included "Communication about error," "Overall perceptions of patient safety and quality," "Communication openness," "Owner/Managing Partner/Leadership support for patient safety," and "Work pressure and pace." The researchers concluded that assessing and improving the culture around patient safety is paramount if a primary healthcare center aims to improve the quality and safety of the clinical services it provides.

8.3.1.2 Emergency Departments, Operating Rooms, and ICUs

Alshyyab et al. [31] researched the factors that influence patient safety culture in two emergency departments in Australian hospitals by interviewing 12 staff and thematically analyzing the data. Their findings revealed four superordinate themes that influence the development of a patient safety culture: (i) environmental and organizational barriers, (ii) healthcare professional considerations, (iii) managerial factors, and (iv) patient factors. In addition, 19 categories were identified for attention because of their possible impact on patient safety culture. The researchers consolidated these 19 factors into two categories: outer (those relating to the external environment) and inner (those relating to the internal environment of the emergency department). The key factors noted as promoting a patient safety culture in the inner environment of the emergency department included effective communication, a commitment to organizational learning, transparent reporting, teamwork, and management support. Inclusions in the outer, contextual environment that impacted the hospital's ability to develop a patient safety environment in emergency departments related to factors beyond their control to influence or affect such as social systems, the economy, policies, laws, and legislation [40]. They reaffirmed Armstrong et al.'s [41] 2007 call for the redesign of the healthcare system to overcome the negative repercussions of sociopolitical influences, particularly in relation to shortages in staffing levels, access blocks, and associated overcrowding, which affect the healthcare practice environment and consequently patient safety culture. They called for closer working relationships to be established between politicians and healthcare leaders to overcome this situation, noting that political and social advocacy is a necessary skill for emergency department leaders so that they can lobby politicians and system managers for the resources they need to keep patients safe. As had

Mendel et al. [42] in earlier research, Alshyyab et al. [31] recommended that funding should address the reporting systems and infrastructure required to enable efficient and safe clinical practice within emergency departments.

In Tunisia, Aouicha et al. [26] investigated patient safety culture within 12 operating rooms with different surgical specialties in two public university hospitals using the French version of the HSOPSC. Survey feedback was provided by 297 professionals, representing a response rate of 85.6%. The highest scoring dimension contributing to a patient safety culture was "Teamwork within units." The three lowest scores negatively impacting patient safety culture were "Nonpunitive response to error," "Frequency of adverse events reported," and "Communication openness." The qualitative data provided a more detailed picture of patient safety issues such as underreporting, absence of an effective reporting system, lack of freedom of expression, and a blame culture in operating rooms. In a similar study in Tunisia conducted by Tlili et al. [27], all 10 dimensions of the HSOPSC had low scores (below 50%) and were considered for improvement [27]. The highest score was for "Teamwork within units" (45%). The lowest scores were for "Nonpunitive response to error" (22.9%), followed by "Frequency of adverse events reported" (25.6%) and "Communication openness" (26.3%). They suggested improvement strategies such as incident reporting, the use of error reporting systems, workload changes, quality management systems, and cultural change to eliminate a blame culture.

Nurses have consistently complained about the lack of a blame-free environment. In a study by Chegini et al. [43], patient safety culture was measured using the HSOPSC to determine perceptions of culture among 256 nurses in the emergency departments of 18 public and private hospitals in Tabriz, northwestern Iran. Nurses who reported a high level of patient safety culture were more likely to report errors, a finding that reflects the results of an earlier Israeli study that confirmed that a readiness to report errors was influenced by an organization's safety culture [44]. Chegini et al. [43] concluded that a culture that sees errors as an opportunity to improve a system should replace a blame culture in which errors are deemed personal failures. However, to implement a patient safety culture, there needs to be continuous educational advancement at every level of the healthcare organization and the provision of the necessary infrastructure, resources, and procedures necessary to support its growth (human, financial, technological, and material) [45].

8.3.1.3 Pediatric Hospitals

"Teamwork within units" was found to be the main determinant of an adverse patient safety culture and a significant contributor to burnout in a pediatric hospital in Brazil, where both the HSOPSC questionnaire and the *Maslach Burnout Inventory (MBI)* [46] were used to evaluate the occurrence of burnout [47].

8.3.1.4 Nursing Homes

Patient safety culture does not only apply to hospitals. It also applies to all forms of inpatient and outpatient care including nursing homes, residential, and aged care communities. Kim et al. [32] reviewed the extant literature on the development of a patient safety culture in nursing homes, which is particularly important given the increase in the number of people living longer and the concomitant likelihood of increasing comorbidity issues. The researchers examined 25 studies that used 7 different tools to measure patient safety in nursing homes, but principally the Nursing Home version of the HSOPSC (NHSPSC—China). In addition, the *Safety Attitudes Questionnaire* (SAQ) and its *Skilled Nursing Facility and Ambulatory* versions were also used. Patient safety culture was found to be an important factor affecting the safety of nursing home residents. Interestingly, nursing homes generally scored lower than hospitals when using the NHSPSC to measure patient safety culture. The researchers posited that this may be due to the nonmandatory nature of adverse event reporting in nursing homes, e.g., of patient abuse or mistreatment by staff or other patients, or of injuries from an unknown source [48]. Kim et al. [32] concluded that (i) staff in nursing homes need to be educated in the importance of reporting adverse events and how to use an adverse event reporting system, and (ii) the appropriate staff composition should be put in place in nursing homes to establish a patient safety culture supported by appropriate policies.

A study by Andersson et al. [49] investigated 173 Swedish nursing homes and reported that 89% of serious adverse reactions occurred due to medication errors, falls, delays or improper interventions, and neglect of care. The researchers posited that the lower scores may be due to the composition of facility staff (nursing assistants rather than registered nurses) which was not recorded since this dimension is not included in the NHSPSC. Studies have reported that the greater the number of registered nurses, the better the indicators of patient safety and quality care [50, 51].

8.3.1.5 Interdisciplinary Teams

Healthcare staff often work in interdisciplinary teams depending on their expertise and what is required to administer patient care. de Brito Passos et al. [28] assessed patient safety culture from the perspective of an interdisciplinary team of 284 professionals using the HSOPSC adapted to Brazil. The dimensions that best supported the development of a patient safety culture were found to be "Supervisor/Manager expectations and actions promoting patient safety" (68.0%) and "Organizational learning" (67.0%). The aspects requiring improvement were "Nonpunitive response to error" (20.0%) and "Staffing" (31.0%). Factors working against the development of a patient safety culture included organizational weaknesses in relation to infrastructure, work processes, and management support, which can have repercussions on the adoption of safe practices.

In a validation study of the Brazilian version of the HSOPSC in 2018, Reis et al. [52] administered the questionnaire to 2702 staff members of a large general hospital with a response rate of 56%. They found that the lowest percentage of positive responses were scored in the "Staffing and work pace" dimension (54%) which they suggest illustrates the extent to which working conditions (in terms of human resources and workload) are essential to ensuring quality healthcare and patient safety. This finding is consistent with that of other HSOPSC studies that have found the "Staffing and work pace" dimension to be weak in approximately 60% of cases [52], confirming that personnel feel overloaded for staffing-related reasons. This scenario became especially acute during the COVID-19 pandemic. Significantly, this dimension scored the lowest percentage of positive responses in both a US validation study [53] in 2019 and a Korean study in 2021 [54]. The dimension that returned the second largest percentage of positive responses in the Reis et al. [52] study was "Handovers and information exchange" (61%) which was a similar result to that recorded in the US study. Moreover, Reis et al. found this dimension to be weak in 30% of the studies that used HSOPSC 1.0. "Response to error"[1] was the dimension with the third lowest percentage of positive responses in the Reis et al. study (62%) which was similar to the US study [53]. Therefore, "Staffing and work pace," "Handovers and information exchange," and "Response to error" appear to be universal indicators of a lack of patient safety culture in interdisciplinary teams.

8.3.1.6 Nurses

In Iran, Kakemam et al. [24] reported on the impact of nurses' perceptions of patient safety culture on the occurrence of adverse events. A total of 2295 nurses employed in 32 teaching hospitals in Iran were surveyed using the Persian version of the HSOPSC. The findings showed that nurses' perceptions of a patient safety culture were associated with higher levels of the following six dimensions which resulted in a lower occurrence of adverse events: "Staffing," "Hospital handovers and transitions," "Frequency of event reporting," "Nonpunitive response to error," "Supervisor expectation and actions promoting safety," "Communication openness," "Organizational learning," "Teamwork within units," and "Hospital management support patient safety." They concluded that the conventional culture of blaming or punishing healthcare professionals for adverse events should be replaced with a nonpunitive culture so that nurses will initiate the reporting of adverse events voluntarily. Management can provide support by encouraging adverse event reporting and holding training courses for nurses to improve their communication skills. They suggested that hospitals install an electronic medical records (EMRs) system for easy and quick reporting and monitoring of adverse events.

[1] *In the original HSOPSC 2.0 model, this dimension, now called "Response to error," was labeled as "Nonpunitive response to error"; that is, the questionnaire asked if the organization had a nonpunitive approach to staff in the event of error. The revised "Response to error" (Version 2.0) dimension encourages staff to consider how the organization responds to issues related to culture (non-blame), fairness (treating staff fairly in the event of errors), and learning from errors/mistakes (Sorra* et al., *2021).*

Another study in Iran by Hafezi et al. [25] investigated the association between nurses' perceptions of patient safety culture and adverse events. Questionnaires were used to assess the perceptions of 338 nurses in three university hospitals regarding the factors that support the development of a patient safety culture. Results linked the occurrence of specific adverse events with items on the HSOPSC questionnaire. For example, medication errors were significantly associated with "Frequency of events reported," "Supervisor/Manager expectations and actions promoting patient safety," and "Management support for patient safety." Pressure ulcers were significantly associated with "Supervisor/Manager expectations and actions promoting patient safety," "Handovers and transition," and "Comfort speaking up about patient safety." Falls were significantly associated with "Teamwork within units," "Feedback and communication about error," and "Handovers and transition." Deterrents to the development of a patient safety culture were noted as a lack of "Staffing" and "Nonpunitive response to error." As a nurse competency, inability to "Speak up" was found to be the factor associated with a poor patient safety culture. They recommended that hospital executives improve patient safety by encouraging staff to frequently report adverse events and provide appropriate feedback on reported errors, conduct handovers and transitions correctly, support teamwork within units, and promote speaking up about patient safety.

Based on existing evidence of a positive correlation between nursing competence and patient safety, Zaitoun et al. [34] reviewed 117 studies aiming to identify the relationship between the level of nursing competence and nurses' perception of the degree to which a patient safety culture had developed in their work unit. In these studies, measures of safety culture, nursing competency, and perception of a patient safety culture were assessed using various instruments. Overall, safety culture was generally perceived as positive. However, no unique tool has been developed to investigate the effect of safety competency on the perception of a safety culture in a standardized way. The researchers concluded that since unsafe health practices are one of the leading causes of disability and even death, competent nurses are crucial for ensuring safe and high-quality healthcare services. A high level of nursing competence ensures the achievement of, and compliance with, a patient safety culture goal.

Patient safety culture is crucial for health staff retention, particularly for nurses. When they surveyed nurses in Jordanian hospitals, Oweidat et al. [16] found a significant negative relationship between patient safety culture and staff intention to leave. They recommended several strategies to ameliorate this effect including: "providing continuing education programs; improving managerial commitment and support; developing administrative policies to improve staff outcomes; increasing staff motivation through recognition of early catchers for near misses, safety heroes, paying more salaries and incentives to nurses, sending simple 'thank you' messages; and establishing a supportive organizational culture that magnets them to their organization" [16].

The results from Malinowska-Lipień et al.'s research [13] indicate the need for management actions aimed at improving working conditions and reducing work stress within the hospital. They particularly noted that it is necessary to recognize the competencies and responsibilities of individual team members as well as improve communication and cooperation within treatment teams. They expect that these improvements will contribute to an attitudinal change toward a more positive patient safety culture among nurses and physicians employed in hospitals.

8.3.2 Summary of Issues Relating to Patient Safety Culture

From the above studies, it is clear that the leading factors that contribute to the development of a patient safety culture are "Frequency of events reported," "Feedback and communication about error," "Handovers and transition," "Teamwork within unit," "Nonpunitive response to error," "Supervisor/Manager expectations and actions promoting patient safety," and "Management support for patient safety." This means that a positive patient safety culture will develop in work units that conduct effective handovers and transitions, communicate effectively about patient progress and treatment care needs, and report adverse events so that staff can learn from debriefing the incident. These teams work *well* as one unit focused on patient care and treatment. They have managers who respond favorably to the reporting of adverse incidents and, in fact, promote reporting. Once reported, managers take immediate and appropriate action to remedy the situation by stabilizing the patient, supporting the team, and respecting individual professionalism.

This accumulation of research findings shows that the development of a patient safety culture is inhibited by a number of factors. It indicates that the underlying reasons for an underdeveloped patient safety culture are consistent with poor teamwork and communication. In relation to communication, the primary inhibitor is when staff feel unable to report adverse events because of fear of a punitive response from their manager; hence, they may fail to speak up and report a near miss which may escalate into an adverse event possibly even death. A second key inhibitor is when staffing issues result in increased workload and/or an inappropriate mix of staff given their clinical expertise or experience. Both of these issues create stress and are directly related to the psychological safety that staff experience in the work unit. Staff stress can lead to burnout which may impact patient safety. At the edge, when communication between a staff member and their manager fails and they cannot express their concerns or how they feel, they may decide that their only way of regaining control over their work and life is by exiting the system. Hence, being able to speak up about adverse events and being heard is very important, especially at times when staff feel least able to do so. This ability to speak up is critical to staff well-being as well as to the retention of competent staff in the healthcare system.

8.4 Other Surveys to Measure Patient Safety

A number of other validated measurement instruments are available for use by healthcare organizations worldwide to assess patient safety culture. In particular, these include the *Safety Attitudes Questionnaire* and the *Manchester Patient Safety Framework*. In some countries such as Australia, state authorities and local hospitals have teamed up with university departments to create their own measurement instrument that best suits their population needs.

8.4.1 Safety Attitudes Questionnaire

The *Safety Attitudes Questionnaire* (SAQ) [55] is the second most common instrument used in conjunction with the HSOPSC to assess patient safety culture [56]. It was developed in 2004 by researchers at the University of Texas and continues to be widely used internationally to measure patient safety culture. The full version of the questionnaire includes 60 items, 30 of which are standard and identical across all settings. The *generic SAQ short-form version* includes these 30 standard items from the full SAQ plus an additional six items and three demographic items, providing a total of 39 items. The generic SAQ is comprised of six factors:

1. Teamwork climate
2. Safety climate
3. Job satisfaction
4. Perceptions of management
5. Working conditions
6. Stress recognition

8.4.2 Manchester Patient Safety Framework

The *Manchester Patient Safety Framework* (MaPSaF) is a validated measurement instrument [57] widely used in a number of countries and healthcare settings [58–62]. It was originally designed specifically for use in the UK NHS in 2009 [63]. Rather than collecting information from a survey, it uses a card sorting activity and facilitated discussion to support units to understand their culture. The implementation is ideally facilitated by a person within the healthcare organization with teams who have a lead role in the patient safety agenda. The framework proposes an improvement process that is designed to guide frontline staff through several steps to assess and improve safety culture within their work unit. The steps include leading and supporting staff, promoting incident reporting, involving patients and the public, and learning and sharing lessons. The framework is presented as a grid for healthcare organizations to assess themselves against five increasing levels of maturity in 10 dimensions of a patient safety culture, namely:

1. Pathology: Why waste time on patient safety?
2. Reactive: We take it seriously and do something after an incident.
3. Bureaucratic or Calculative: We have systems in place to manage patient safety.
4. Proactivity: We are always on the alert thinking about safety issues that might emerge.
5. Generative: Managing patient safety is an integral part of everything we do.

The 10 dimensions are as follows:

1. Overall commitment to continuous improvement
2. Priority given to patient safety
3. System errors and individual responsibility/perception of causes of incidents
4. Recording incidents and best practices
5. Evaluating incidents and best practices
6. Learning and effecting change
7. Communication about safety issues
8. Personnel management and safety issues
9. Staff education and training about safety
10. Team working around safety issues

The results of the grid assessment produce a profile of the areas of relative strength and challenge in relation to patient safety culture for that healthcare organization, which can be used to identify issues for change and improvement.

8.4.3 Australian Measures of Patient Safety Culture

Since the release of the HSOPSC by the AHRQ in 2004, many countries have used the survey to measure patient safety culture in their hospital wards and departments and in other healthcare settings. Before doing so, each country would have examined the instrument and made version modifications as necessary, e.g., to language. As an example, the ACSQH conducted a validation and approval process before its introduction into the Australian healthcare system.

HSOPSC 2.0 was selected by the ACSQH *Safety Culture Measurement Expert Advisory Group* as the most suitable survey for the measurement of patient safety culture in both public and private hospitals in Australia, since it measures the most contemporary view and key aspects of patient safety culture. It is easy to complete and can be implemented in a range of hospital types. The Commission developed the Australian version of the survey (*Australian Hospital Survey on Patient Safety Culture Version 2* (A-HSOPSC 2.0) in 2021, based on the advice of the expert advisory group which evaluated the modifications through cognitive testing and undertook a pilot survey in nine hospitals. The A-HSOPSC 2.0 is shorter to be more user-friendly and promote uptake, while maintaining sufficient detail to be actionable. It includes a total of 35 questions. There are 26 items across nine composites, as per the following list. The remaining nine questions include two overarching items (rating patient safety for their unit/work area and likelihood of recommending their unit/work area to a friend or family member), one open-ended item, and six demographic items.

1. Supervisor, manager, or clinical leader support for patient safety (3 items)
2. Teamwork (3 items)
3. Communication/openness (3 items)
4. Reporting patient safety events (2 items)
5. Organizational learning—continuous improvement (3 items)
6. Communication about errors (3 items)
7. Hospital management support for patient safety (3 items)
8. Response to error (3 items)
9. Handovers and information exchange (3 items).

Subsequently, the ACSQH developed the *Patient Safety Culture Measurement Toolkit,* which provides information to support hospitals in the collection, interpretation, discussion, and actioning of results from surveys of patient safety culture, principally the A-HSOPSC 2.0. It includes a suite of templates and supporting resources to assist healthcare organizations in undertaking a quality improvement process across all levels of the healthcare system [64].

While the A-HSOPSC 2.0 is the recommended survey tool for Australian hospitals to measure patient safety culture, healthcare organizations are also encouraged to collect data and examine trends in relation to a number of other patient safety indicators such as the following:

- Complications acquired while in hospital
- Serious in-hospital incidents
- Mortality rate
- Patient-reported experience and outcome measures
- Accreditation outcomes

Other surveys may be used to obtain measurements in a particular specialty or in a certain setting or to focus on a specific element of patient safety culture in more detail. For example, some Australian hospitals have developed their own surveys, such as the following:

- The *Staff Survey on Patient Safety* was developed by South Australia Health, working with researchers at Macquarie University, to adapt the SAQ to Australian hospitals. This survey was used in a statewide study in 2009 [65] and repeated in some SA local health networks in 2013.
- The *Safety Climate Survey* was developed by the Victorian Managed Insurance Authority and the Victorian Quality Council, working with consultants to adapt the SAQ. This survey was piloted in six hospitals in Australia in 2010. A guide and a range of templates to support implementation were also developed for use in hospitals. The modified version of the SAQ continues to be used in Australia to monitor patient safety culture and measure the impact of improvement projects.

Using a modified version of the SAQ, Long et al. [66] investigated the impact of the pace of the work environment on patient and staff outcomes in Australian hospitals. Their version combined two subscales to form a composite measure of culture: teamwork culture (six items) and safety culture (seven items). Example items included "Nurse input is well received in this clinical area" (Teamwork) and "In my work area, it is difficult to discuss errors" (Safety). Questions were measured on a five-point Likert-type scale (1 –strongly disagree to 5 –strongly agree) with an option for "neutral." Responses to each item were summed to create an overall "Hospital Culture" score in the range of 0–100. Higher scores indicated a more positive perception of hospital culture. Qualitative culture measurements were obtained from observational data. They also measured staff job satisfaction using five items from the *Job Diagnostic Survey* (JDS) [67, 68] and staff burnout using two subscales of the *MBI* [46]: emotional exhaustion (five items) and depersonalization (five items) [46, 69, 70]. A sample item is "I feel emotionally drained from my work." The items were measured on a seven-point Likert scale (1 –strongly disagree to 7 –strongly agree) with an option for "neutral." Scale scores were calculated by averaging items for each subscale, with higher scores indicating greater burnout. The results revealed that a faster perceived pace significantly predicted negative perceptions of organizational culture, greater burnout, and lower job satisfaction. Different perceptions of hospital pace of life were found between different clinical settings and the type of care delivered. For example, staff working in emergency departments reported significantly "faster-paced" work environments than staff working in palliative, aged care, or rehabilitation wards. However, perceived pace did not predict perceptions of patient safety.

8.5 Strategies to Develop a Patient Safety Culture

A number of frontline strategies have traditionally been used to ensure quality and patient safety in clinical units. Interventions such as clinical training and establishing unit-based safety teams have been associated with lower error rates and improvements in safety culture. Another proven method of developing a strong patient safety culture is senior leader walk-rounds [71]. Rapid response teams and structured communication methods have also been found to be useful for addressing rigid hierarchies and communication problems. Realist evaluation helps clarify what does not work. For example, in a study that introduced safety huddles as a forum for the discussion of patient safety issues, care processes, troubleshooting, and the prevention of harm, the findings revealed that when quality clinical leadership was absent, there was a clear negative consequence for the success of the patient improvement initiative [72].

Many commercial risk management tools are available to reduce the incidence of adverse events occurring in hospitals (e.g., surgical safety checklists and handover programs). Research studies have shown that appropriate risk management tools significantly reduce the occurrence of adverse events [73–75]. However, in some settings, the introduction of these measures has not led to better patient safety outcomes [76, 77]. From their research, Draganović and Offermanns [9] proposed that the reason for this was that the use of these tools had not been embedded into the hospital's culture; staff were not informed of the importance of their use, so the tools were neglected shortly after their introduction.

The majority of strategies to keep patients safe from harm are based on a Safety-1 philosophy of determining what went *wrong* and then finding ways to *fix* it. Since adverse events continue to occur, the outcomes of these "fix" interventions suggest that piecemeal approaches to improving patient safety are insufficient to avoid future patient harm. Instead, what is needed is a holistic approach that spans all levels of the healthcare organization in terms of philosophy toward, and understanding of, the importance of patient safety. Developing a culture of safety is integral to any sustainable change efforts toward patient safety improvement. At times, policy decisions and legislative interventions may be necessary to facilitate an environment in which a patient safety culture will flourish. Ultimately, however, a culture of safety must become embedded in the attitudes, beliefs, values, skills, and practices of healthcare leaders and staff and integrated into the overall culture of healthcare organizations. The need for cultural change, not just process change, has been supported by researchers [78, 79]. A Safety-11 approach [1] is needed to develop a patient safety culture.

Although individual healthcare organizations must identify their own optimal ways of achieving a culture of patient safety, certain intervention strategies remain the same and are essential. These include leadership commitment, transparency, open and respectful communication, learning from errors and best practices, and a just culture [80]. A strong patient safety culture is not only central to reducing patient harm; it is critical to providing a safe working environment for staff in which they can speak up regarding patient safety issues and any other concerns without fear of negative consequences.

There are a number of systemic factors that may hinder the development of a patient safety culture, such as a lack of or conflicting policies and procedures, or unclear goals and directions. Conversely, from a positive perspective, there are a number of enablers that support its development. Research has shown that a patient safety culture grows when the following characteristics exist within the organization [72]:

- Leadership that develops workforce capability
- Teams that work *well* together
- Systems that are coordinated
- Organizational values that are both expressed and lived by leaders
- The organization is ready for cultural change (Fig. 8.1)

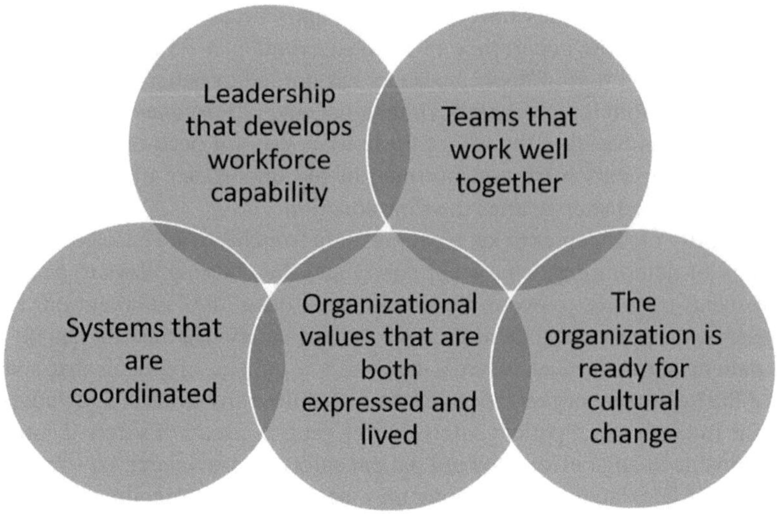

Fig. 8.1 Enabling the development of a patient safety culture

8.5.1 Leadership that Develops Workforce Capability

The first enabler of a patient safety culture is leadership which develops capability in its workforce. At all levels of healthcare, problems with organizational commitment to establishing a culture of patient safety have been noted. Commitment to a patient safety culture will only result from a combination of purposeful leadership and supportive management championing a program of improvement that frontline practitioners understand and can subscribe to in their everyday work practices. Developing and sustaining a patient safety culture requires strong leadership at all levels. There is a need for a new generation of patient safety leaders who are skilled and passionate about creating the conditions in which a patient safety culture can grow. This new generation of leaders will ensure that *excellent* clinical practices are emulated, learnings from near misses underpin system and process improvements, procedures comply with the highest standards, and staff are guided and motivated to deliver the best possible care [80]. Effective communication with everyone feeling listened to, clarity of roles and expectations, and a focus on collaborative solutions are characteristics of this new generation of leadership. At both clinical and organizational levels, excellent leadership is a core component of governance which ensures that the necessary processes are in place to improve patient care, including the establishment and maintenance of a no-blame learning culture [72]. Leadership is recognized as the main strategy for developing and embedding workplace cultures that are safe and effective and in which learning is valued [81].

Person-centered leadership ensures that staff are consistently listened to and heard, resulting in empowerment and improved experiences. Staff who are heard and have positive work experiences are more fulfilled at work and, consequently, deliver positive patient care. Leaders who use the coaching skills of curious enquiry and genuine support encourage team members to ask questions regardless of their status or role, and everyone feels safe reporting errors or near misses. Staff with the confidence to challenge and question each other, even across professional boundaries, ensure that safety issues and quality of care are addressed proactively.

Research has shown that when leaders are coached in an organization, the well-being of others connected to those leaders also improves. This ripple effect [82] was discovered using social network analysis which identified connectivity by the quality and frequency of interactions that a team member had with the team leader being coached. This relatedness influences the degree to which team members' own well-being improves. That is, the more connected team members are to a leader who is being coached, the more likely they are to improve their own well-being without even attending a coaching session. Effective leadership has been found to be an important element of patient safety culture among nurses [83, 84], with a leader's attitude being reported as a contextual factor in a healthcare professional's decision to raise issues in relation to patient safety [85].

8.5.2 Teams that Work Well Together

The second enabler of a patient safety culture is teams working *well* together to support cultural change. Evaluating how teams function is important because poor team functioning can lead to patient harm [86]. Research has shown that ineffective team factors contribute to 32% of patient care incidents [87]. Less successful team outcomes were explained by less collaborative approaches when not all parties were actively or voluntarily involved; there was a lack of focus on consistent sustainable action and a reluctance to speak out [72].

Quality clinical leadership has been linked to two themes relevant to developing a patient safety culture in teams: (i) shared meanings, and (ii) observations of clinical practice followed by constructive feedback to make improvements and support team functioning. Research has identified the strategies that optimize safe clinical decision-making for patient and team well-being: clear communication; clarity of purpose; respectful interdisciplinary relationships formed through shared team values; the ability to act on feedback for improvement; and listening to and valuing the contributions of team members to collaboratively developed, holistic, action plans for patients [72]. When team values are focused on improving practice, learning is experienced through the transformational leadership approaches of clinical leaders.

Team culture is experienced as values in action based on the observable behaviors of leaders and team members. If personal values and behaviors are aligned with these of the team, the culture is supportive of team members. However, if personal motivations and aspirations are misaligned to the team culture or in conflict with it, it is likely that individuals will experience a state of internal dissonance. Moreover, if the values in action of the team leader are misaligned with those of team members, harmonious relationships are unlikely to develop within the team.

Frontline teams working to achieve a patient safety culture through quality clinical leadership are empowered when they are able to make their own choices about projects rather than being told what to do. Such a situation highlights the opportunity for organizations to look at culture within teams and consider a different way of establishing it across the organization—from the bottom up! When quality clinical leadership and proactive behaviors coexist with shared values, there is the greatest potential for embedding a patient safety culture within teams and organization-wide.

8.5.3 Coordinated Systems

The third enabler of a patient safety culture is the presence of coordinated systems to support cultural change [72]. Healthcare organizations with an integrated systems approach enable safety, quality improvement, learning, and governance to flourish in unison. Those lacking a coordinated approach run the risk of error and omission. For example, Auraanen et al. [88] reported that lapses in primary care are common and represent approximately half of the global causes of patient harm. They argued that integrated information systems, patient involvement in measurement, and increased teamwork were essential conditions for improving safety in primary care. Their conclusion was that positive outcomes flow from coordinated systems that provide stability, certainty, and reliability.

8.5.4 Organizational Values that Are "Lived" by Leaders

The fourth enabler of a patient safety culture is when organizational values are not only expressed but also "lived." When this occurs, leaders create a psychologically safe workplace that supports cultural change. Feeling psychologically safe is critical to the delivery of safe and effective care within a complex, dynamic, and high-stakes work environment such as healthcare. Staff who feel psychologically safe are comfortable expressing themselves without fear of embarrassment or criticism from others. Unfortunately, a culture of fear and low psychological safety still exists within many healthcare organizations [89]. Given the important outcomes associated with patient care, there is a need to develop and implement interventions to improve psychological safety at both the individual and team levels.

The culture of the healthcare organization dictates the psychological environment in which the clinical team functions. If the environment is perceived to be supportive, team members will thrive and high performance will result. Alternatively, if the environment is not conducive to team members' well-being, performance and quality of care will be reduced, eventually resulting in deleterious effects on patients.

Patient safety coaching helps individuals and teams create a culture in which ideas, challenges, and concerns can be freely voiced—in which everyone feels safe to take personal risks such as asking for help, admitting errors, and challenging others. Since cultures are socially constructed from the collection of behaviors within the team and organization, culture can be changed by changing the behavior of individuals. In an environment in which staff are able to experiment and make small-scale changes autonomously, individuals know that it is okay to try, even if they "fail."

When leaders are trained in patient safety coaching,[2] they are in a much stronger position to influence culture so that it is more psychologically safe for staff to report errors or near misses. They possess all the knowledge and skills about human motivation and endeavor, which is crucial when helping others to find their passion for patient safety and take action. Coaching skills are transformational when the individual or team is ready to make significant changes in how they work and deliver care to patients. Other skills that are specifically relevant to leaders who deliver patient safety coaching are their ability to develop clarity of purpose "in the moment" of practice in different contexts, integrate multiple agendas, and support staff on their personal and professional journeys [90]. Leaders who are coached become advocates for a patient safety culture and begin the cultural transformation process at whatever level the organization is ready to undertake change.

8.5.5 The Organization Is Ready for Cultural Change

The fifth enabler of a patient safety culture is that the organization is ready, willing, and able to take action to change the organizational culture. In a patient safety culture, leaders have a growth mindset and an integrated approach to learning, development, and improvement. Education and training equip staff with an understanding of how harm occurs in healthcare, how systems fail, and how the impact of both can be reduced. Learnings may be of a technical and practical nature, such as how to address recurring incident reports that make visible the sources of actual and potential risk and harm to patients. Alternatively, they may be of a nontechnical nature, such as how to manage the pressure generated from increased workloads when working in high-stress environments to keep patients safe and retain staff.

When healthcare organizations have learned how to create a patient safety culture through a process of individual, collective, and systemic learning, staff will embrace patient safety values, behaviors, and *excellent* clinical practices, which together bring about sustained cultural transformation.

---

[2] The *Australian Institute of Professional Coaches* delivers coaching education programs in patient safety coaching. www.professionalcoachtraining.com.au

Key Takeaways

- Before starting a cultural change program, it is important to measure where the organization is now and identify the areas in which it needs to make improvements.
- Measurement instruments may be quantitative or qualitative. Quantitative measures include surveys. Qualitative measures include focus groups and brainstorming workshops. Ideally, both forms of measurement are conducted to identify areas for intervention and determine the extent of the cultural change required.
- The HSOPSC is the most commonly used instrument to identify areas for cultural improvement in relation to patient safety. It provides data across 10 patient safety dimensions at various levels of an organization, e.g., ward or department, occupation, position, or seniority.
- Results from research using the HSOPSC have identified the factors that contribute to the development of a patient safety culture: effective leadership; clear and detailed communication especially at times of handover and transition; teamwork; patient safety values that are "lived"; a psychologically safe workplace in which staff feel able to speak-up and report near misses; nonpunitive response to error; and management support for patient safety including action taken when a near miss is reported.

8.6 Case Study 8: Measuring a Patient Safety Culture Using HSOPSC

A large regional 800-bed hospital has faced several adverse events over the past 12 months including several potentially preventable patient deaths. These incidents have attracted significant media attention as this region is undergoing a change of local government, and healthcare has been firmly on the election agenda.

As a result of the media attention, online forums have been bombarded with negative community feedback about the hospital, highlighting the urgent need for a change in the hospital's patient safety culture. To address these concerns, the hospital administration decided to undertake a comprehensive assessment of its current patient safety culture using the Hospital Survey on Patient Safety Culture (HSOPSC) developed by the Agency for Healthcare Research and Quality (AHRQ), to establish a baseline and then action plan the areas for improvement to move it into its future state.

The survey was distributed electronically to all hospital staff including physicians, nurses, administrative staff, and support personnel. It was delivered by an external group who spent much time and effort guaranteeing the confidentiality of the data. Participation was voluntary and anonymous to encourage honest and candid feedback. The survey was available for 4 weeks, with weekly reminders sent to encourage participation.

The overall response rate was 62%, with the largest groups represented being nursing staff, operational staff, and allied health staff. Of note, the most significant issues were the following:

1. "Nonpunitive response to error": Lower scores suggested a fear of blame and punishment existed within the hospital when reporting errors.
2. "Communication openness": Mixed responses indicated that some staff felt hesitant to speak up about safety concerns.
3. "Supervisor/Manager expectations and actions promoting safety": Leadership's role in promoting safety practices needed evaluation.

Regular training sessions on patient safety best practices and the importance of reporting errors and near misses were conducted. Hospital leadership attended these and began to speak at each of these sessions to the actions they were taking as a result of the HSOPSC survey findings. Over the first 4 months, these training sessions became hospital-wide grand-rounds designed to promote learning from feedback.

In addition, leadership coaching was introduced, whereby leaders received patient safety coaching after a series of workshops for supervisors and managers were conducted. These workshops emphasized the importance of a nonpunitive approach to error reporting and encouraged open communication. The coaching that followed assisted them to change their leadership practices to become more supportive and collaborative in patient safety-related matters.

The hospital planned to readminister the HSOPSC 9 months' post-intervention to evaluate the effectiveness of the changes.

For Discussion

1. Discuss the various ways in which a patient safety culture can be measured in a healthcare organization.
    - What happened in this case study, and what could have been done differently?
2. What strategies can be used to develop a patient safety culture within teams?
    - What happened in this case study, and what could have been done differently?
3. What strategies can be used to develop a patient safety culture within a healthcare organization?
    - What happened in this case study, and what could have been done differently?
4. For what other purposes can coaching be used?

References

1. Hollnagel, E., Wears, R., & Braithwaite, J. (2015). *From safety-I to safety-II: A white paper*. University of Southern Denmark, University of Florida, USA, and Macquarie University, Australia.
2. Frankel, A., et al. (2017). *A framework for safe, reliable, and effective care.*
3. Foundation, N.P.S. (2015). *Free from harm: Accelerating patient safety improvement fifteen years after to err is human.*
4. Muthulingam, D., et al. (2019). Using nominal group technique to identify barriers, facilitators, and preferences among patients seeking treatment for opioid use disorder: A needs assessment for decision making support. *Journal of Substance Abuse Treatment, 100*, 18–28.
5. Gallagher, M., et al. (1993). The nominal group technique: A research tool for general practice? *Family Practice, 10*(1), 76–81.
6. Rafikul, I. (2010). Group decision making through nominal group technique: An empirical study. *Journal for International Business and Entrepreneurship Development, 5*(2), 134–153.
7. Hellings, J., et al. (2007). Challenging patient safety culture: Survey results. *International Journal of Health Care Quality Assurance, 20*(7), 620–632.
8. Kohn, L. T., et al. (1999). *To err is human: Building a safer health system*. Institute of Medicine.
9. Draganović, Š., & Offermanns, G. (2022). Patient safety culture in Austria and recommendations of evidence-based instruments for improving patient safety. *PLoS One, 17*(10), 1–17.
10. IOM. (2001). *Crossing the quality chasm: A new health system for the 21st century*. Institute of Medicine Committee on Quality of Health Care in America.
11. Santana, M. J., et al. (2018). How to practice person-centered care: A conceptual framework. *Health Expectations, 21*(2), 429–440.
12. Hedsköld, M., et al. (2021). Acting between guidelines and reality- an interview study exploring the strategies of first line managers in patient safety work. *BMC Health Services Research, 21*(1), 1–10.
13. Malinowska-Lipień, I., et al. (2021). Nurses and physicians attitudes toward factors related to hospitalized patient safety. *PLoS One, 16*(12), 1–13.
14. Grindean, A., & Domnariu, C. D. (2022). Study on the organizational culture of patient safety. *Acta Medica Transilvanica, 27*(2), 1–6.
15. Fassi, C. F., et al. (2023). Patient safety culture perception among Moroccan healthcare professionals: Cross-sectional study in public hospitals. *Ethiopian Journal of Health Sciences, 33*(2), 273–280.
16. Oweidat, I., et al. (2023). The association of patient safety culture with intent to leave among Jordanian nurses: A cross-sectional study. *BMC Nursing, 22*(1), 1–11.
17. Abraham, V., et al. (2022). Perceptions of managerial staff on the patient safety culture at a tertiary hospital in South Africa. *International Journal of Qualitative Studies on Health & Well-Being, 17*(1), 1–13.
18. Binkheder, S., et al. (2023). The relationships between patient safety culture and sentinel events among hospitals in Saudi Arabia: A national descriptive study. *BMC Health Services Research, 23*(1), 1–15.
19. Beyene Shashamo, B., et al. (2023). Patient safety culture and associated factors among nurses working at public hospitals in Gamo Zone, Southern Ethiopia. *BMC Health Services Research, 23*(1), 1–12.
20. Lee, S. E., Dahinten, V. S., & Lee, J. H. (2023). Testing the association between the enabling and enacting factors of patient safety culture and patient safety: Structural equation modeling. *BMC Nursing, 22*(1), 1–8.
21. Noviyanti, L. W., Ahsan, A., & Sudartya, T. S. (2021). Exploring the relationship between nurses' communication satisfaction and patient safety culture. *Journal of Public Health Research, 10*(2), 125–128.
22. Abuosi, A. A., et al. (2022). Safety culture and adverse event reporting in Ghanaian healthcare facilities: Implications for patient safety. *PLoS One, 17*(10), 1–18.

23. Tenza, I. S., et al. (2022). Hospital managers' views on the state of patient safety culture across three regions in Ghana. *BMC Health Services Research, 22*(1), 1–14.
24. Kakemam, E., et al. (2021). Nurses' perception of patient safety culture and its relationship with adverse events: A national questionnaire survey in Iran. *BMC Nursing, 20*(1), 1–10.
25. Hafezi, A., et al. (2022). The relationship between patient safety culture and patient safety competency with adverse events: A multicenter cross-sectional study. *BMC Nursing, 21*(1), 1–13.
26. Aouicha, W., et al. (2022). Patient safety culture as perceived by operating room professionals: A mixed-methods study. *BMC Health Services Research, 22*(1), 1–12.
27. Tlili, M. A., et al. (2022). Assessing patient safety culture in 15 intensive care units: A mixed-methods study. *BMC Health Services Research, 22*(1), 1–9.
28. de Brito Passos, A. C., dos Santos, D. B., & de França Fonteles, M. M. (2021). Patient safety culture: From perception to assessment. *Journal of Young Pharmacists, 13*(3), 291–297.
29. Reis, C. T., et al. (2023). Cross-cultural adaptation and validation of the hospital survey on patient safety culture 2.0—Brazilian version. *BMC Health Services Research, 23*(1), 1–12.
30. Alfadhalah, T., et al. (2021). Baseline assessment of patient safety culture in primary care centers in Kuwait: A national cross-sectional study. *BMC Health Services Research, 21*(1), 1–18.
31. Alshyyab, M. A., et al. (2022). Safety culture in emergency medicine: An exploratory qualitative study. *International Journal of Risk & Safety in Medicine, 33*(4), 365–383.
32. Kim, K.-A., et al. (2022). Patient safety measurement tools used in nursing homes: A systematic literature review. *BMC Health Services Research, 22*(1), 1–12.
33. Zabin, L. M., et al. (2023). The relationship between job stress and patient safety culture among nurses: A systematic review. *BMC Nursing, 22*(1), 1–7.
34. Zaitoun, R. A., Said, N. B., & de Tantillo, L. (2023). Clinical nurse competence and its effect on patient safety culture: A systematic review. *BMC Nursing, 22*(1), 1–10.
35. Vikan, M., et al. (2023). The association between patient safety culture and adverse events—A scoping review. *BMC Health Services Research, 23*(1), 1–27.
36. NPSA, National Patient Safety Agency. (2006). *Manchester patient safety framework (MaPSaF)*. National Patient Safety Agency.
37. Churruca, K., et al. (2021). Dimensions of safety culture: A systematic review of quantitative, qualitative and mixed methods for assessing safety culture in hospitals. *BMJ Open, 11*(7), e043982.
38. Halligan, M., & Zecevic, A. (2011). Safety culture in healthcare: A review of concepts, dimensions, measures and progress. *BMJ Quality Safety, 20*(4), 383–343.
39. Sorra, J., Yount, N., & Famolaro, T. (2019). *AHRQ Hospital survey on patient safety culture version 2.0: User's guide*. Agency for Healthcare Research and Quality.
40. Squires, J. E., et al. (2015). Understanding context in knowledge translation: A concept analysis study protocol. *Journal of Advanced Nursing, 71*(5), 146–155.
41. Armstrong, B. K., et al. (2007). Challenges in health and health care for Australia. *Medical Journal of Australia, 187*(9), 485–489.
42. Mendel, P., et al. (2008). Interventions in organizational and community context: A framework for building evidence on dissemination and implementation in health services research. *Administration and Policy in Mental Health, 35*(1–2), 21–37.
43. Chegini, Z., et al. (2020). The impact of patient safety culture and the leader coaching behavior of nurses on the intention to report errors: A cross-sectional survey. *BMC Nursing, 19*(1), 1–9.
44. Kagan, I., & Barnoy, S. (2013). Organizational safety culture and medical error reporting by Israeli nurses. *Journal of Nursing Scholarship, 45*(3), 273–280.
45. Silva, N. D., et al. (2016). Patient safety in organizational culture as perceived by leaderships of hospital institutions with different types of administration. *Revista da Escola de Enfermagem da USP, 50*(3), 490–497.
46. Maslach, C., & Jackson, S. (1981). The measurement of experienced burnout. *Journal of Occupational Behavior, 2*, 99–113.
47. de Lima Garcia, C., et al. (2019). Association between culture of patient safety and burnout in pediatric hospitals. *PLoS One, 14*(6), 1–14.

48. Administration, A.f.H.C. *Nursing Home Federal reporting*. 1989; Available from: https://ahca.myflorida.com/MCHQ/Field_Ops/CAU/Federal_Reporting
49. Andersson, Å., et al. (2018). Factors contributing to serious adverse events in nursing homes. *Journal of Clinical Nursing, 27*(1–2), e354–e362.
50. Lee, H. Y., Blegen, M. A., & Harrington, C. (2014). The effects of RN staffing hours on nursing home quality: A two-stage model. *International Journal of Nursing Studies, 51*(3), 409–417.
51. Spilsbury, K., et al. (2011). The relationship between nurse staffing and quality of care in nursing homes: A systematic review. *International Journal of Nursing Studies, 48*(6), 732–750.
52. Reis, C. T., Paiva, S. G., & Sousa, P. (2018). The patient safety culture: A systematic review by characteristics of hospital survey on patient safety culture dimensions. *International Journal of Quality Health Care, 30*(9), 660–677.
53. Sorra, J., et al. (2019). *Pilot test results from the 2019 AHRQ surveys on patient safety cultureTM(SOPSTM) hospital survey version 2.0—Part1: Overall results*. Agency for Healthcare Research and Quality.
54. Lee, S. E., & Dahinten, V. S. (2021). Adaptation and validation of a Korean-language version of the revised hospital survey on patient safety culture (K-HSOPSC20). *BMC Nursing, 2021*(20), 12.
55. Sexton, J. B., et al. (2006). The safety attitudes questionnaire: Psychometric properties, benchmarking data, and emerging research. *BMC Health Services Research, 6*(1), 1–10.
56. Bartonickova, D., Kalankova, D., & Ziakova, K. (2021). How to measure patient safety culture? A literature review of instruments. *Acta Medica Martiniana, 21*(2), 69–79.
57. Ashcroft, D., et al. (2005). Safety culture assessment in community pharmacy: Development, face validity, and feasibility of the Manchester patient safety assessment framework. *BMJ Quality & Safety, 14*(6), 417–421.
58. Sari, A. A. (2017). Assessing patient safety culture in the hospital: A pilot study using a modified Manchester Patient Safety Framework (MaPSaF). *JMMR (Jurnal Medicoeticolegal dan Manajemen Rumah Sakit), 6*(3), 159–168.
59. Wallis, K., & Dovey, S. (2011). Assessing patient safety culture in New Zealand primary care: A pilot study using a modified Manchester Patient Safety Framework in Dunedin general practices. *Journal of Primary Health Care, 3*(1), 35–40.
60. Wang, L. J., et al. (2023). Assessing patient safety culture in obstetrics ward: A pilot study using a modified Manchester Patient Safety Framework in China. *Nursing Open, 10*(2), 658–664.
61. Marshall, M., et al. (2017). Assessing the safety culture of care homes: A multimethod evaluation of the adaptation, face validity and feasibility of the Manchester Patient Safety Framework. *BMJ Quality & Safety, 26*(9), 751–759.
62. Braithwaite, J., et al. (2009). *Staff survey on patient safety*. Centre for Healthcare Resilience and Implementation Science, UNSW for the South Australian Council for Safety and Quality in Health Care and South Australian Department of Health.
63. Parker, D. (2009). Managing risk in healthcare: Understanding your safety culture using the Manchester Patient Safety Framework (MaPSaF). *Journal of Nursing Management, 17*(2), 218–222.
64. NSQHS. (2021). *National safety and quality health service standards. Second edition*. Australian Commission on Safety and Quality in Health Care.
65. Öhrn, A., Rutberg, H., & Nilsen, P. (2011). Patient safety dialog: Evaluation of an intervention aimed at achieving an improved patient safety culture. *Journal of Patient Safety, 7*(4), 185–192.
66. Long, J. C., et al. (2021). The pace of hospital life: A mixed methods study. *PLoS One, 16*(8), 1–12.
67. Bowling, N. A., & Hammond, G. D. (2008). A meta-analytic examination of the construct validity of the Michigan organizational assessment questionnaire job satisfaction subscale. *Journal of Vocational Behavior, 73*, 63–77.

68. Hackman, J., & Oldham, G. (1975). Development of the job diagnostic survey. *Journal of Applied Psychology, 60*(2), 159–170.
69. Schaufeli, W., Enzmann, D., & Girault, N. (1993). Measurement of burnout: A review. In W. B. Schaufeli, C. Maslach, & T. Marek (Eds.), *Professional burnout: Recent developments in theory and research* (pp. 199–215). Taylor & Francis.
70. Maslach, C., Schaufeli, W., & Leiter, M. P. (2001). Job burnout. *Annual Review of Psychology, 52*, 397–422.
71. WHO. (2015). *Patient safety tool kit*. World Health Organization, Regional Office for the Eastern Mediterranean.
72. Manley, K., & Jackson, C. (2019). Microsystems culture change: A refined theory for developing person-centered, safe and effective workplaces based on strategies that embed a safety culture. *International Practice Development Journal, 9*(2), 1–21.
73. Valentin, A., et al. (2006). Patient safety in intensive care: Results from the multinational Sentinel Events Evaluation (SEE) study. *Intensive Care Medicine, 32*(10), 1591–1598.
74. Valentin, A., et al. (2009). Errors in administration of parenteral drugs in intensive care units: Multinational prospective study. *BMJ, 338*, b814.
75. Pronovost, P. J., et al. (2010). Sustaining reductions in catheter related bloodstream infections in Michigan intensive care units: Observational study. *BMJ, 340*, c309.
76. Urbach, D. R., et al. (2014). Introduction of surgical safety checklists in Ontario, Canada. *New England Journal of Medicine, 370*(11), 1029–1038.
77. Reames, B. N., et al. (2015). A checklist-based intervention to improve surgical outcomes in Michigan: Evaluation of the Keystone Surgery program. *JAMA Surgery, 15*(3), 208–215.
78. Sorra, J. S., & Dyer, N. (2010). Multilevel psychometric properties of the AHRQ hospital survey on patient safety culture. *BMC Health Services Research, 10*, 199.
79. Sexton, J. B., et al. (2006). The safety attitudes questionnaire: Psychometric properties, benchmarking data, and emerging research. *BMC Health Services Research, 6*, 44.
80. WHO. (2021). *Global patient safety action plan 2021–2030:Toward eliminating avoidable harm in health care*. World Health Organization, License: CC BY-NC-SA 3.0 IGO.
81. Manley, K., et al. (2011a). Effective workplace culture: The attributes, enabling factors and consequences of a new concept. *International Practice Development Journal, 1*(2), Article 1.
82. O'Connor, S., & Cavanagh, M. (2013). The coaching ripple effect: The effects of developmental coaching on wellbeing across organisational networks. *Psychology of Well-Being: Theory, Research and Practice, 3*(2), 1–23.
83. Sammer, C. E., et al. (2010). What is patient safety culture? A review of the literature. *Journal of Nursing Scholarship, 42*(2), 156–165.
84. Chegini, Z., Arab-Zozani, M., & Janati, A. (2019). Patient and health professional perspectives about engaging patients in addressing patient safety: A systematic review protocol. *Journal of Medical Science, 7*(9), 1561–1565.
85. Okuyama, A., Wagner, C., & Bijnen, B. (2014). Speaking up for patient safety by hospital-based health care professionals: A literature review. *BMC Health Services Research, 14*(1), 61.
86. Rosen, M., et al. (2018). Teamwork in healthcare: Key discoveries enabling safer, high-quality care. *American Psychologist.*
87. Dietz, A. S., et al. (2014). A systematic review of teamwork in the intensive care unit: What do we know about teamwork, team tasks, and im provement strategies? *Journal of Critical Care, 29*(6), 908–914.
88. Auraaen, A., Slawomirski, L., & Klazinga, N. *The economics of patientsafety in primary and ambulatory care- Flying blind.* 2018, OECD Health Working Papers(No. 106).
89. Moore, L., & McAuliffe, E. (2012). To report or not to report? Why some nurses are reluctant to whistleblow. *Clinical Governance: An International Journal, 17*(4), 332–342.
90. Martin, A., & Manley, K. (2017). Developing standards for an integrated approach to workplace facilitation for interprofessional teams in health and social care contexts: A Delphi study. *Journal of Interprofessional Care, 32*(1), 41–51.

Chapter 9
Governance in Healthcare

Executives in healthcare organizations are responsible for the effective and efficient operation of their facility. They must ensure compliance with all government legislation and associated regulations. They have a fiduciary duty of care as well as a moral obligation to manage the best possible healthcare system for their patients. Society expects that patients can turn to healthcare staff to look after them in their hours of need. However, managerial and clinical staff perceptions of patient safety may vary significantly in terms of prioritizing interventions that can improve patient care and safety, as well as in relation to their perceived roles in establishing and maintaining a patient safety culture [1, 2]. Research has shown that hospital executives and managers, by failing to recognize their role in supporting patient safety, may actually hinder error reporting and learning from *excellence*, particularly at critical times such as patient handovers [3, 4].

The World Health Organization (WHO) defined *organizational governance* in 2007 through a policy-focused lens as "the ability to achieve intended outcomes and the tasks and processes necessary to do so" [5]. They drilled down to describe *healthcare governance* as referring to the rules and norms that shape roles and responsibilities, incentives, and interactions within that sector [6]. Through the exercise of their governance functions, healthcare providers, both public and private, are essential in the establishment and maintenance of healthcare systems that ensure compliance with all legal, ethical, and moral obligations and the achievement of targeted outcomes in relation to patient care and safety.

In an address on 13th July 2023, the Director-General outlined the WHO's priorities for universal health coverage (UHC) post-pandemic for all countries—to promote, protect, provide, power, and perform for health—a shift to a Safety-11 [7] preventative approach to keeping patients safe from harm.

1. *Promote health* by shifting the focus to prevention and promotion rather than root cause analysis of diseases and injuries. Making this paradigm shift means that health is not only the business of state health departments but also a societal priority for the whole of government.

© The Author(s), under exclusive license to Springer Nature Switzerland AG 2024

S. Knowles, *Patient Safety Coaching*,
https://doi.org/10.1007/978-3-031-68722-8_9

2. *Protect health* by establishing a new Accord that applies to all Member States to strengthen the global architecture for health emergency preparedness and response to events such as pandemics. The Accord is governed by key proposals for stronger governance, financing, and systems and tools for health security.
3. *Provide health* by reorienting service delivery toward primary healthcare systems as the main vehicle to promote, protect, and provide health.
4. *Power health* by partnering with scientific research associations and exploiting data, digital technologies, and artificial intelligence into healthcare innovations.
5. *Perform for health* by building a stronger WHO and the combined strength of the local health workforce and infrastructure. Providers are thus better able to deliver an impact where it matters most—in healthier people, families, communities, and nations.[1]

The Director-General mused that investments in the health workforce and infrastructure would likely account for at least one-third of the investment needed to achieve the WHO's health-related targets, as reported in their *Sustainable Development Goals* [8]. He emphasized that capital investment in facilities and equipment allows the health workforce to perform its jobs *well,* as an *investment* to be nurtured, not a *cost* to be contained. Furthermore, he asserted that health financing must be provided by domestic, public funding, not private financing, so that spending will be aligned with government priorities. He announced that, in the previous month (June 2023), a group of multilateral development banks launched the *Health Impact Investment Platform* which aims to attract investment from development banks to deliver country-led health projects, with technical support from the WHO.

9.1 Organizational Governance

Organizational governance in healthcare relates to the goals and priorities that organizations put in place to ensure that the system of providing healthcare for patients through the personal efforts of staff is fit for purpose and sustainable. It encompasses "the system by which an organization is controlled and operates, and the mechanisms by which it and its people are held to account. Ethics, risk management, compliance and administration are all elements of governance."[2] Overall, the primary objective of governance in healthcare is to ensure that the organization functions effectively and efficiently, providing services that meet patient needs in accordance with applicable laws and regulations.

In healthcare, organizational governance systems monitor financial viability, risk, and the allocation and management of resources. Governance processes

[1] Appendix 9.1. Readers may like to estimate the degree to which their healthcare organization promotes, protects, provides, powers and performs for health.

[2] https://www.governanceinstitute.com.au/resources/what-is-governance/

coordinate the collective efforts of multiple stakeholders to ensure the quality, safety, and effectiveness of services to patients while also making efficient use of resources. Organizational governance is assured by adherence to the following:

- *The rules* of law and accountability which operate to ensure the financial viability of the organization.
- *Effective relationships* within the organization and between management and the board, as well as with key stakeholders.
- *Processes* that direct activities to meet the organization's strategic objectives and monitor its performance.
- *Coordinated systems* that govern the way in which the organization is controlled and operates, including the mechanisms by which it and its people are held accountable, e.g., for ethical management, compliance, and risk management.

The concept of organizational governance has four key components: accountability, transparency, stewardship, and integrity.

9.1.1 Accountability and Transparency

Accountability was introduced into the healthcare sector in the 1990s following public demands for greater transparency regarding the expenditure of government funds, health sector performance, and responsiveness to concerns about service provision in relation to public healthcare providers [9]. Accountability and transparency are two of the most important aspects of healthcare, and they are critical to ensuring that healthcare systems are cost-effective, efficient, and compliant with regulations. Good governance is embodied not only in the systems by which organizations operate but also in the mechanisms by which organizational representatives who implement them are held accountable.

Accountability is the responsibility of healthcare providers, administrators, and other stakeholders to ensure that they are providing the best possible care for patients. They are responsible for significant strategic and operational decisions and for putting meaningful mechanisms in place to ensure adherence to all applicable laws and regulations. As public funds are expended, healthcare providers must be held accountable for their organization's performance both in terms of quality service provision and cost. This includes ensuring that services are delivered in a timely manner, that patients receive appropriate care, and that healthcare workers are competent and deliver to professional standards.

Transparency from a governance perspective is about having clarity of executive roles and responsibilities, explicit procedures for exercising power and making decisions, and timely means of communicating or reporting these decisions to the appropriate people or authorities. It includes making information readily available about the cost and quality of care, the nature and outcomes of service provision, and the performance of healthcare providers. From an organizational perspective, transparency ensures that healthcare providers are held accountable for their performance. From a person perspective, transparency is essential for improving the quality of care, as it allows patients to make informed decisions about the care they receive.

The executive team is accountable for the design and operation of governance arrangements and practices within its healthcare organization. They need to provide visibility of results to the board, government, legislators, and the community. To meet all applicable legislative and policy obligations as well as public expectations of openness and transparency, executives need to:

- Establish clear roles, responsibilities, and accountabilities for decisions and actions.
- Set clear expectations regarding transparency when reporting on performance and operations.
- Build relationships with stakeholders to ensure that services are fit for purpose.
- Exhibit high standards of probity and integrity in providing services, including managing conflicts of interest.

Gurung et al. [10] found that social auditing plays a positive role in organizational responsiveness by increasing the transparency, accessibility, and quality of services. They proposed that social auditing can be used as a complementary accountability mechanism (a "voice") to support traditional bureaucratic accountability processes as well as to develop "partnership with the notion of joint problem-solving and emphasis on relational elements of accountability which hold promise for building trust and responsiveness" [10].

9.1.2 Stewardship and Integrity

Stewardship and integrity are two other important principles in healthcare. They are essential for the provision of quality, systemic care, and delivery of the best possible outcomes for patients. It was in 2000 when the WHO first assigned responsibility to national entities to advance global health initiatives such as UHC that the principle of stewardship was included as one of the four key functions underpinning a well-performing health system [11].

Key stakeholders in the development of an effective governance system within the health sector include healthcare provider organizations, regulatory bodies, professional groups, and professional educational institutions. Each of these groups has differing interests, and strategic stewardship is required to align operational imperatives with government policies to achieve state and national health objectives. Within the government, there is a need to coordinate across ministries accountable for meeting fiscal responsibilities, legal compliance, and professional and educational standards of care. The department responsible for health in each state or nation must take the lead in providing stewardship of the governance process to ensure political commitment to the strategic health agenda at the highest level of government.

Executives with a governance responsibility exert stewardship when they organize and manage the delivery of key healthcare functions to achieve an overarching vision, direction, and goals for the organization. Stewardship also holds executives responsible for the effective and efficient use of resources, materials, and labor to achieve the best possible healthcare outcomes for patients. This involves balancing the needs of patients, providers, and the community, considering the cost-effectiveness of services, and ensuring that all resources are used responsibly.

Integrity is about acting impartially, ethically, and in the best interests of the public and health system. It is the adherence to ethical and moral principles even when no one is looking. Healthcare providers are expected to be honest and forthright in all their communications and dealings with patients, staff, and relevant authorities. They are expected to take responsibility for their actions, keep their promises, and never compromise their values or standards. Integrity in healthcare is essential for creating a safe and trusted environment for everyone involved.

9.1.3 Leadership, Efficiency, and Performance

Some healthcare systems add three further dimensions to these governance principles [12]:

- Leadership—achieving good governance through leadership from the top.
- Efficiency—ensuring the best use of resources to further the aims of the public health system.
- Performance—designing and managing governance arrangements and practices that shape and enable overall performance and delivery of effective, efficient, and economical patient services. This relates to how healthcare systems:
  - Plan for high performance through strategic and operational planning supported by robust financial management.
  - Clearly define outcomes and improve results through effective use of performance information.
  - Engage with and strategically manage risks and take advantage of opportunities.
  - Evaluate and review programs to build on strengths and improve outcomes for the community.
  - Drive continuous improvement by supporting the implementation of best practices and innovation.

A number of key stakeholders work together to ensure the effective and efficient delivery of healthcare services. These include board directors, the executive team, clinicians, patients, and other stakeholders such as regulatory bodies and organizations. Each of these stakeholders has distinct roles and responsibilities. Governments are responsible for regulating healthcare services, healthcare providers are responsible for providing high-quality care, and patients are responsible for making informed decisions.

Within each healthcare organization, the governing board is responsible for setting the strategic direction and overseeing its performance. The executive team establishes structures, policies, and procedures to ensure the efficient and effective delivery of healthcare services. The senior leadership team is responsible for the day-to-day management of the organization and for implementing the strategies set by the executive team. The roles and responsibilities of various actors vary depending on the level of governance but typically include developing policies, ensuring compliance with laws and regulations, setting objectives, and monitoring performance. To ensure ongoing governance, healthcare executives and boards must regularly review their policies and procedures to ensure compliance with any changes in healthcare legislation or regulations.

9.2 Clinical Governance

Clinical governance has been defined as "the set of relationships and responsibilities established by a health service organization between its state or territory department of health, governing body, executive, workforce, patients, consumers and other stakeholders to ensure good clinical outcomes".[3] In 2022, the Australian Commission on Safety and Quality in Healthcare (ACSQH) launched a clinical governance framework that is distinct from other governance frameworks but just as important.[4] To deliver *excellence* in patient care, a clinical governance framework must be integrated into the overarching organizational governance framework, be embedded in the culture of the organization, and be clearly linked with other governance aspects such as risk management and financial probity [13].

9.2.1 Process or Outcome Driven

In the health workforce literature, governance is conceptualized as *process driven, outcome focused*, or both [14]. As a process-oriented function, governance is described as a set of processes by which directives and responsibilities are distributed among different actors to achieve goals. As an outcome-oriented function, it is described according to the administrative and policymaking aspects of an executive's role that are required to align policies with the healthcare organization's goals and objectives. These two characterizations are neither mutually exclusive nor mutually complementary; they are just different perspectives on the concept of clinical governance.

---

[3] https://www.safetyandquality.gov.au/standards/primary-and-community-healthcare/guide-primary-and-community-healthcare-standards/glossary

[4] https://www.safetyandquality.gov.au/newsroom/national-standards-updates/launch-national-clinical-trials-governance-framework

A study by Draganović and Offermanns [15] in 2022 investigated the outcomes of a patient safety culture in Austrian hospitals. They analyzed the correlation between ten patient safety culture factors, three background characteristics (descriptive variables), and three outcome variables (patient safety grade, number of adverse events reported, and influence on patient safety). Using the Austrian Patient Safety Climate Inventory (A-PaSKI), their findings revealed that the factors most highly rated as likely to produce the outcome of a patient safety culture were "Communication openness" and "Supervisor/Manager's expectations and actions promoting safety." The factor least likely to deliver the desired outcome was "Nonpunitive response to error." In addition, they compared the value that various professional groups placed on developing a patient safety culture which revealed significant differences among nurses, doctors, and other groups. The outcome factors of a patient safety culture that professionals thought important were "Frequency of event reporting" (although 68% of the staff stated they had not reported a single event in the year before), "Support of management," "Teamwork," "Communication openness," and "Feedback within the clinics." The researchers concluded that if a culture of blame within hospitals is replaced with one that does not sanction errors, patient safety will improve.

Although management issues are often highlighted within the health sector governance literature, Dieleman et al. [16] noted that less attention is given to political considerations.

9.2.2 Political Dimension

Decision-making in organizations is highly complex and involves a number of political and economic considerations. Healthcare organizations must make decisions that are ethical, in the best interests of their patients, and based on evidence-based practice. This involves balancing the needs of patients with the political interests of governing authorities, plus a realistic assessment of what can be done given the finances available to the healthcare organization at that time. Decisions can be influenced by a variety of external factors, including state and federal regulations, public opinion, and the political views of healthcare professionals.

Political considerations often influence decisions about the allocation of resources, the types of services offered, and the standards of care. For example, decisions about healthcare funding and resource allocation can be influenced by the political views of elected officials. Similarly, decisions about the types of services offered and the standards of care can be influenced by public opinion and the political views of healthcare professionals, private sector providers, professional associations, and health-related networks.

Governments play a major role in establishing governance arrangements in the healthcare sector. They act through a broad range of legal, policy, planning, and monitoring instruments. In addition to these formal instruments available to the government, a variety of conventions, norms, cultural traditions, forms of persuasion, economic pressure, and other mechanisms are increasingly shaping governance arrangements and health system performance. O'Keefe et al. [24] cite the International Bureau of Education (2019) as reporting that "For many, considerations of governance are intimately related to considerations about how power is distributed and shared, how policies are formulated, priorities set, and stakeholders made accountable". This is what Brinkerhoff and Bossert [17] describe as governance with a political dimension, notably that of authority, power, and decision-making in shaping policy. Lim and Lin [14] believe that the fundamentally political nature of health workforce issues should not be seen as a barrier to discussing governance issues but rather as an opportunity for improving the conceptualization of governance within a health workforce context. Executives must carefully evaluate the implications of their decisions and ensure that they deliver the best possible outcomes in relation to patient care.

9.2.3 The Role of Executives

Although clinical managers play an important role in maintaining the quality of care for patients in wards and promoting a safety culture within teams [18], it is ultimately the responsibility of healthcare executives to ensure that organizational policies and systems support and promote a patient safety culture within the facility they govern. The patient safety culture of an organization is established by senior executives; clinical managers are tasked with delivering a positive and just patient safety culture within their units [19]. The consequences of not providing a safe patient environment were made clear by the US government in 2008 when Medicare stopped paying hospitals for errors deemed preventable; the hospital was considered liable for any litigation payments that arose as a result of errors, including for the cost of any additional procedures and/or extended hospital stays [20]. This situation has caused many health systems to introduce or re-think their quality of care and safety standards to better manage patient safety incidents within their organization. In some instances, financial disincentives have been imposed on healthcare organizations to ensure that they successfully implement patient safety initiatives [21]. Executive and managerial support and engagement can help reduce the risks associated with medical liabilities at the unit level and, conversely, substantially improve quality patient outcomes [1, 22].

Unfortunately, there are many occasions when organizational duty of care to patients has failed, resulting in major impacts on patients and their families. In the past, when adverse events occurred, they were typically blamed on the individual—the last person in the delivery chain. This is the Safety-1 view of how to keep patients safe. The more contemporary view is to prevent errors from occurring by putting mechanisms in place to: (i) recognize when the system components are approaching failure, and (ii) relieve the pressure on extended health systems so that the limits of their operability are not breached or broken [23].[5] This is a Safety-11 [7] approach to patient safety.[6]

9.3 Governance Principles

Across all types of healthcare delivery services (national and state governments, private, and not-for-profit organizations), there are shared foci in terms of person-centered care, evidence-based clinical practice, workforce sustainability, and the use of innovative technology [24]. In complex environments such as combined university and healthcare services in hospitals, while many interrelated systems coexist to support and improve patient care, different priorities may, at times, cause tension in interdisciplinary teams, presenting opportunities for discipline-specific and joint learning. Overall, joint agreement is usually focused on high standards of patient care based on principles similar to the following:

- Healthcare organizations are committed to providing quality care to patients and measuring outcomes to ensure that standards are met.
- Communication between clinicians, staff, and patients is open, honest, and effective.
- Patient data are securely stored, and privacy is respected.
- Patients are informed of their rights and encouraged to participate in decisions about their care.
- Healthcare leadership is competent, ethical, and accountable.
- Healthcare organizations are accountable for their actions and decisions, and executives ensure that they follow the standards of care and regulations set by governing bodies.
- Healthcare organizations strive to be transparent in their operations and decision-making processes, including financial dealings, organizational policies, and patient care practices.[7]

[5] You can read more about the 'boundary of acceptable performance' in Chap. 3.

[6] You can read more about Safety-1 and Safety-11 approaches to better manage patient care in Chap. 2.

[7] Appendix 9.2. Readers may like to consider whether these principles apply in a healthcare organization with which you are familiar.

9.4 Governance Issues in Healthcare

The function of governance is a management issue. Barbazza and Tello [25] describe the dimensions of governance as comprising three categories: fundamental *values*, *subfunctions*, and *outcomes*. These categories represent the compositional makeup of governance and how the delivery of health services is operationalized as the "components, elements, principles, or attributes" of governance [25]. The role of executives and clinical leaders is to ensure that the *values* are "lived," that the *subfunctions* are operationalized, and that the *outcomes* are achieved.

In healthcare settings where patient safety is a lived *value*, good governance creates a patient safety culture in which all people involved in patient care (providers, staff, administrators, and patients/families) are engaged, encouraged, and supported to make care safer. According to their research, Beyene et al. [26] recommended that hospital administrators, nurses, doctors, directors, and healthcare policymakers work together in collaboration to improve every healthcare organization's culture to create a blame-free environment that promotes event reporting. Psychological safety is essential if healthcare staff are to feel free to speak up about adverse events or near misses.

The *subfunctions* of good governance have been described as the "actionable processes for which the system's steward has oversight" [25]. The two critical subfunctions identified in Lim and Lin's [14] research are *stakeholder participation* and *strategic direction*. They found that these two elements were the only two subfunctions consistently mentioned when discussing the governance of the health workforce in the extant literature. These two subfunctions are considered to be essential for enabling governance improvements in the health workforce.

The *outcomes* to be achieved by good governance include: (i) improved patient care, (ii) a reduction in adverse events, and (iii) the establishment of a patient safety culture. These quality and safety outcomes can only be achieved by the dedication and commitment of healthcare staff to the services they deliver to patients. Support from management and organizational executives is critical to achieving these outcomes.

The sections that follow discuss six issues that have been highlighted in recent research as contributing to good governance in healthcare. These are usually standard inclusions on the executive governance agenda:

1. Strategic planning
2. Workforce planning
3. Resource optimization
4. Technology, AI, patient data, data privacy and storage, data sharing
5. Stakeholder participation and social accountability
6. Organizational culture

9.4.1 Strategic Planning

Strategic planning in relation to healthcare governance focuses on ensuring consistent quality of care across the organization and implementing measures to improve quality over time. This involves identifying and mitigating risks to patient safety. Strategic planning is important because it helps the organization plan for the future and ensure that it is in a position to provide the best possible care for patients. It also helps to identify areas where improvements can be made. It is an important part of the overall management of a healthcare organization because it helps to ensure that resources are allocated efficiently to achieve desired outcomes. By taking into account the current and future needs of healthcare organizations as well as the changing needs of patients, strategic planning helps to ensure that resources are used in the most effective way.

During strategic planning, the healthcare organization clarifies its vision, mission, and values, establishes priorities and goals, identifies strategies to meet objectives, and determines actions to implement the plan. The process involves in-depth analysis of the internal and external environment, consultation with key stakeholders, and consideration of current and future needs and aspirations. It typically begins with an analysis of the current state of the organization including its financial position, operational plans, and objectives.

When conducting strategic planning, several organizational factors need to be considered including high-level goals and priorities, available resources and infrastructure, current and emerging patient needs and expectations, and technological advances. In addition, external factors such as the goals and priorities of regulatory, professional, and political stakeholders need to be considered. An important part of the planning process is the determination of reporting measures that show when strategic goals and priorities have been achieved.

Once the strategic plan has been developed, it is shared with all stakeholders, internal and external, to ensure that everyone is able to comment on what is proposed. This process involves gathering feedback from stakeholders, discussing the goals and objectives with them, and gaining their commitment to the proposed strategies and actions. The focus on publicizing strategic health plans has grown in recent years in response to stakeholder expectations of accountability and transparency, and to anchor the strategic vision based on analysis and evidence with indicators of success. It is important that the executive team engage in ongoing evaluation and monitoring of the plan's progress, which involves measuring performance against the stated goals and adjusting objectives as necessary.

Finally, it is important to ensure that the strategic plan is supported by the organization's culture. This involves focusing on the organization's core values and associated behaviors that all staff are expected to display in their interactions with colleagues and patients. Best practice is to embed the organization's mission, vision, and values into a Code of Conduct that is socialized through Town Hall meetings and training programs, so that everyone understands where the organization is going and what is expected of them. Sufficient resources and equipment must be available to ensure the success of the plan.

The key accountabilities of healthcare executives may be summarized as follows:

1. Setting and managing organizational goals and objectives
2. Establishing financial and operational performance targets
3. Developing policies and procedures to ensure compliance with healthcare regulations
4. Developing strategies to increase access, quality, and cost-effectiveness of care
5. Managing and controlling the healthcare organization's budget
6. Identifying and managing risks

A key accountability of healthcare executives is also adequately staffing, developing, and effectively managing clinical and operational teams to maximize patient treatment and care.

9.4.2 Workforce Planning

With increasing complexity in the healthcare environment and the organizations that deliver healthcare, regulatory power over issues is often shifted away from the direct control of state or health authorities [27]. That is, health workforce policies may be more influenced by local factors such as fiscal availability, employment practices, and health workforce resistance to change [28]. Government agendas and priorities inevitably lead to challenges in implementing and operationalizing local health workforce policies and planning [29].

Workforce governance in healthcare is a technical process requiring expertise in planning, education and management, and strategy "rooted in a long-term vision for the health system" [30]. Sales et al. [31] believe that it is also a political process "requiring the will and the capacity to coordinate efforts on the part of different sectors and constituencies in society and different levels of government." Because power is shared among a diverse array of stakeholders in healthcare organizations [14], coordinating and implementing policies for the health workforce may require governance that is divergent from the usual top-down hierarchical governance process. Rather, what is needed is a combination of top-down and bottom-up stakeholder participation and consensus-building within the policymaking process. This dual approach acknowledges and addresses the increasingly diverse stakeholder groups within healthcare, all with different workforce needs.

The aim of workforce planning is to ensure that the right people receive the right services at the right place at the right time from those with the right skills and at the right cost [32, 33]. This task has become increasingly challenging for workforce planners as healthcare embraces integrated care, which is broadly considered to be an inter-sectoral approach that aims to align the healthcare system with other human service systems to improve outcomes for targeted populations, enhancing their quality of life and improving consumer satisfaction. New models of care include in-home and community care, residential and nursing home care, and aged care [34]. Integrated care can be provided for individuals (using case management or care plans), groups (e.g., for chronic care or for the frail and elderly), or categories (e.g., of patients with specific long-term conditions such as diabetes or cardiovascular disease) [35].

By proactively planning for future workforce needs, organizations are better able to meet their goals and objectives. This includes ensuring that they have sufficient resources to recruit and retain the right talent, maintain appropriate staffing levels, and develop the right mix of skills and competencies. The workforce planning process identifies key skills gaps and develops strategies to address them. This ultimately leads to increased efficiency of delivery, as well as improved customer service and satisfaction. The following issues may need to be considered in clinical workforce planning:

- Shortage of qualified staff
- Difficulty recruiting and retaining qualified staff
- High turnover of staff
- Inadequate staffing levels
- Disproportionate skills mix
- Distribution imbalance

Tackling these key systemic workforce issues requires a cohesive and strategic governance approach centered around coordinating and implementing policies to improve workforce performance [14].

Martineau et al. [36] believe that key considerations in developing and maintaining a fit-for-purpose health workforce require a long-term planning and financing agenda informed by labor market analysis. The challenge is to conduct a well-informed dialog with a sufficient range of stakeholders, building investment in long-term health plans while appreciating the short-term needs of some stakeholders, and navigating an ever-changing external environment (e.g., brought about by pandemics, political unrest). They suggest that the keys to this process are as follows:

- Leadership that recognizes the health workforce as essential to UHC, and the need for a financial plan for long-term investment in the health workforce.
- Robust and transparent mechanisms that promote political and social accountability and responsibility for performance and results (i.e., health workforce outcomes).
- Well-informed stakeholders and decisionmakers through the provision of good health workforce information and the construction of "health workforce literacy" which enables them to plan for and understand changing health workforce dynamics.
- A unified approach to the coordination of stakeholders who support the timely development and oversight of an appropriate and costed health workforce strategy, subsequently implemented and monitored by a human resource unit.
- Adaptable and flexible health workforce governance arrangements and policies that can respond to shocks and emergencies.
- Reliable, timely, and comprehensive health workforce data available at all levels to inform evidence-based decision-making.

In addition to a sustainable workforce, patient outcomes will only be achieved when clinicians have ready access to all the resources, equipment, and technology they need to ensure patient care.

9.4.3 Resource Optimization

Resource optimization in healthcare is the practice of making the most efficient use of resources such as staff and equipment to deliver quality care. By optimizing available resources, healthcare organizations can reduce costs, improve patient outcomes, and increase the availability of care. To optimize patient care, they need to ensure that they have the right number and mix of competent staff to meet patient needs. Resource optimization requires policies to retain existing staff, prepare to hire additional staff, cross-train existing staff if necessary, and, at times, reallocate staff to alternate areas of need. Organizations also need to optimize equipment use and ensure that the right equipment is available for patient treatment when needed. Importantly, they need to invest when they can in new and upgraded equipment as well as ensure that existing resources are properly maintained.

Hospital congestion has become a major concern in many healthcare settings. The incidence of ambulance ramping continues to receive increasing attention, and patients are increasingly turning to the media to bring about changes in hospital systems, particularly within emergency departments. Longer waiting times and queuing lengths have been associated with a number of factors including a greater risk of patient death while ramping or waiting for bed access, hospital-acquired infections, public complaints, and negative impacts on staff mental health [37, 38].

Traditional resource modeling has not improved this situation. Hou et al. [39] researched an alternative model of resource optimization in hospitals. Rather than using the traditional congestion prevention method that estimates the hospital congestion risk level (R) and activates minimum intervention when R is above a certain threshold, they created a virtual hospital by simulation modeling, which included a traffic light color-coded system to indicate the level of bed congestion. They showed that small adjustments that are less disruptive to current practices than traditional methods can be made to reduce bed congestion. Specifically, their findings revealed the following:

- Discharging patients had fewer effects because it involved only certain numbers of discharged patients but saved money.
- Discharging an extra two medical inpatients rather than surgical patients, a day earlier on days when R is above the threshold, was more beneficial in terms of congestion reduction for the hospital (because medical patients contribute to hospital congestion more significantly than other types of patients).
- Adding beds, especially in the medical department, brought the expected benefits in congestion reduction, but opening a bed costs more money.

- Adding two beds greatly decreased the number of high-congestion days compared with adding four or six beds, as these beds were quickly taken by patients waiting in the queue.
- When interventions were implemented for medical patients and medical departments, the reduction in the number of red days was more obvious.

Hou et al. [39] concluded that applying a less disruptive intervention is often enough and more cost-effective to reduce the risk of hospital congestion. That is, adding a small number of extra beds (two), particularly in medical wards, is a superior solution compared with discharging patients to reduce crowding in hospitals.

Another key accountability of healthcare executives is evaluating and selecting new technologies.

9.4.4 Technology and Artificial Intelligence

Technology has become an increasingly important part of hospital life. It has revolutionized how healthcare is delivered, providing both patients and healthcare professionals with access to information and services that were previously unavailable. As technology continues to evolve, it is becoming increasingly important for healthcare organizations to take advantage of the opportunities that technology provides. For example, technology and artificial intelligence can be used to predict staffing needs and improve scheduling processes. Moreover, the growth and adoption of artificial intelligence (AI) tools and systems has the potential to transform the health and wellness of those who are ill. However, that potential also brings certain challenges, especially in relation to ethical issues such as data protection and privacy, equitable access, and appropriate uses and users of AI [40].

In 2020, the WHO embarked on an 18-month process to develop guidelines for the use of AI in healthcare settings, which resulted in the publication of the *Global Strategy on Digital Health 2020–2025* [41]. The aim of the Global Strategy is multipurposed:

- Accelerate the development and adoption of appropriate, accessible, affordable, scalable, and sustainable person-centric digital health solutions to prevent, detect, and respond to epidemics and pandemics.
- Develop infrastructure and applications that enable countries to use health data to promote health and well-being.
- Achieve the WHO's health-related *Sustainable Development Goals* and the *Triple Billion* targets of the WHO's *Thirteenth General Program of Work, 2019–2023*.

The Global Strategy has four objectives intended to provide guidance and coordination on digital health transformation, and strengthen synergies between initiatives and stakeholders to improve health outcomes and mitigate associated risks at all levels.

1. Promote global collaboration and advance the transfer of knowledge on digital health.
2. Advance the implementation of national digital health strategies.
3. Strengthen governance of digital health at the global, regional, and national levels.
4. Advocate for people-centered health systems that are enabled by digital health.

The WHO's expert panel developed a set of principles to encourage governments, programmers, and associated organizations to adopt ethical guidelines for the appropriate use of AI in healthcare. These principles are the first to be specifically geared toward AI in health with international scope. They are as follows:

- Protecting human autonomy
- Promoting human well-being and safety and the public interest
- Ensuring transparency, interpretability, and intelligibility
- Fostering responsibility and accountability
- Ensuring inclusiveness and equity
- Promoting AI that is responsive and sustainable

One of the most significant ways in which technology can be used in healthcare is with patients in hospitals. For example, many hospitals now utilize electronic medical records (EMRs) to track patient data, eliminating the need for paper-based records. EMRs also make it easier for healthcare providers to access and share patient information, which can help improve communication and coordination of care. When staff are provided with access to vital information such as patient health records and medication doses, they can deliver better and faster care, more quickly, and can more accurately respond to questions or requests.

In addition to EMRs, hospitals can take advantage of a number of other technologies to improve patient care. For example, many hospitals use telemedicine systems to connect patients with remote healthcare providers. This enables patients to receive care from specialists who may not be available in their local area and allows them to access care without having to travel to a hospital.

Wearable technology has become increasingly popular in recent years, and its use continues to grow in both the consumer and business markets. Devices such as fitness trackers and heart monitors can be used to monitor patient vital signs and provide real-time alerts to staff if a patient is in distress, allowing for a quick and appropriate response. Another benefit of wearable technology is improved communication; wearables can be used to quickly and easily communicate with other staff members, allowing for more efficient and effective communication.

9.4.5 Stakeholder Participation and Social Accountability

Another key accountability of healthcare executives is to establish, manage, and maintain effective relationships with other healthcare authorities, jurisdictions, and organizations. Stakeholders play a vital role in holding healthcare organizations accountable for the effective and efficient operation of health facilities. Governance is enhanced when stakeholders are consulted about major reforms or key initiatives, as they are the ones who will most likely be affected by changes. Consultation with stakeholders is important when significant decisions need to be made that will affect the health of individual patients, patient groups, and healthcare staff.

Healthcare organizations typically seek feedback from stakeholders using both formal and informal means to discover what is working *well* and what needs improvement. Lim and Lin [14] argue that governance is not simply an ad hoc consideration of ways to improve the implementation of health workforce policies but rather a "distinct process through which networks of conflicting stakeholder interests influence the formation and implementation of policy decisions." Key challenges to intersectoral governance and coordination efforts among stakeholders have been identified by the WHO as willingness, commitment, technical capacity, financial mobilization (often in a fiscally constrained space), operational accountability, and effective leadership [30].

Engaging stakeholders across multiple contexts and levels is a quintessential aspect of the governance process. The government sets policy in relation to the health agenda (legislation, financing and stewardship) but devolves other responsibilities to local stakeholders. This approach has two key elements: a *network-based* dimension and a *stakeholder-driven* dimension [14]. The network-based dimension emphasizes *connections* between stakeholders. The stakeholder-driven dimension legitimizes the bottom-up participatory approach that builds *consensus* and improves the health system's performance. Hence, the focus of a network governance-based approach is to encourage stakeholders to work together to influence from the bottom-up while also acknowledging and accounting for the power dynamics and vested interests of stakeholder groups.

Stakeholders can participate in the governance of health organizations through a variety of methods such as providing feedback on strategic plans, attending local forums and Town Hall meetings, and providing input on decisions made by the organization. Key stakeholders may be invited to join advisory boards and committees to provide expertise and insight into the organization's operations; some may serve on the board of directors to provide oversight and guidance. Stakeholders can also participate in public forums and meetings to express their opinions and concerns regarding the health agenda. As a last resort, they may contact their local political representative to provide input on issues that affect their local health organization or to raise matters of importance to them that they do not believe have been adequately addressed by the health system.

Existing professional governance bodies such as registration boards, professional accreditation councils, and university faculties and schools traditionally focus on regulating their own profession. As a consequence, it is up to the healthcare organization to ensure that the guidelines and standards set by these entities are strictly adhered to in the daily treatment and care of patients. This level of governance is above and beyond what is required from an administrative, structural point of view yet essential given the delicacy of patient concerns and treatment regimens. Healthcare organizations also need to consider the vested interests and significant resources of some very powerful health professional bodies [42] as well as the power differential among interdisciplinary teams (e.g., physicians often exert dominance over other health professionals) [43]. Thus, governance issues are structurally entrenched within a networked, web-like system of heterogeneous stakeholders within and outside the health sector [44]. It is therefore necessary to consolidate stakeholder involvement before seeking any policy changes due to extensive stakeholder influence. If the governance process is adaptive and flexible to stakeholder demands, a consensus can be reached.

In a healthcare setting, an interdisciplinary team works best when there is collaboration across professions and respect for professional disciplines. Since teams are formed for a specific purpose (as a "one off" to treat one patient), it is not always clear who has governance responsibility or if this responsibility is covered by the healthcare organization's existing governance system. The recognition of healthcare organizations as interdisciplinary teams operating under interdisciplinary models of collaborative practice [45] challenges traditional governance frameworks [24] because the greater the level of interdisciplinary collaboration, the greater the complexity. Hence, in an interdisciplinary context, there is a need to ensure agreements concerning the involvement of all the professions, a commonality of shared language, and a distribution of leadership with a clear focus at all times on the end user or patient [24].[8]

9.5 Cultural Issues in Healthcare

At the most fundamental level, a key accountability of healthcare executives is to ensure that a patient safety culture operates within their organization. Culture in healthcare facilities refers to the values, beliefs, and standards shared by the workforce that influence their care provision actions and conduct [46]. Healthcare organizations that make the strengthening of their organizational culture a priority improve the quality and safety of patients in their care.[9] Measuring patient safety culture through validated instruments such as the *Hospital Survey of Patient Safety Culture* (HSOPSC) is a strategy applied worldwide.[10]

Vikan et al. [47] mapped the characteristics of a patient safety culture and concluded that, consistent with previous research [48], "Teamwork climate" and "Safety climate" were the most frequent dimensions of the HSOPSC associated with reduced adverse event rates. Less visible dimensions that support a culture of patient safety included "Leadership," "Supervisor/Manager action promoting patient safety," "Management support," "Communication openness," "Organizational

[8] Appendix 9.3. Readers may like to complete the Survey of Governance Issues to identify areas for improvement in their healthcare organization.

[9] Organizational culture is discussed in Chap. 8.

[10] Ways to measure a patient safety culture are discussed in Chap. 8.

learning," and "Nonpunitive response to errors." These findings infer that accountability for the development of a patient safety culture lies squarely with the executive leadership of healthcare organizations [49].

It is unfortunate that a culture of individual blame is still found in traditional healthcare organizations [50]—a Safety-1 approach to patient safety. A responsible healthcare organization acknowledges when patient safety failures are the result of weak systems—a Safety-11 approach [7]. The WHO recommends the establishment of a "just" culture [19] that recognizes the complexity of situations and events, and the possibility of both system and human error. In such a culture, the response to an error or near miss is predicated on the type of behavior associated with the error and not on the severity of the event. However, there may be occasions when an individual should be held accountable, e.g., where there has been reckless behavior or willful misconduct such as refusing to perform a "time-out" prior to surgery. In these situations, the reckless behavior would warrant punitive action even if patients were not harmed, or the instigation of procedures as per the guidelines for managing poor performance published by professional associations and regulatory bodies.

A significant cultural issue that contributes to staff stress, affecting their well-being and performance when delivering patient care, is the bullying and harassment they experience or witness on-the-job. When not addressed, bullying and harassment leads to a psychologically unsafe workplace in which staff fear giving voice to near misses from which staff can learn.

9.5.1 Bullying and Harassment

A significant stressor in healthcare systems is bullying and harassment which is rapidly being recognized as a cultural issue in the healthcare environment and a systemic failure of the hospital system [51, 52]. It is endemic in systems that, over the past few decades, have not challenged bad behavior which can take many forms and be exhibited in many ways—verbally (criticism, sarcasm, nasty comments), physically (poking, jabbing, aggression), or sexually (unwanted touching) [53]. An inverse relationship between personal experiences of disengagement from work and psychological safety has been found following staff being personally bullied as well as from witnessing others being bullied [52]. Although the legal definition of bullying in some jurisdictions requires repeated incidences [54], in others, a single incident of abusive treatment of a staff member is regarded as harassment. Unfortunately, bullying and harassment in many healthcare organizations is "swept under the rug" so that individuals do not lose their jobs. Whistleblowers are reluctant to speak out until they can no longer contain their concerns. They want the culture to change to one in which there is respect and social connectivity, and organizational values are upheld not just espoused.

There are extensive references in the literature to bullying in healthcare [55, 56]. As early as 1999, a research survey revealed that 38% of the staff in an NHS Community Trust reported being subjected to bullying, while 42% had witnessed the bullying of others [57]. A 2014 report from the UK General Medical Council showed that 8% of doctors in training had experienced bullying (down from 16.5% in 2006), while another 13.6% had witnessed bullying [58]. These incidents were most frequently reported by consultants (70%) rather than by nurses or midwives (10%) since they tend to have a better overview of the system. In the USA in 2012, a Joint Commission report examined the damage that can be caused by the intimidating and disruptive behaviors of fellow workers, which undermine a culture of safety. It concluded that such behaviors can foster medical errors and contribute to preventable adverse events [59].

In Australia, a 2005 report of the *Victorian Taskforce on Violence in Nursing* revealed that nurses are frequently subject to occupational violence and bullying in their workplace from other health professionals, supervisors, and nursing peers [20]. The bullying of nurses by other nurses is known as *horizontal violence*; it is the second most common form of bullying experienced by nurses [23, 24]. A survey conducted in 2017–2018 with all staff at seven Australian hospitals investigated the prevalence of 26 unprofessional behaviors, ranging from rudeness to physical assault between staff [60]. Thirty-nine percent ($n = 2009$) of the staff reported experiencing one or more of these behaviors in the previous week.

Challenges in relation to nurse–doctor interactions are often the subject of bullying or harassment investigations. Arnetz et al. [52] researched the experience of workplace bullying among 331 registered nurses in an American regional healthcare system and reported that 36.9% of respondents were bullied in the preceding 6 months. The social complexity of nurse–doctor relationships suggests that demarcations between nurses and doctors may be viewed as expressions of knowledge and power [61, 62].

9.5.2 Communication

A second cause of cultural stress in healthcare organizations that has a major impact on patient care, staff well-being, and collegial relationships is communication. How staff speak to one another, how they communicate with patients, and how they interact as members of an interdisciplinary team are all reinforced by the culture in which the workforce operates. Sociological studies of nurse–doctor power relationships are particularly germane as policymakers, researchers, and healthcare centers advance interdisciplinary care as a way of delivering quality patient care and ensuring patient safety [63].

Hierarchy has been cited in the literature as supporting bullying behavior in the workplace. Appelbaum et al. [64] investigated the influences of power distance and leader inclusiveness on psychological safety among 106 medical residents. A greater perceived power distance predicted lower levels of psychological safety, while leader inclusiveness was positively correlated with psychological safety. Higher levels of psychological safety were positively correlated with intentions to report adverse medical events, further highlighting the importance of mitigating barriers to psychological safety to maintain and improve patient safety. If *respect* is a value that is operationalized, everyone benefits from knowing that they are valued both as a person and as a clinician. In turn, they start to model respect for others and value their contributions to the team in promoting patient health. Conversely, if disrespectful behaviors are evident in the workplace, such as bullying and harassment, unconditional regard for others fails [65]. Multiple research studies have identified effective communication as a key component of patient safety culture.[11] Clear communication is vital in the diagnosis and treatment of patients in healthcare settings and is one of the key factors that research has identified as a pivotal indicator of patient safety culture [66–69]. The lack of clear, detailed, and relevant information about patients and their care is one of the key factors contributing to the occurrence of adverse events that may cause them harm [70–73].

Effective communication is a two-way process that involves one person sending a clear and appropriate message to another that is received, accepted, and understood. In a healthcare setting, communication needs to be effective between staff members and patients, among staff members within a team, and among and across interdisciplinary teams [74]. When communication is effective, it reduces the risk of avoidable incidents and fragmentation of patient care resulting from loss of important information about treatment [75, 76]. Effective communication between nurses and doctors has been found to positively affect the quality of patient outcomes such as satisfaction and length of stay, and reduce adverse events [77, 78].

A lack of communication, or miscommunication, is the main cause of most adverse events in hospitals which lack a systematic, universal method for accurately communicating important information [79]. Inadequate communication leads to dissatisfaction and a lack of nurse autonomy [80]. Other disincentives for communication include the cultural hierarchy of professional groups, which can result in staff being afraid to speak up, and disrespectful behavior [81, 82]. Hence, it is essential to identify and address disrespectful behaviors in healthcare settings when they occur [15].

In 2013, the US Joint Commission report stated that poor communication accounted for two-thirds of sentinel incidents in healthcare [59]. In 2017, the American College of Healthcare Executives recommended three key strategies for leaders to foster strong teams and good communication: making oneself approachable, inviting everyone into the conversation, and establishing shared goals [83]. However, poor communication is still responsible for approximately 10% and 16.6%, respectively, of adverse events in the UK and Australia [84]. A study by Abuosi et al. [85] affirms the importance of communication between healthcare providers in preventing errors. They advise dialog between the health workforce and the rest of the healthcare team, as well as the active participation of the patient where possible, to develop an action plan to address their care needs and give them confidence in the workforce. Evidence-based tools and approaches such as briefings and debriefings have been recommended to improve communication within teams.

[11] See the discussion on how leaders can communicate more effectively to avoid adverse events in Chap. 3 and the evidence from research studies in Chap. 8.

Communication is particularly important during handovers and transitions as this is the time when details significant to the patient's condition and treatment can be missed or passed over. It can be measured using the "Handovers and transitions/ Information exchange" dimension in the HSOPSC to identify the safety culture shared among hospital staff. In their research, Draganović and Offermanns [15] found that poor handovers and transitions may be related to a lack of nonstandard, nonwritten handover and transition procedures, different documentation systems, and nonstandardized technical terms. They recommended the use of accepted handover protocols such as "I pass the baton" [86] to overcome the loss of information between healthcare professionals at these times and promote more successful sharing of information, thus improving the outcomes for patients, providers, and organizations.

Noviyanti et al. [84] found a significant relationship between nurse communication satisfaction and the quality of patient safety culture in Indonesian hospitals; the greater the nurses' level of communication satisfaction, the better the applied quality of patient safety culture. Communication satisfaction was described as consisting of eight dimensions: the organization's general perspective, organizational integration, personal feedback, relationships with superiors, horizontal and informal communication, media quality, communication climate, and staff relations [87]. According to their research, communication is a determining factor in the provision of quality services in a hospital. Nurse communication satisfaction affects the provision of effective healthcare in that it builds cooperative relationships and fosters trust between professionals to improve the quality of service delivery and patient safety.

The role of the nursing unit leader is to use effective communication processes to foster learning through supervision, motivation, and encouragement, and to provide information that will improve staff work capabilities and increase team effectiveness [88]. The leader is responsible for building a collaborative workplace and creating a psychologically safe environment in which staff have freedom of speech regarding emotional events, teamwork, roles, and organizational aspects affecting their ability to provide excellent patient care. Clinical leaders help team members better understand their roles and responsibilities and solve problems among team members through effective communication. Responsible and respectful communication between nurses, doctors, and other health workers enhances cooperative relations and increases trusting relationships between related professions [80].

Effective communication is needed in all hospital units to improve service quality and patient safety. When a unit team's effectiveness increases, its performance in implementing a patient safety culture increases, maximizing the positive services provided. The role of hospital executives is to support clinical teams wherever possible within budgetary constraints while also achieving organizational goals. This often requires a significant degree of communicative tact, diplomacy, and influence [84] so that trust and relationships are not eroded.

9.6 Recommendations for Healthcare Executives

Several research teams have focused on how hospital managers can develop, implement, and support a patient safety culture within their facilities. The findings of research by Hedsköld et al. [89], Abraham et al. [21], and Fassi et al. [90] are summarized below. These recommendations are then combined with the findings of the HSOPSC research into a comprehensive table of actions that executives can take within their healthcare organization to ensure that patients remain safe from harm.

9.6.1 Strategies to Develop a Patient Safety Culture

In their 2021 research, Hedsköld et al. [89] focused on exploring how frontline managers in intensive care units in eight Swedish hospitals perceive their role and how they promote patient safety and a patient safety culture within their units. From their analysis of findings, they deduced five themes describing strategies that managers used to promote a patient safety culture within their units:

- Valuing and developing healthcare professionals' expertise
- Organizing for resilience
- Being "present" and setting a good example in daily work
- Encouraging individual and organizational learning from incidence reporting
- Balancing adherence to, with questioning of, standardized operative procedures

Overall, in relation to the role of managers in developing and sustaining a culture for patient safety, they recommended the following strategies:

- Maintaining correct routines and constantly encouraging incidence reporting.
- Speaking up about adverse events to increase staff attention to the risks in daily work environments and to underline the necessity of adhering to safe work practices.
- Developing a blame-free environment that does not condemn errors and mistakes, by role modeling how staff could approach a situation where they felt uncertain about the correct way of doing things.
- Emphasizing patient safety as everybody's responsibility and recognizing patient safety aspects in every detail of the job.
- Promoting a positive and supportive working climate in which staff who have been involved in adverse events feel supported, by having routines and a structure in place to debrief the event and learn from it.

Specific strategies related to each theme were also recommended for managers to adopt. These are Safety-11 [7] strategies that may be implemented separately or in combination to more quickly develop a patient safety culture with a team or organization:

Valuing and developing healthcare professionals' expertise

- Actively support the development of healthcare professionals' competencies to promote staff resilience.
- Support the continuous development of staff members in relation to both medical care and inpatient safety issues.
- Conduct daily respectful conversations between managers and unit staff, with the manager offering constructive suggestions as appropriate and inviting reciprocal recommendations from staff for professional growth.
- Use the expertise of staff members to promote improvements in change routines and, at times, invite experts to present new evidence or information.

Organizing for Resilience

- Ensure that enough staff are present during each shift.
- Make sure that the necessary competences are present within the team for each shift.
- Schedule the right competencies for a shift so that the team is capable of managing everyday work, as well as being able to reorganize and respond to a variety of expected and unexpected situations without deviating from safe practice.

Being "Present" and Setting a Good Example in Daily Work

- Be "present" within work units and, as much as possible, take part in the daily work of clinical teams, which will enable them to do the following:
  - Identify potential problems not normally communicated to them as well as potential risks.
  - Role model effective ways of acting and reacting in routine work as well as in critical situations.
  - Exert a direct influence on the attitudes and manners of team members.

Encouraging Individual and Organizational Learning from Incidence Reporting

- Foster active incidence reporting, preferably via an electronic system.
- Share information on adverse events.
- Provide staff with feedback from analyses of adverse events.
- Involve staff in group discussions to develop their capacity to solve problems, stimulate their creativity, and find ways to provide safer care.

Balancing Adherence to, with Questioning of, Standardized Operative Procedures

- Ensure that constantly updated documents on evidence-based, standard operative procedures are available and adhered to in daily work, and use discretion when these procedures, in their opinion, are not applicable to a certain situation of patient care.
- When written guidelines are lacking, encourage staff to use their own initiative to focus on the best way of solving the situation without harm to the patient.

- Thereafter, to prevent maverick behavior, decide whether the current guideline is obsolete and needs updating, or a new guideline is needed, and formulate an explicit process for dealing with uncontrolled methods and ways of working.[12]

9.6.2 Implementation of a Patient Safety Culture

In 2022, Abraham et al. [21] investigated the perceptions of managerial staff regarding patient safety culture at a leading tertiary public hospital in South Africa. They identified four main themes with underpinning subthemes that emerged from the interview data provided by ten managers within the Clinical Services Directorate (Fig. 9.1).

First, when *implementing* patient safety, measures must be in place to ensure patients' physical security such as the use of access codes to enter and exit high-risk areas including pediatric wards and intensive care units. Policies and procedures regarding patient safety should be consistent with national safety guidelines, well-established and followed throughout the hospital. Similarly, clinical guidelines should be followed at all times. They recommended that in certain units such as pediatrics, internal medicine, and family medicine, weekly mortality and morbidity meetings take place to address potential issues that could have caused errors or adverse events and learn from them to make improvements. They noted that

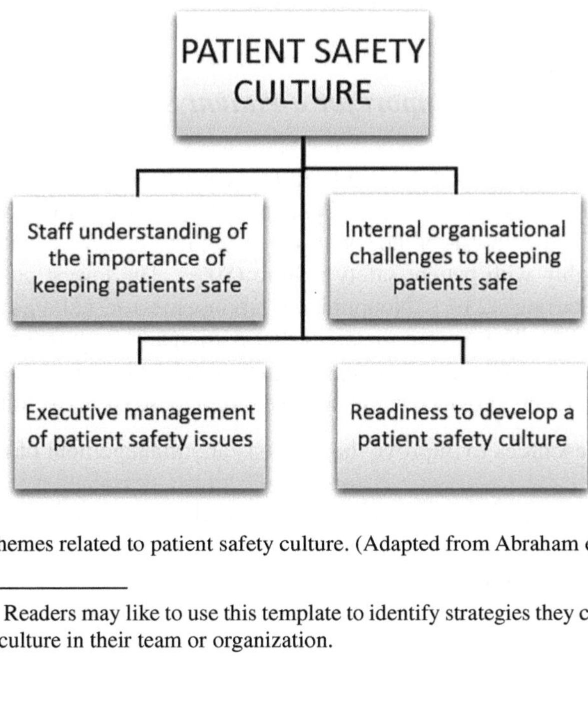

Fig. 9.1 Four themes related to patient safety culture. (Adapted from Abraham et al. [21])

[12] Appendix 9.4. Readers may like to use this template to identify strategies they can use to develop a patient safety culture in their team or organization.

interdisciplinary committees such as the Adverse Event Committee and Quality Assurance Committee are important sources of information and support when implementing a patient safety culture within hospitals.

Second, several challenges to the implementation of a patient safety culture were mentioned by participants in their study, principally: infrastructure deficiencies and lack of resources, poor staff attitudes and lack of patient safety awareness, and poor reporting of adverse events. These factors were thought to impede the establishment of a positive patient safety culture in hospitals.

Third, participants believed that proactive measures were needed to increase patient safety awareness within the entire hospital and to prevent patient safety issues from occurring. They recommended that reporting systems be implemented to create a culture of reporting, individual/team learning, and organizational learning. This finding supports those of previous research [91–93]. The benefit of reporting is that adverse events are less likely to occur, thus circumventing possible litigation claims for compensation. Richter et al. [4] suggested that hospitals incentivize good safety performance among staff because, for a positive patient safety culture to exist, all staff and the hospital as a whole must be proactive about patient safety rather than reactive.

Fourth, as patient care is the core business of the hospital and for all clinical and nursing staff, each team member needs to embrace patient safety as a personal priority. Participants in the study noted that a patient safety culture would improve if staff were more caring, empathetic, and respectful to patients and one another, similar to how they would want to be treated themselves or how they would treat their relatives. Moreover, when staff act in this way, hospital management should have a way of recognizing this respectful behavior [21].

9.6.3 Management Support for a Patient Safety Culture

In 2023, Fassi et al. [90] used the validated French version of the HSOPSC to study physicians' and nurses' perceptions of patient safety culture within two university Moroccan hospitals. Analysis of the results revealed that "Teamwork within units" correlated most highly with patient safety culture (80%). The lowest positive response rates were for "Staffing" (23%), "Nonpunitive response to error" (31%), and "Teamwork across units" (47%). These were the areas that participants recommended healthcare executives and managers address to improve patient safety culture within their organization. The researchers provided strategies to address these issues as follows:

- Allocating resources to improve the analysis and management of risk and medical errors.
- Providing training to raise staff awareness of the culture of patient safety and their ability to report adverse events.
- Encouraging staff to propose actions for improvement.
- Eliminating a blame culture by taking collective responsibility for a multifactorial and interdisciplinary approach to patient care.

- Involving administrative staff in the problems of the units.
- Improving communication between administrators and clinical staff so that human resources can be adapted in number and availability as necessary to ensure quality patient care.
- Seeking continuous improvement of teamwork both within and across professional units and teams.
- Fostering improved quality of life at work for professionals by implementing a better communication system to narrow the gap across department units.

In summary, implementing these strategies to develop a patient safety culture, fostering the spread of this culture across teams and departments, and managing its sustainability throughout the entire organization, will ensure that patient safety becomes a *priority* for, and a *value* held by, every healthcare professional and clinician, as well as every organizational executive [90]. Since hospital management support has been identified as an essential factor for establishing and embedding a patient safety culture [94, 95], executives are encouraged to use a participative, coaching leadership style that positively impacts culture [15].[13]

Key Takeaways

- Organizational governance is concerned with how the healthcare facility is operated in relation to its structure, financial affairs, workforce, resource allocation, use of technology, risk management, legal compliance, and regulatory obligations.
- Clinical governance is concerned with how the healthcare facility cares for its patients, providing the best possible treatment while keeping them safe from harm.
- Executives are responsible for both organizational and clinical governance of the healthcare facility, engaging in strategic and workforce planning to ensure that patients receive the correct clinical treatment when needed from the right mix of professionally trained staff effectively and efficiently.
- The involvement of stakeholders is sought when undertaking strategic planning to determine the issues of concern to the greater community and specific patient populations.
- Cultural change to a patient safety culture requires executive support for, and commitment to, a range of interventions including creating a psychologically safe workplace, encouraging speaking-up, addressing adverse events as they occur, and capitalizing on individual and collective learnings to make changes in organizational policies and procedures.

[13]A coaching leadership style is discussed in Chap. 5. This leadership style supports the development of a patient safety culture in healthcare organizations. It can be developed through coach education and training delivered by the Australian Institute of Professional Coaches. www.professionalcoachtraining.com.au

9.7 Case Study 9: Governance and the Cultural Change Agenda

Over the last two decades, a regional hospital in a geographically diverse state has been plagued with media reports of adverse events. Whistleblowers have resorted to the media to precipitate investigation into significant events that may have been preventable. Escalating claims from unions of poor working conditions have also received local media coverage. The hospital has instigated multiple reviews and investigations which have highlighted several significant issues, but despite this, and efforts to resolve them, there has been little improvement in patient care or staff conditions.

The hospital is currently dealing with multiple probes into possible surgical and obstetric malpractice. The government minister responsible for health has agreed to make public the findings of these investigations, indicating an effort towards transparency and accountability; however, this dialog has not changed over the last two decades, with little difference resulting in the management of the hospital or the occurrence of adverse events—which seem to be increasing.

The hospital also faces calls from the nurses' association to halt elective surgeries due to concerns over patient safety and operational issues.

These incidents have raised significant concerns about the hospital's management and the quality of care provided, leading to increased public and governmental scrutiny. This scrutiny follows a broader review last year that revealed a culture of bullying and instances of clinical negligence.

When analyzed, it is clear that the last two decades have proven difficult for this hospital, which has faced a number of challenges:

1. A rapid turnover of senior leadership, management, and key healthcare executives.
2. The diversity of services offered has been hampered by economies of scale in relation to nearby tertiary hospitals. Being peripheral to three larger metropolitan hospitals has meant that they have been chosen last for the development of specialist services.
3. Difficulty in recruiting permanent specialist staff, and a heavy reliance on locums and international medical graduates, has led to cultural clashes.
4. Being located in a growth corridor has meant significant population growth nearby with no commensurate growth in hospital services or funding; demand has outpaced supply.
5. Perpetual redevelopment which is slow and lags behind population needs. This is historical and also political in nature; health funding is unfortunately linked to the political term which is up for renewal every 3 years. This leaves the hospital in a state of perpetual redevelopment from a lack of consistent vision, commitment, and funding. Hospital services are consistently being updated but insufficiently in type and extent to meet demand. This contributes to change fatigue in staff and potential errors.

There is a significant hospital redevelopment currently in place with services being redistributed among several sites. Long-term planning remains an issue, and a hospital identity that attracts dedicated permanent staff remains elusive. The hospital relies on forced rotation of junior medical and nursing staff in order to survive.

For Discussion

1. What kind of governance issues need to be addressed within a healthcare organization?
    - What governance issues are exposed in this case study?
    - How can they be rectified to ensure patient safety?
2. Discuss the concept of clinical governance. What does it mean in terms of everyday practice?
    - What clinical governance issues are exposed in this case study?
    - How can they be remedied to ensure patient safety?
3. How can good governance principles and practices promote a patient safety culture within a healthcare organization?
4. In what ways can coaching and coaching programs be used to address governance issues and bring about cultural change to ensure patient safety?

Appendices

Appendix 9.1: Healthcare Performance Scorecard

On a scale of 1 (low) to 10 (high), what is your estimate of the degree to which your healthcare organization performs the following functions? Make comments as to what needs to change or can be improved.

1. Promote health
2. Protect health
3. Provide health
4. Power health.
5. Perform for health (Adapted from WHO [6])

Function	Your assessment (1–10)	What needs to change or be improved?
1. *Promote health*, by shifting the focus to prevention and promotion rather than root cause analysis of diseases and injuries.		
2. *Protect health*, by strengthening the organization's infrastructure for health emergency preparedness and response.		

Function	Your assessment (1–10)	What needs to change or be improved?
3. *Provide health*, by reorientating service delivery towards primary healthcare systems.		
4. *Power health* by partnering with scientific research associations to drive innovation and exploit data, digital technologies and artificial intelligence, in healthcare applications.		
5. *Perform for health*, by building a stronger local health system, health workforce, and health infrastructure		

Appendix 9.2: Principles Guiding Operational Governance

Comment and provide examples of how the following principles [45] guide executive decision-making and are operationalized in your healthcare organization.

Are there any other guiding principles that operate in your organization? Add these with examples.

#	In my healthcare organization …	Comments and examples
1	Executives are committed to providing quality care to patients and measuring outcomes to ensure that standards are being met	
2	Communication between clinicians, staff, and patients is open, honest, and effective	
3	Patient data is securely stored and privacy is respected	
4	Patients are informed of their rights and encouraged to participate in decisions made about their care	
5	Healthcare leadership is competent, ethical, and accountable	
6	The organization is accountable for its actions and decisions, and executives ensure that they are following the standards of care and regulations set by governing bodies	
7	The organization strives to be transparent in its operations and decision-making processes, including financial dealings, organizational policies, and patient care practices	

Appendix 9.3: Survey of Governance Issues in Healthcare

Instructions In the table below, indicate if any of these areas are hindering the development of a patient safety culture within your organization (Yes/No) and, if so, what START-STOP-CONTINUE strategies/actions can be put in place to remove any barriers and promote *excellence* in terms of:

1. Strategic planning
2. Workforce planning
3. Resource optimization
4. Technology and artificial intelligence
5. Stakeholder participation
6. Organizational culture

START: What strategies/actions can you put in place to begin developing a patient safety culture?

STOP: What does the organization need to stop doing to relieve the pressure on staff, resources, and facilities so that staff can have the space to develop a patient safety culture?

CONTINUE: What is the organization currently doing *well* that can continue and be expanded on to develop a patient safety culture?

#	Governance issue	Yes/No	What can be done to …
1	Strategic planning		START: STOP: CONTINUE:
2	Workforce planning		START: STOP: CONTINUE:
3	Resource optimization (incl. equipment access and availability)		START: STOP: CONTINUE:
4	Technology and artificial intelligence		START: STOP: CONTINUE:
5	Stakeholder participation (patients and others e.g., regulators, professional bodies)		START: STOP: CONTINUE:
6	Organizational culture (patient safety culture) (organizational communication)		START: STOP: CONTINUE:

Appendix 9.4: Strategies to Develop a Patient Safety Culture

Instructions On the left-hand side of this table are the strategies and actions that research has identified as positively contributing to the development of a patient safety culture. Reflect on each category and the strategies therein and then determine how your organization can adopt these strategies or learn from them to improve on what is currently happening in your organization. Insert your reflections on what you and your executive team can do differently or in addition to current practices on the right-hand side to stimulate the development of a patient safety culture in your organization. (Adapted from Hedsköld et al. [89]).

#	Strategies identified in the research	Strategies that your organization can do to develop a patient safety culture
1	*Risk management* Request resources to improve the analysis and management of risk and medical error. Encourage managers to be present within work units and, as much as possible, take part in the daily work of clinical teams, which will enable them to: Identify potential problems not normally communicated to them, as well as potential risks. Role model effective ways of acting and reacting in routine work as well as in critical situations. Exert a direct influence on the attitudes and manners of team members.	START: STOP: CONTINUE:
2	*Workforce* Ensure that enough staff are present during each shift. Ensure that the necessary competences are present within the team for each shift so that the team is capable of managing everyday work as well as being able to reorganize and respond to a variety of expected and unexpected situations without deviating from safe practice. Improve communication between administrators and clinical staff so that human resources can be adapted in number and availability as necessary to ensure quality patient care.	START: STOP: CONTINUE:
3	*Interdepartmental/Interdisciplinary communication* Involve administrative staff in the problems of the units. Seek continuous improvement of teamwork both within and across professional units and teams. Improve the quality of life at work for professionals by implementing a better communication system to narrow the gap across department units.	START: STOP: CONTINUE:

#	Strategies identified in the research	Strategies that your organization can do to develop a patient safety culture
4	*Adverse event reporting* Eliminate a blame culture by encouraging managers to take a nonpunitive approach to error reporting (e.g., adopt a "learning from" approach) and role model how staff can approach a situation where they feel uncertain about the correct way of doing things. Encourage staff to speak up about adverse events to raise their awareness of the risks in daily work environments. Implement an adverse events reporting system—preferably electronic—and constantly encourage incidence reporting. Raise staff awareness of their ability to report adverse events and the necessity to do so. Emphasize patient safety as everybody's responsibility. Encourage staff to propose actions for improvement so they take collective responsibility for a multifactorial and interdisciplinary approach to patient care. Promote a positive and supportive working climate in which staff who have been involved in adverse events feel supported by having routines and a structure in place to debrief the event and learn from it. Share information on adverse events and provide staff with feedback from analyses of adverse events so they can learn. Analyze an incident to stimulate creativity among staff members, develop their capacity to solve problems, and find ways to provide safer care.	START: STOP: CONTINUE:
5	*Policies and procedures* Keep up correct routines and underline the necessity of adherence to safe work practices while being vigilant to situations where alternative approaches may need to apply. When written guidelines are lacking, encourage staff to use their own initiative to focus on the best way of solving the situation without harm being done to a patient. Ensure that constantly updated documents on evidence-based, standard operative procedures are available and adhered to in daily work (Safety-1); also use discretion when these procedures do not seem applicable to a certain situation of patient care (Safety-11). Thereafter, to prevent maverick behavior, decide whether a new guideline is needed or the old one is obsolete and in need of updating, and formulate an explicit process for dealing with uncontrolled methods and ways of working so they do not override current procedures.	START: STOP: CONTINUE:

References

1. Parand, A., et al. (2014). The role of hospital managers in quality and patient safety: A systematic review. *BMJ Open, 4*(9), e005055.
2. Quenon, J.-L., et al. (2020). Exploring the role of managers in the development of a safety culture in seven French healthcare facilities: A qualitative study. *BMC Health Services Research, 20*(1), 517.

3. Richter, J. P., McAlearney, A. S., & Pennell, M. L. (2016). The influence of organizational factors on patient safety: Examining successful handoffs in health care. *Health Care Management Review, 41*(1), 32.
4. Richter, J. P., McAlearney, A. S., & Pennell, M. L. (2015). Evaluating the effect of safety culture on error reporting: A comparison of managerial and staff perspectives. *American Journal of Medical Quality, 30*(6), 550–558.
5. WHO. (2007). *Everybody's business—Strengthening health systems to improve health outcomes: WHO's framework for action*. World Health Organization.
6. WHO. (2023). *Health governance in the Western Pacific*. Available from: https://www.who.int/westernpacific/health-topics/health-systems-governance
7. Hollnagel, E., Wears, R., & Braithwaite, J. (2015). *From safety-I to safety-II: A white paper*. University of Southern Denmark, University of Florida, USA, and Macquarie University, Australia.
8. WHO. (2023, July 13). *Director-General's keynote speech at the international conference on health infrastructure investment "investing to achieve universal access in health services"*. Available from: https://www.who.int/director-general/speeches/detail/who-director-general-s-keynote-speech-at-the-international-conference-on-health-infrastructure-investment%2D%2Dinvesting-to-achieve-universal-access-in-health-services%2D%2D%2D%2D13-july-2023
9. Brinkerhoff, D. W. (2004). Accountability and health systems: Toward conceptual clarity and policy relevance. *Health Policy & Planning, 19*(6), 371–379.
10. Gurung, G., et al. (2020). The role of social audit as a social accountability mechanism for strengthening governance and service delivery in the primary health care setting of Nepal: A qualitative study. *Critical Public Health, 30*(5), 612–623.
11. WHO. (2000). *The World Health Report 2000: Health systems, improving performance*. World Health Organization.
12. Government, Q. (2019). *Department of health governance framework*. State of Queensland (Queensland Health).
13. Government, Q. (2020). *Good practice guide for boards* (Vol. 2). State of Queensland (Queensland Health).
14. Lim, M. Y. H., & Lin, V. (2021). Governance in health workforce: How do we improve on the concept? A network-based, stakeholder-driven approach. *Human Resources for Health, 19*(1), 1–10.
15. Draganović, Š., & Offermanns, G. (2022). Patient safety culture in Austria and recommendations of evidence-based instruments for improving patient safety. *PLoS One, 17*(10), 1–17.
16. Dieleman, M., Shaw, D. M., & Zwanikken, P. (2011). Improving the implementation of health workforce policies through governance: A review of case studies. *Human Resource Health, 9*, 10.
17. Brinkerhoff, D. W., & Bossert, T. (2008). *Health governance: Concepts, experience, and programming options*. USAID.
18. Pierre, M. S. (2013). Safe patient care–safety culture and risk management in otorhinolaryngology. *GMS Current Topics in Otorhinolaryngology, Head and Neck Surgery, 12*, Doc09.
19. WHO. (2021). *Global Patient Safety Action Plan 2021–2030: Toward eliminating avoidable harm in health care*. World Health Organization, License: CC BY-NC-SA 3.0 IGO.
20. Brooks, J. (2007). US Medicare will stop paying for preventable errors. *Canadian Medical Association Journal, 177*, 841.
21. Abraham, V., et al. (2022). Perceptions of managerial staff on the patient safety culture at a tertiary hospital in South Africa. *International Journal of Qualitative Studies on Health & Well-Being, 17*(1), 1–13.
22. Parand, A., Dopson, S., & Vincent, C. (2013). The role of Chief Executive Officers in a quality improvement initiative: A qualitative study. *BMJ Open, 3*(1), e001731.
23. Cook, R., & Rasmussen, J. (2005). Going solid: A model of system dynamics and consequences for patient safety. *Quality Safety Health Care, 14*, 130–134.

24. O'Keefe, M., et al. (2020). Governance options for effective interprofessional education: Exposing the gap between education and healthcare services. *Medical Teacher, 42*(10), 1148–1153.
25. Barbazza, E., & Tello, J. E. (2014). A review of health governance: Definitions, dimensions and tools to govern. *Health Policy & Planning, 116*(1), 1–11.
26. Beyene Shashamo, B., et al. (2023). Patient safety culture and associated factors among nurses working at public hospitals in Gamo Zone. *Southern Ethiopia. BMC Health Services Research, 23*(1), 1–12.
27. Mitchell, A., & Bossert, T. J. (2013). *Politics and governance in human resources for health, in The Labor Market for Health Workers in Africa: A new look at the crisis*. The World Bank.
28. Cometto, G., et al. (2019). Analyzing public sector institutional capacity for health workforce governance in the South–East Asia region of WHO. *Human Resource Health, 2019*, 17–43.
29. Witter, S., et al. (2013). Implementing the Agenda for Global Action on human resources for health: Analysis from an international tracking survey. *Journal of Hospital Administration, 2013*(2), 1.
30. WHO. (2016). *Global strategy on human resources for health: Workforce 2030*. World Health Organization.
31. Sales, M., et al. (2013). Human resources for universal health coverage: From evidence to policy and action. *Bulletin of the World Health Organization, 9*(11), 798–798A.
32. Hurst, K., & Patterson, K. D. (2014). Health and social care workforce planning and development–an overview. *International Journal of Health Care Quality Assurance, 27*(7), 562–572.
33. Birch, S., et al. (2009). Health human resources planning and the production of health: Development of an extended analytical framework for needs-based health human resources planning. *Journal of Public Health Management Practice, 15*(6), 556–561.
34. Rees, G. H., et al. (2020). Rethinking workforce planning for integrated care: Using scenario analysis to facilitate policy development. *BMC Health Services Research, 20*(1), 1–12.
35. WHO. (2016). *Integrated care models: An overview. Working document*. World Health Organization: Copenhagen: WHO Regional Office for Europe.
36. Martineau, T., et al. (2022). Improving health workforce governance: The role of multistakeholder coordination mechanisms and human resources for health units in ministries of health. *Human Resources for Health, 20*(1), 1–12.
37. Sprivulis, P., et al. (2006). The association between hospital overcrowding and mortality among patients admitted via Western Australian emergency departments. *Medical Journal of Australia, 184*(5), 208–212.
38. Virtanen, M., et al. (2008). Overcrowding in hospital ward as a predictor of antidepressant treatment among hospital staff. *American Journal of Psychiatry, 165*, 1482–1486.
39. Hou, W., Qin, S., & Thompson, C. H. (2022). A virtual evaluation of options for managing risk of hospital congestion with minimum intervention. *Scientific Reports, 12*(1), 1–8.
40. Goodman, K. W., et al. (2023). Global health and big data: The WHO's artificial intelligence guidance. *South African Journal of Science, 119*(5/6), 6–9.
41. WHO. (2020). *Global strategy on digital health 2020–2025*. World Health Organization.
42. Kuhlmann, E., & Burau, V. (2018). Strengthening stakeholder involvement in health workforce governance: Why we need to talk about power. *Journal of Health Services Research & Policy, 23*(1), 66–68.
43. Schoeb, V. (2016). Healthcare service in Hong Kong and its challenges: The role of health professionals within a social model of health. *China Perspective, 2016*, 51–58.
44. Fox, D. M. (1996). From piety to platitudes to pork: The changing politics of health workforce policy. *Journal of Health Politics, Policy & Law, 21*(4), 823–842.
45. Kuipers, P., Ehrlich, C., & Brownie, S. (2014). Responding to health care complexity: Suggestions for integrated and interprofessional workplace learning. *Journal of Interprofessional Care, 28*(3), 246–248.

46. Reis, C. T., et al. (2023). Cross-cultural adaptation and validation of the Hospital Survey on Patient Safety Culture 2.0 – Brazilian version. *BMC Health Services Research, 23*(1), 1–12.
47. Vikan, M., et al. (2023). The association between patient safety culture and adverse events – A scoping review. *BMC Health Services Research, 23*(1), 1–27.
48. Alsabri, M., et al. (2022). Impact of teamwork and communication training Interventions on safety culture and patient safety in emergency departments: A systematic review. *Journal of Patient Safety, 18*(1), e351–e361.
49. Sammer, C. E., et al. (2010). What is patient safety culture? A review of the literature. *Journal of Nursing Scholarship, 42*, 156–165.
50. Tenza, I. S., et al. (2022). Hospital managers' views on the state of patient safety culture across three regions in Ghana. *BMC Health Services Research, 22*(1), 1–14.
51. Davis, E., & Beale, N. (2015). It is time: The poor culture regarding safety and quality in Australian hospitals must be addressed! Asia Pacific. *Journal of Health Management, 10*(3), GS36–GS41.
52. Arnetz, J. E., et al. (2019). Organizational determinants of bullying and work disengagement among hospital nurses. *Journal of Advanced Nursing, 75*(6), 1229–1238.
53. Kieseker, R., & Marchant, T. (1999). Workplace bullying in Australia: A review of current conceptualizations and existing research. *Australian Journal of Management & Organisational Behavior, 2*(5), 61–75.
54. PSC. (2004). *Behavior and culture: People matter survey*. Victorian Public Sector Commission.
55. Rosenstein, A. H., & O'Daniel, M. (2005). Disruptive behavior and clinical outcomes: Perceptions of nurses and physicians. *American Journal of Nursing, 105*(1), 54–65.
56. Porto, G., & Lauve, R. (2006). *Disruptive clinical behavior: A persistent threat to patient safety*. Patient Safety and Quality Healthcare.
57. Quine, L. (1999). Workplace bullying in NHS Community Trust: Staff questionnaire survey. *British Medical Journal, 318*, 228–232.
58. General Medical Council UK. (2014). *National training surveys*. General Medical Council UK.
59. Commission, J. (2013). *Behaviors that undermine a culture of safety* (Sentinel event alert number 40). Joint Commission.
60. Westbrook, J., et al. (2021). The prevalence and impact of unprofessional behavior among hospital workers: A survey in seven Australian hospitals. *Medical Journal of Australia, 214*(1), 31–37.
61. Schlitzkus, L. L., et al. (2014). Workplace bullying of general surgery residents by nurses. *Journal of Surgical Education, 71*(6), e149–e154.
62. Stein-Parbury, J., & Liaschenko, J. (2007). Understanding collaboration between nurses and physicians as knowledge at work. *American Journal of Critical Care, 16*(5), 470–477.
63. Fernando, O., et al. (2016). Interprofessional communication between surgery trainees and nurses in the inpatient wards: Why time and space matter. *Journal of Interprofessional Care, 30*(5), 567–573.
64. Appelbaum, N. P., et al. (2016). The effects of power, leadership and psychological safety on resident event reporting. *Medical Education, 50*(3), 343–350.
65. Rogers, C. (1956). Client-centered theory. *Journal of Counseling Psychology, 3*(2), 115–120.
66. Sammer, C. E., et al. (2010). What is patient safety culture? A review of the literature. *Journal of Nursing Scholarship, 42*(2), 156–165.
67. Alsabri, M., et al. (2022). Impact of teamwork and communication training interventions on safety culture and patient safety in emergency departments: A systematic review. *Journal of Patient Safety, 18*(1), e351–e361.
68. Lawati, M. H. A., et al. (2018). Patient safety and safety culture in primary health care: A systematic review. *BMC Family Practice, 19*, 1–12.
69. El-Jardali, F., et al. (2011). Predictors and outcomes of patient safety culture in hospitals. *BMC Health Services Research, 11*, 1–12.
70. Bartlett, G., et al. (2008). Impact of patient communication problems on the risk of preventable adverse events in acute care settings. *CMAJ, 178*(12), 1555–1562.

71. Schrimpff, C., et al. (2023). Communication matters in regard to adverse events: Associations of adverse events during implant treatment with patients' communication quality and trust assessments. *Patient Education and Counseling, 110*, 107675.
72. Guijarro, P. M., et al. (2010). Adverse events in hospitals: The patient's point of view. *BMJ Quality & Safety, 19*(2), 144–147.
73. Duclos, C. W., et al. (2005). Patient perspectives of patient–provider communication after adverse events. *International Journal for Quality in Health Care, 17*(6), 479–486.
74. Brady, A. M., et al. (2017). Barriers to effective, safe communication and workflow between nurses and nonconsultant hospital doctors during out-of-hours. *International Journal of Quality Health Care, 29*, 929–934.
75. Lee, S.-H., et al. (2016). Handoffs, safety culture, and practices: Evidence from hospital survey on patient safety culture. *BMC Health Services Research, 16*, 254.
76. Blazin, L. J., et al. (2020). Improving patient handoffs and transitions through adaptation and implementation of I-PASS across multiple handoff settings. *Pediatric Quality & Safety, 5*(4), e323.
77. Larrabee, J. H., et al. (2004). Predictors of patient satisfaction with inpatient hospital nursing care. *Research in Nursing & Health, 27*, 254–268.
78. Tschannen, D., & Kalisch, B. J. (2009). The impact of nurse/physician collaboration on patient length of stay. *Journal of Nursing Management, 17*, 796–803.
79. Commission, J. (2017). Inadequate hand-off communication. *Sentinel Event Alert, 58*, 1–6.
80. Wang, Y. Y., et al. (2018). Interventions to improve communication between nurses and physicians in the intensive care unit: An integrative literature review. *International Journal of Nursing Science, 5*, 81–81.
81. Leape, L., et al. (2012). A culture of respect, Part 1: The nature and causes of disrespectful behavior by physicians. *Academic Medicine, 87*, 1–8.
82. Leape, L., et al. (2012). A culture of respect, Part 2: Creating a culture of respect. *Academic Medicine, 87*, 853–858.
83. Executives, A.C.o.H. (2017). *Leading a culture of safety: A blueprint for success*. IHI/NPSF Lucian Leape Institute.
84. Noviyanti, L. W., Ahsan, A., & Sudartya, T. S. (2021). Exploring the relationship between nurses' communication satisfaction and patient safety culture. *Journal of Public Health Research, 10*(2), 125–128.
85. Abuosi, A. A., et al. (2022). Safety culture and adverse event reporting in Ghanaian healthcare facilities: Implications for patient safety. *PLoS One, 17*(10), 1–18.
86. Keebler, J. R., et al. (2016). Meta-analyses of the effects of standardized handoff protocols on patient, provider, and organizational outcomes. *Human Factors, 58*(8), 187–205.
87. Donchin, Y., et al. (1995). A look into the nature and causes of human errors in the intensive care unit. *Critical Care Medicine, 23*, 294–300.
88. Silla, I., Navajas, J., & Koves, G. K. (2017). Organizational culture and a safety-conscious work environment: The mediating role of employee communication satisfaction. *Journal of Safety Research, 61*, 121–127.
89. Hedsköld, M., et al. (2021). Acting between guidelines and reality- an interview study exploring the strategies of first line managers in patient safety work. *BMC Health Services Research, 21*(1), 1–10.
90. Fassi, C. F., et al. (2023). Patient safety culture perception among Moroccan healthcare professionals: Cross-sectional study in public hospitals. *Ethiopian Journal of Health Sciences, 33*(2), 273–280.
91. Katusiime, B., Semakula, D., & Lubinga, S. J. (2015). Adverse drug reaction reporting among health care workers at Mulago National referral and teaching hospital in Uganda. *African Health Sciences, 15*(4), 1308–1317.
92. Shamim, S., et al. (2016). Adverse drug reactions (ADRS) reporting: Awareness and reasons of underreporting among health care professionals, a challenge for pharmacists. *Springerplus, 5*(1), 1778.

93. Parand, A., et al. (2011). The disparity of frontline clinical staff and managers' perceptions of a quality and patient safety initiative. *Journal of Evaluation in Clinical Practice, 17*(6), 1184–1190.
94. Zaheer, S., et al. (2021). Acute care nurses' perceptions of leadership, teamwork, turnover intention and patient safety – A mixed methods study. *BMC Nursing, 20*(1), 1–14.
95. Zaheer, S., et al. (2018). Importance of safety climate, teamwork climate and demographics: Understanding nurses, allied health professionals and clerical staff perceptions of patient safety. *BMJ Open Quality, 7*(4), e000433.

Index

© The Editor(s) (if applicable) and The Author(s), under exclusive license to Springer Nature Switzerland AG 2024
S. Knowles, *Patient Safety Coaching*,
https://doi.org/10.1007/978-3-031-68722-8

MIX
Papier aus verantwortungsvollen Quellen
Paper from responsible sources
FSC® C105338

If you have any concerns about our products,
you can contact us on
ProductSafety@springernature.com

In case Publisher is established outside the EU,
the EU authorized representative is:
Springer Nature Customer Service Center GmbH
Europaplatz 3, 69115 Heidelberg, Germany

Printed by Libri Plureos GmbH
in Hamburg, Germany